Design for HEALTH

SCHOOL AND
COMMUNITY

Health Education, Physical Education, and Recreation Series

RUTH ABERNATHY, Ph.D.

EDITORIAL ADVISER
Chairman, Department for Women, School of Physical and Health Education
University of Washington, Seattle

Design for HEALTH

SCHOOL AND COMMUNITY

JOHN J. HANLON, M.D., M.S., M.P.H.
Assistant Surgeon General, Public Health Service U.S. Dept. of Health, Education and Welfare, Washington, D.C.

ELIZABETH McHOSE, ED.D.
Professor Emeritus of Health, Physical Education, and Recreation, Temple University, Philadelphia, Pennsylvania

Second Edition

I L L U S T R A T E D

LEA & FEBIGER *Philadelphia • 1971*

ISBN 0-8121-0308-4

Library of Congress Catalog Card Number 71:146023

Published in Great Britain by Henry Kimpton, London

Printed in the United States of America

Preface

An endless and constantly swelling stream of new young faces appears over our horizon. Beyond them, still unborn are countless more. Like all living things, they are endowed with an almost insatiable eagerness for learning, experience and living. Yet they can be deprived of these, as all too many are, by the absence of health. What can be done to assure them of this birthright? While society may provide many safeguards and services, in the final analysis it is the acquired knowledge and attitude of the individual regarding healthful living that makes the critical difference. Some of this knowledge and attitude is absorbed from the family, acquaintances and the environment. A dominant source can and should be the school. But this in turn depends upon knowledgeable teachers who play such an important role in the lives of all of us.

Recent years have seen the appearance of a plethora of textbooks on health for use by students on the elementary, secondary and college levels. The majority of these deal essentially with the important subject of personal health. Few of them, however, have been developed specifically with the teacher and the community as the prime foci. It was with this lack in mind that the book at hand was prepared,—to provide for the person who is now being trained and educated to enter teaching as a career a book on community health problems and programs and the teacher's important continuing role in relation to them. For the most part, the approach has been based upon fundamental principles and time-proven patterns, rather than upon details and methods which have a tendency to become obsolescent. It is hoped that this effort will contribute to the teacher's broadened horizon, and assist in the transmission of useful knowledge to those who are so eager to live and learn.

During the few years since the foregoing was written to describe the essential purpose of this book, remarkable advances have occurred in public health and school health. Health and educational legislative action on all levels of government have been extensive, resulting in many significant progressive programs. Meanwhile scientific and technological progress has been breathtaking;—on the one hand, the structure of the molecule has been unravelled and on the other man has walked on the moon. It is hoped that for its part, this second edition will be found by the reader to have kept properly apace.

John J. Hanlon
Elizabeth McHose

Washington, D.C.
Philadelphia, Pa.

Acknowledgments

Grateful acknowledgment is made for permission to use the following:

To the United States Public Health Service for figures 1, 2, 6, 7, 9, 11, 15, 30, 32, 38, 42, 43, 46, 47, 48, 49 and 60;

To the Philadelphia Department of Public Health for figures 28, 29, 34, 35, 36, 45, 51, 52, 53 and 61;

To the Pennsylvania Department of Public Health for figures 12, 24 and 50;

To the Pan American Health Organization for figures 13, 14 and 27;

To the Pfizer Laboratories for figures 44, 56, 57 and 58;

To the Temple University Alumni Review for figures 26 and 33;

To the American Medical Association for figure 54;

To the Merck Sharp and Dohme Co. for figure 37;

To the Grolier Society for figure 59;

To the Pennsylvania Tuberculosis and Health Society for figure 55.

Particular appreciation is expressed to the C. V. Mosby Company for permission to use figures 16, 17, 18 and 19, as well as adaptations of certain material presented in *Principles of Public Health Administration* by John J. Hanlon, M.D.

Contents

PART III. THE PLAYERS: PEOPLE

Tables

Illustrations

PART I
Prologue

A star, a world, a land, a town, a child is born. How seldom it is realized how closely related they are. Each in turn derives from the others, each in turn depends upon the others. Each arises in much the same way, is conceived, develops, achieves a zenith of vigor and power, then wanes,—phenomena of nature. In a true sense each one of them represents a different manifestation of the same fundamental inexorable process. The appearance or birth of anything necessarily introduces a new factor into the cosmic, community or family scene. Merely by virtue of its existence it upsets some previously established balance. It generates its own set of problems. It must be contended with,—it cannot be ignored. In turn, it stimulates solutions to problems, usually in the form of natural adaptations, and often by meaningful contributions from its own inherent force. This is one of the greatest enigmas, yet, at the same time, one of the greatest glories of nature. Through eons, nature has worked out a most intricate and elaborate organization of its innumerable interrelated forces. This has reached its apogee in man in a conscious and deliberate form. Thus, while a number of the other creatures of the earth have achieved the ability to form organized communities, only man, on the basis of his superior brain, has done this on the conscious sphere by planned solutions to the problems of his society and his communities. The first section of this book is devoted to a brief presentation of some of these considerations with emphasis upon their relation to health.

Chapter 1

The Emerging Community

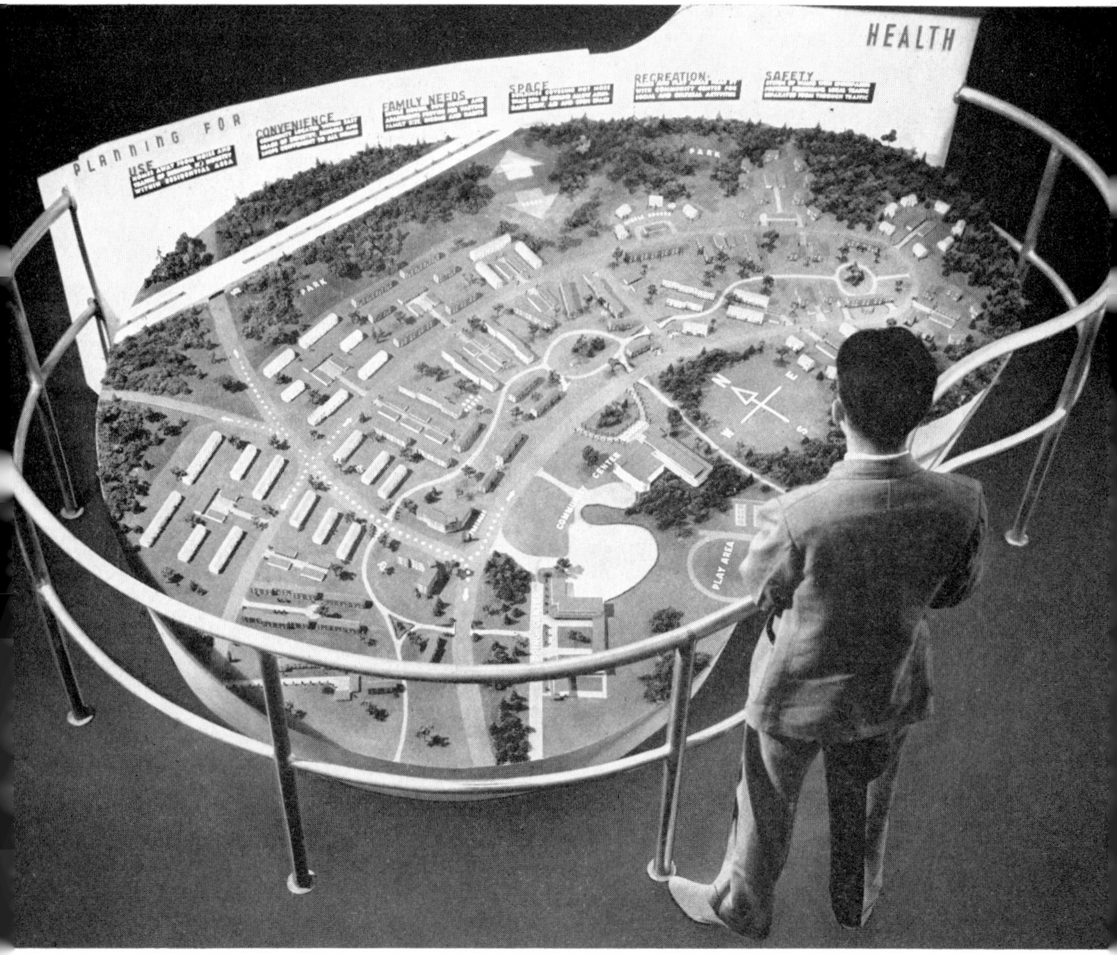

FIG. 1. The emerging community.

The Community is Born

Choose any empty spot on the landscape. Through time, it may remain unused, it may be farmed or it may become the center of a teeming metropolis. What determines its fate? If it becomes a center of population, how does it get that way and what problems are inherent to its development? For sake of illustration, consider a site on the bank of a river. At first there was nothing. Gradually, explorers, missionaries and traders came through the forests or by boat. For some it was a convenient spot to camp overnight. Gradually a few remained to fish and hunt, to clear the land and plant corn, to raise barns and rear herds and children. This embryonic settlement, if now with a permanent root in farming, mining, trade or otherwise, attracted more and more of the restless. Docks were built and so were streets and roads, the latter gradually linked with an ever widening network.

For a while this community was isolated and its problems were restricted to itself. In surviving and flourishing, however, it had to look increasingly outward. Steam power brought the railroad which not only connected it with other communities, but also provided a means of travel onward. For a while a simple ferry gave access to the other side of the river. This was eventually replaced by a bridge for the railroad as well as for wagons and foot passage.

By now, this location had developed its own personality. It had a name. The residents identified with it and with each other. There were romances, marriages, followed by children and later by death. These gave reason to the development of a number of the basic components of any stable community,—churches, schools, stores, banks, and graveyards. In fact, early in its history, there came hard on the heels of the farmers and the traders three important and related professionals,—the physician, the teacher and the clergyman.

As long as the community exists, its coordinated guidance by these three is crucial. The first makes physical existence possible. The second transmits the cultural gains of the past to the young and stimulates them to further thought and action. The last serves as catalyst in the development of a relationship between the physical world and that which transcends it. Each, in his way, augments the work of the others in serving what by now is clearly a community.

It is well at this point to consider the meaning of the word community. Webster defines it as, "A body of people having common organization or interests or living in the same place under the same laws; hence, an assemblage . . . living in a common home under similar conditions." It is convenient and pertinent to think of the life cycle of a community as analogous to that of an individual or even of a cell. It has a conception, a birth, a period of growth and maturation, followed eventually by degeneration, senility and even death.

At first, the single cell has its environment to itself with no competition. It multiplies with a purpose and the resultant cells become mutually supportive. Some specialize, also having as a purpose mutual organic support and development. This process proceeds to a point when certain undesirable phenomena may occur. There may arise competition for survival among the cells or organs. Some cells may become cancerous and continue existence at the expense of others. So inter-dependent do the parts become that, if anything goes wrong with a group of cells or an organ, there results a deleterious if not disastrous effect on all of the others. Concerted mutual defense by healthy cells or organs may overcome these threats. If not, mutual support may be superseded by overwhelming mutual threat leading to degeneration and death, not only of the cells, but also of the organs and even of the total biological being.

Problems Appear

Similarly, and in a very correct sense, a community may be regarded as a biological entity. In fact, this is what it is. Individuals take the place of cells, and specialized groups of individuals are analogous to organs. As in biology, they are first mutually supportive but later some may become competitive, and even threatening. What one does begins to affect all for good or ill. At various times, certain of these individuals or groups may become aberrant or antisocial, and like cancerous cells act to the detriment of the whole organism. During the mutually supportive phase of a community's life, growth occurs economically, intellectually and in many other ways. At some point, however, competition, distraction and other influences become so great that a state of imbalance results. There follow such phenomena as "central rot of cities," unmanageable delinquency, a flight of industry, and other undesirable social and economic consequences. If these proceed unchecked, the senility and death of the community are inevitable.

The field of public health provides many examples of these interrelationships. At first, when the evolving or emerging community had but few people and families, they dwelt somewhat apart from each other. They met various needs on a strictly individualistic basis. Each family dug its own well for water and its own privy for the disposal of waste. Since space was no problem, they could be sufficiently separated so that no threat arose. As more people settled, more wells and privies were dug, necessarily closer together. Eventually, therefore, a breaking point was reached, manifest by repeated outbreaks of disease caused by the contamination of the many sources of drinking water by the many sites of excreta disposal. Similarly, the introduction of respiratory or other types of disease could easily cause a rapid widespread epidemic like a brush fire. If steps to solve and prevent such situations are not taken, the premature demise of the community may result.

A Time for Action

A time is reached, therefore, in the life history of a modern community when responsible citizens face up to the situation and decide that it would be safer, more convenient, and eventually less expensive to take whatever steps are necessary. They do away with individual wells and privies and replace them with self-contained, closed systems for the adequate provision of safe water and for the safe removal of waste. Regulations are passed and implemented to protect the group against the introduction of communicable diseases and other threats to life and well being.

The same series of events occurs with regard to many other things. Milk is required as part of the diet. At first it is produced on individual small farms and peddled by small entrepreneurs. If one or a few of these small sources of milk become contaminated, the number of people affected tends to be small and perhaps unnoticed. As the community grows, however, and the consumers of milk and other dairy products become greater in number, the consequences of even a single hygienic accident are too great socially and economically for the community to tolerate. Typically, therefore, and by common consent, there are developed controls of various sorts to assure the safety and salubrity of particular products. These controls may take various forms such as legislation, regulation, prohibition, standards, inspections, pasteurization and the like.

In other words, as these few general examples indicate, from the hygienic as well as from other points of view, there comes a time when the members of the community of necessity are indeed their brother's keepers. They must be, if individually and collectively they are to survive. It is out of such problems of community evolution that public health activities derive.

The Cast of Characters

Brief passing mention has been made of the types of individuals who may enter or develop in a community. As background for subsequent exposition, it would be well to consider in more detail the human components of a community. A population may be classified in a great many ways. One way to categorize people is as dependents, learners or trainees, and producers. In the final analysis, at any given point in time it is the last of these, the producers, who maintain the life of the community. They consist essentially of two subgroups, wage earners and housewives. For convenience, professionals who work in personal service fields such as teachers, physicians and the like are included among wage earners. The proportion of producing wage earners in the total population is surprisingly small. Wage earners, and indeed most of the other components of the community, are sustained by productive housewives. In the category of learners are included all of those who, while not yet producers, are actively engaged in the process of preparing to enter that category,–school children, those in colleges and universities and those attending various professional, technical and trade schools. At the present time this category makes up approximately 30 per cent of the total population. It is comprised of a variety of interesting groups. As in the case of learners, all of these must be supported by the producers in one way or another. For some dependents, the expense is greatly justified. These are infants and pre-school children, about 11 per cent of the population. At the other end of the age scale are the retired and elderly, those over 65 years of age, who comprise almost 10 per cent of the population.

On the other hand there are large numbers of dependents whose existence is unfortunate and regrettable. At any given time in any community there are individuals who are ill, acutely or chronically, physically or mentally. Some have been subjected to physical injury, while others have been trapped by various addictive diseases. Certain aspects of these are discussed in subsequent chapters. Suffice to say here that in the United States at any given moment about 2 per cent of the population falls in the category of those who are ill.

A very significant group of dependents are those commonly referred to as multi-problem or hard-core individuals or families They consist for the most part of persons or groups who are disadvantaged for one or a variety of socio-economic reasons such as recent immigration, prejudice, inadequate education, chronic ill-health or genetic defects,–all essentially representing faults or failures of society. Out of these groups come significant numbers of special subgroups of dependents such as chronic criminals, prostitutes, derelicts and other types of social delinquents. Generally they tend to concentrate in slum districts of center cities because of economic or discriminatory reasons and because of their dependence upon the social services of the community.

Family Types

Generally speaking, there are three types of families or situations (Fig. 2). The first is the well established, self-sufficient and independent family. An occasional difficulty may arise and, either through its own resources and efforts or with assistance from others, the individual or family gets back on its feet relatively promptly and retains its self-sustaining characteristics. The second type of family gets along reasonably well most of the time. It wants to be self-sufficient and self-sustaining but somehow does not have much "staying power." As a result, every once in a while it slips into difficulty and becomes relatively helpless. It requires outside assistance which gets it back on its feet for a while longer until it slips again and repeats the cycle. The third situation is the true hard core or multi-problem family. Trouble and difficulty appear to be a continuous inherent part of its life. It is almost impossible to get it on its feet and to make it self-sufficient because of repeated overwhelming crises and catastrophes or because it is intrinsically defective. Occasionally a wish for recovery or a different way of life is actually lacking, unacceptable or incomprehensible. The roots of the problems go very deep. Such persons or families seem almost irrevocably or irretrievably caught in an exceedingly complex and difficult vortex of trouble that might be referred to as the "syndrome of the seven D's;"—Disease, Deficiency (often both mental and nutritional), Destitution, Dependency, Despondency, Delin-

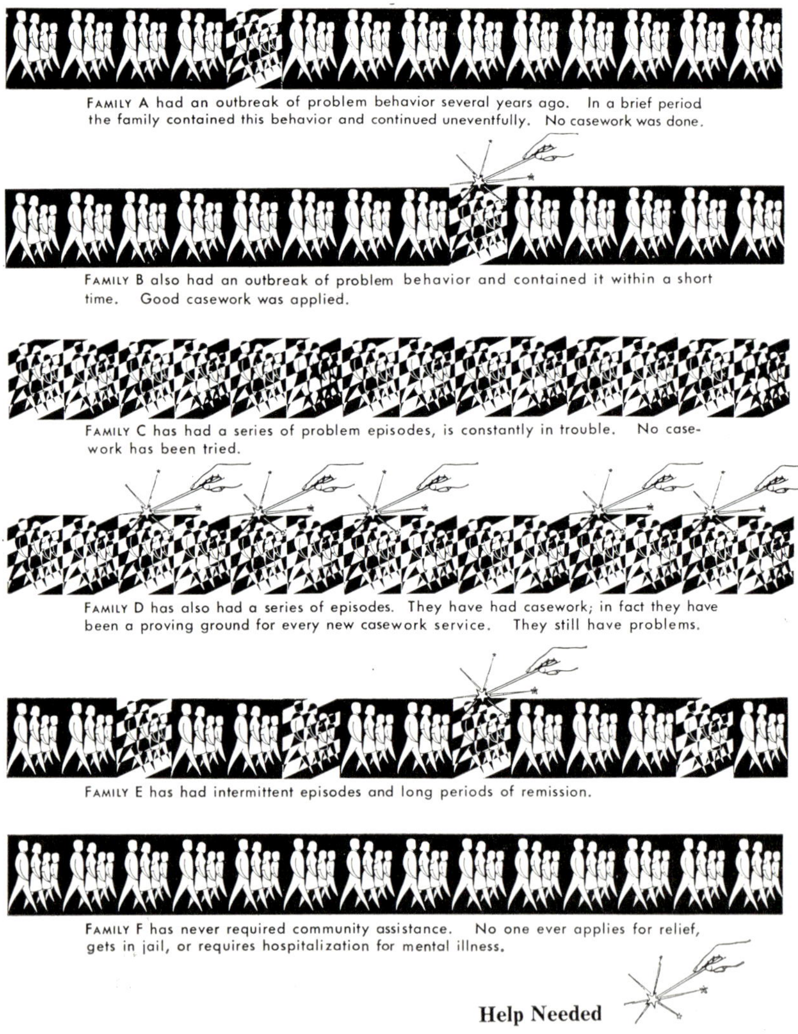

FIG. 2. Different families have different needs.

quency and Degeneracy.[1] Where one of these stops and the next one begins, or which is cause and which is effect is more or less academic. However, it is known that lack of education and opportunity or ill health play dominant initiating and continuing roles.

For example, in a classical study of St. Paul, Minnesota,[2] some years ago, it was found that only 4 per cent of hard core, multi-problem families were dependent financially because of unemployment, whereas 58 per cent were dependent because of ill health and/or mal-adjustment which prevented their being or becoming self-sufficient. This group of families, while proportionately small, gives rise to a major part of the social problems of the present-day community, including of course, the problems that confront the educational system. Again, referring to the St. Paul study, it was found that 6500 families or 6 per cent of the total suffered from a continuing complex of problems which absorbed 46 per cent of the community's health and medical services, 55 per cent of the social adjustment services, and 68 per cent of the dependency and welfare services of the community.

Contemporary surveys in Great Britain indicated a multi-problem family incidence of 3 per 1000 families. Whatever the intrinsic causes of such families, the typical slum environment in which they ordinarily live is not conducive to an improvement of the situation. In fact, the physical environment in which they are trapped, or which they choose, tends to promote further spiralling degradation. Even the most cursory observation shows a relationship between undesirable living conditions and various types of social problems. This is especially true and evident in crowded urban situations and is most readily seen in their slum or substandard sections. Here houses are small and crowded together with a maximum area devoted to living space at profitable rents to absentee owners. Industry is usually near this convenient supply of unskilled or semiskilled labor. The crowding of buildings, the generally narrow streets, the absence of open recreational areas and the smoke of factories limit the amount of sunshine and fresh air. Cleanliness and sanitation are difficult to maintain. Accidental injury or death are invited by narrow traffic laden streets, rickety abandoned buildings, and poorly planned flammable dwellings. Education and nutrition also tend to be substandard, and combine with insanitation and overcrowing to maintain a high incidence of illness. The lack of privacy due to overcrowding encourages immorality and is conducive to a lowering of self-esteem.

These environmental, social and psychological handicaps to the developing child and adolescent breed attitudes of insecurity, hopelessness, frustration, cynicism, resentment and explosive pent-up hostility. Respon-

[1]Hanlon, John J., *Principles of Public Health Administration,* 5th Ed., St. Louis, C. V. Mosby Co., 1969, p 93.

[2]Buell, Bradley, and others: *Community Planning for Human Services,* New York, Columbia Univ. Press. 1952.

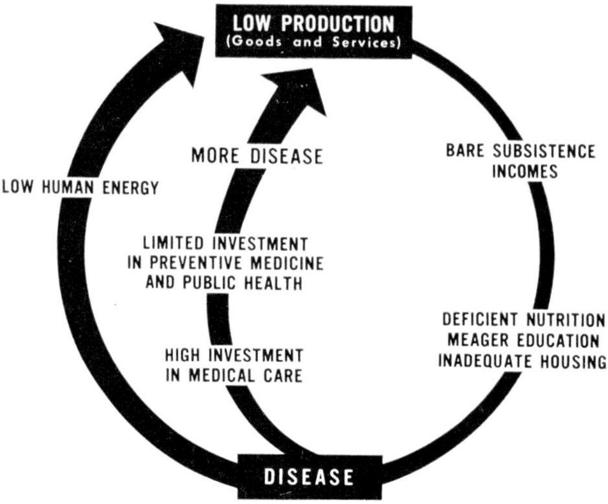

FIG. 3. The interrelationships of social problems.

sibility and initiative appear pointless and what seem to be the only roads to self-expression and escape more often than not are socially undesirable. There tend to occur, therefore, undesirable positive reactions of rebellion such as destructiveness and crime, or negative escapes such as mental and psychological illnesses, addictions or prostitution. These relationships have been repeatedly and conclusively shown to exist both for the individual and the group (Fig. 3).

A study of the slum area of Cleveland, Ohio, some years ago, illustrated the complexity and consequences of this phenomenon. The area included 2½ per cent of the population of the city. However, it produced 21 per cent of the homicides, 26 per cent of prostitution, 12 per cent of the tuberculosis deaths and 10 per cent of the illegitimate births, to list only a few of the many possible social diseases. It required 14.5 per cent of expenditures for fire protection, over 8 per cent of the health and medical expenditures and 4.5 per cent of the police expenditures. At the time of the study this area contributed only $225,000 per year in taxes but required about 2 million dollars a year to sustain it.

A similar recent study[3] by the Sacramento City Planning Commission of that city's substandard housing areas produced the same picture. These sections contained 20 per cent of Sacramento's population and included most of the unemployed. It contributed only 12 per cent of the city's tax income. By contrast, it accounted for 26 per cent of the fires, 36 per cent of juvenile delinquency, 42 per cent of adult crime, and 76 per cent of reported cases of tuberculosis. As a result, it required 25 per cent of the city's fire protection services, 41 per cent of the police protection services,

[3]Osborne, Philip B.: *The War That Business Must Win.* New York, McGraw-Hill Book Co., 1970, pp. 60-61.

and 50 per cent of the municipal health services. By contrast it is pointed out that the average productive person taken off the welfare rolls and placed in a steady self-supporting job will contribute $10,000 per year to the Gross National Product, pay $300 per year in state and federal income taxes, increase purchasing power for goods and services by $3,400 per year, and reduce unemployment costs and the need for welfare and other community services.

The Role of the Teacher in Community Development

Difficult as it may be to improve the plight of those already trapped in such a vortex of trouble, there are in every community certain individuals and agencies constantly trying to help others resist the downward pull. The labors of the physician and the clergyman to raise the health and ethical standards of the community are readily recognized and understood. The role of the teacher, equally essential to the community, is somewhat less tangible and therefore needs to be scrutinized more closely.

The survival of the community depends upon the perpetuation of its culture. Many cultural ideas and practices are absorbed unconsciously by the youth of the society; however, some become outmoded and can no longer prove useful to the developing generation. Heretofore the selection from the cultural heritage of that which appeared sufficiently useful for the present and the foreseeable future as to deserve retention, rested largely with the parent and the teacher. The history of civilization depicts clearly the special contribution of each generation to its culture as well as the gradual cultural changes brought about by each succeeding generation.

Since World War II, however, the world has witnessed in an unbelievably short span of time, a forward surge of discovery, expansion of knowledge and progress in science, technology, and industry without parallel in history. For man the impact has resulted in great and rapid changes in every area of living. Some changes have proved of immeasurable benefit to him, contributing to his health and comfort. But many of the changes have been too sudden and bewildering for his own ability to adjust. The implication for education, therefore, is clearly the urgent need for self-study and total re-appraisal at every level and from every angle: administration, curriculum, methods, practices, and activities. On the part of educators there is need for open-mindedness and receptivity toward new knowledge and techniques, and for objectivity in selection; also, a willingness to relinquish and discard time-honored practices and knowledge which may now be useless. Thus, at the beginning of the seventies education faces a great re-evaluation in terms of relevance to life to-day and in the foreseeable future, with built-in provision for constant and continuing evaluation.

The acuity of the need, the enormity of the problem, the endless ramifications involved in meeting the educational needs of all people of all ages, the absence of tested and proven precedents and answers further confuse the scene. The youth of the world, trapped by time and circumstances in the very center of the maelstrom and sensitive to and well-aware of the multiple facets of their dilemma, have actively protested the situation, questioning and often rejecting present societal practices and cultural values. The earlier maturation of youth, the enormous increase in the numbers to be educated, and the speed in communication intensify the complexities of their plight. Certainly youth needs to be involved as much as possible in the wise solution of existing shortcomings and in the planning of their own future. Obviously, the student, the parent, the teacher, the school, and the community need to work together toward finding workable solutions and in building intelligently for the future. This would mean selecting the best of the new, while retaining a substantial core of values, principles, and practices which time has shown to be indispensable and desirable. Included should be those most likely to help youth to identify with and to understand their role as a part of their cultural milieu, to realize their own powers and tendencies, to judge, to evaluate, and to assume responsibility for the gradual development of their own built-in, dependable value system by which they may live and make decisions.

The teacher's task involves helping young people prepare for their future life roles including those of efficient wage-earners, housewives, and parents. Some of the present wage-earners and housewives are parents who have tried to fulfill their responsibilities of parental teaching during their children's infancy and pre-school years. Therefore, the teacher finds already implanted in his pupils, some of the understandings, attitudes, ways, and aspirations of their parents. Thus, when a child enters school, the parent and the teacher immediately become active partners in the mutual task of educating the young of the community.

It is extremely important that the school emphasize knowledge, attitudes, and practices that will help the rising generation to face and to cope successfully with change itself. Here the teacher serves in the dual role of cultural transmitter and agent of social change. It imposes upon the teacher the ceaseless task of trying to keep abreast with and to evaluate new knowledge of consequence, the even more vital need to understand the inter-play of the many forces (social, economic, and political) which have led to the change, and its short and long-range effects upon the people and the community. The teacher needs a genuine understanding of people—why they think, feel, and act as they do. In the absence of such understanding, he would be at an utter loss to advise upon which portions of culture might merit inclusion in the school curriculum and the lives of his pupils.

The teacher is largely responsible both for what and how the child is taught. The tremendous expansion of knowledge during the past half-century has added to the difficulty of the selection of curriculum content and experience. Today, for example, we are concerned not only with the acquisition of new knowledge, but also with its application. With increasing speed, new discoveries and developments supersede old facts, practices, and time-honored procedures in health and education. This means constant evaluation of both new discoveries and older knowledge to determine which deserve a place in the curriculum from the point of view of value to the generation presently in school. Complicating the situation further is the fact that because of new and improved methods of public communication, much of the new learning is lateral in its spread, with the teacher, parents, and children all learning the facts at the same time. Thus, even small children are as well informed as their elders about astronauts and the space program.

Rapid world change has left few communities and lives untouched. New ways of living have created new needs on the part of the people. Thus, the impact of world change upon health and education has highlighted the need for modification of content, procedures, and in some cases, direction. The teacher today is indeed a prime agent of social change. He is helping children and youth to prepare for adulthood in a world upon whose nature he can for the most part only speculate. Obviously, methods and emphases will need to be in the direction of helping the individual child to develop attitudes, understandings, and skills that will help him to judge, evaluate and cope successfully with the new conditions and unfamiliar situations.

In view of these changes, education needs to focus upon helping the learner

(1) to develop a sound value system of his own and to recognize that individual value systems differ;
(2) to look at situations and events objectively and to try to understand why they happened as they did;
(3) to acquire insight and skills which will be helpful in meeting new situations, solving new problems, and applying the knowledge he obtains throughout his life. Such skills should be based upon principles and concepts rather than upon specific facts or techniques that may soon become obsolete.

Since the development of leaders is one of the desired outcomes of education, the teacher entrusted with this significant task needs to be familiar with community organization, power structure and problems, the governmental and voluntary agencies, resources, institutions, and probable growth trends and developmental directions. These he must envision as affected by and affecting the ethical and cultural patterns of the families whose children he is teaching. If the teacher is to fill his role acceptably, he needs to perceive the interactions of these elements as the framework within which he practices his profession and which will enable him to assist children to perceive their roles and responsibilities as citizens. Few can match the teacher in equipment for community leadership. His role is truly a constructive influence in the community.

Today as never before, the very survival of the human race depends upon a sound value system and the controls which man himself possesses and applies. It is imperative that the teacher realize the full import of his responsibility for influencing the quality of the value system and the outlook of each of his students. He needs to share with the community to the fullest extent, the assets of his personal and professional equipment. He needs to encourage other social institutions in the community to join forces in this significant task. If the teacher would accept this significant role in its fullest implications, the result might be a nation-wide upsurge in character and purpose which could well prove to be the greatest stabilizing force the world has yet witnessed.

Questions for Discussion

1. When was your community founded?
   What were the original reasons for its founding?
   Do those reasons still exist? Are they valid?
   What are its nationalities; when and why did they come?
   Do they still cling together in separate neighborhoods?
2. In what ways have present world affairs affected life in your community?
3. What roles do your schools play in helping the community as a whole to adjust to such changes?
4. Are there centers of special problems such as delinquency, physical deterioration, disease, etc.?
5. In your readings, what families have you discovered that correspond with the types mentioned in this chapter?

Suggested Reading

1. WARREN, R. L.: *The Community in America.* Chicago, Rand, McNally & Co., 1963.
2. NELSON, LOWRY, RAMSEY, CHARLES E., and VERNER, COOLIE: *Community Structure and Change.* New York, The Macmillan Co., 1960.
3. BROWNELL, BAKER: *The Human Community.* New York, Harper and Bros., 1950.
4. GLADSTON, IAGO (Ed.): *The Family in Contemporary Society.* New York, International University, 1958.
5. ROSEN, GEORGE and WELLIN, EDWARD: *A Bookshelf on the Social Sciences and Public Health.* Am. J. Pub. Health, 49:4, 441, 1959.
6. PAUL, BENJAMIN D.: *Health, Culture and Community.* New York, Russell Sage Foundation, 1955.
7. KLUCKHOLN, C.: *Mirror for Man.* New York, Whittlesey House, 1949.

8. Boek, W. E. and Boek, J. K.: *Society and Health.* New York, Putnam's Sons, 1956.
9. Banks, A. Leslie: *Social Aspects of Disease.* London, Edward Arnold, 1953.
10. Buell, Bradley and Associates: *Community Planning for Human Services.* New York, Columbia University Press, 1952.
11. *The Urban Environment* (Editoral Research Reports on) Washington, D.C., Congressional Quarterly, Inc., 1969.
12. McKee, E. M.: *The People Act.* New York, Harper and Bros., 1955.
13. Miller, Paul A.: *Community Health Action.* East Lansing, Michigan State College Press, 1953.

Chapter 2

The Roots of Community Health

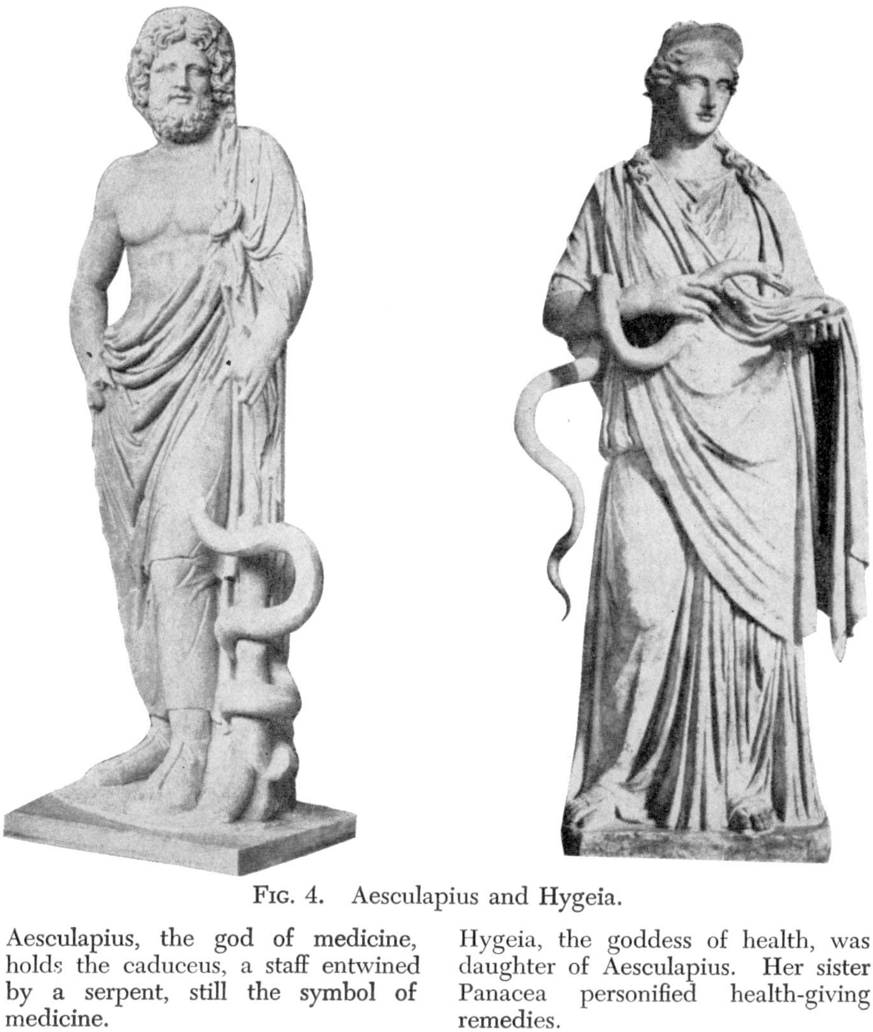

FIG. 4. Aesculapius and Hygeia.

Aesculapius, the god of medicine, holds the caduceus, a staff entwined by a serpent, still the symbol of medicine.

Hygeia, the goddess of health, was daughter of Aesculapius. Her sister Panacea personified health-giving remedies.

The Relation of Health to Total Living

While health and education are common needs, and efforts to achieve them represent common drives, they are actually secondary or intermediate goals. Man, both alone and in his social groups, strives for the achievement of a total or integrated life. From this viewpoint, while it may be a bitter pill for their professional egos, it is important for health workers and educators to recognize that their interests and activities are of significance and value only to the extent that they protect and prepare the individual for accomplishments in other fields. Since the totality of living, even in a primitive society, involves many complex factors, the definition of total or integrated life is not easy. It is possible under certain circumstances, however, to distinguish between factors that are fundamental and those that are secondary in importance. This is especially true when one observes primitive societies, or societies under stress. One can only conclude that although man and his societies are subject to many needs, urges, drives or goals, only a few are primary, and these are for the provision of transitory or temporary benefits and satisfactions. They are the basic biological activities related to the protection of the individual and his species; the urges for food, for shelter, and for sexual expression or propagation.

Conversely, activities that hold promise of long-term or permanent value are generally regarded as of secondary importance. It is among these that efforts for better health and education are found. Indeed, a desire for comfort, for the absence of pain, for a state of physical well being, and for the achievement of knowledge are very relative terms. In the many societies where the majority have malaria or external or internal parasites, for example, or where everyone is ignorant or illiterate, these conditions tend to be accepted as part of the normal pattern of life and are adapted to accordingly. Ill health or intellectual incapacity in effect are interpreted as any condition beyond these. In other words, man ordinarily will always tend to seek food, shelter and sexual expression in the absence of health or knowledge, but he will not and cannot achieve health or education in the absence of the others. This is a simple fact of life. As far as man and his societies are normally concerned, most other needs or goals, including improved health and education, are of interest and concern only to the extent that they assist in the achievement of related goals, particularly the three which are primary in nature.

Some examples may illustrate the point. Visualize a man and a woman cast upon an island. They are confronted with a problem of first things first. The initial necessity is sustenance, and they will seek it even in the face of risks such as disease-infested swamps or dangerous animals. They next must think of shelter to protect themselves from the hazards of the environment. With the darkness and cold of the night their next tendency will be to seek mutual solace and comfort, eventually through sexual intimacy, thereby fulfilling the natural drive for continuation of the species. After achieving these goals to a satisfactory degree, they may then begin to attend to other needs and goals.

The willingness to forego what may appear as nobler or more logical goals is no mere philosophic concept. Many diseases could long since have been eradicated except for this. The venereal diseases, syphilis and gonorrhea, would quickly disappear if all people, at least those infected, would abstain from sexual intercourse for a relatively brief period of time. This has even been suggested and attempted with social delinquents, but with understandably little success. Intestinal infections are a major cause of sickness and death in many countries. In Egypt, much of it is attributable to the drinking of polluted water from the Nile and irrigation canals which lead from it. An attempt was made to remedy the danger and inconvenience by drilling wells in villages. The villagers, however, were reluctant to drink the pure "thin" water from the wells for the interesting reason that "everyone knows that from time immemorial nothing is fertile unless it is touched by the water of the Nile, and we want to be fertile."

Another cause of intestinal infection in Egypt is the myriad number of flies which breed in the dung in and around the houses. It was felt that if the gamoose or water buffalo could be removed from the houses there would be less fly breeding and therefore less dysentery. However, many village women complained that during the day they were left alone and the gamoose was their only company. On the surface this may seem ludicrous until one realizes how many people in our own society keep various types of animals such as dogs, cats, and birds for exactly the same reason. Still another example was observed in certain malarious areas of North Africa where DDT was used to destroy the disease-bearing Anopheles mosquito. To the surprise of western technicians, after a short interval they were asked to stop spraying because a fly which normally carries pollen from the male to the female date palm was also being destroyed. Since the food supply and the economy of the area depended upon the date, the people were willing to risk malaria in order to have food. With reference to educational efforts, there are places even in the United States where the operation of schools is impractical during the planting or harvesting seasons.

The foregoing is not intended to discount, disparage or discourage efforts for the improvement of health and education. The intent is merely to place health and education in their proper perspective. It is to emphasize that they are not necessarily primary or basic goals, that they are relative concepts, that their definition and value vary through time and place, that even in a particular society they represent only two of the many facets of the total life interests of the individual and his society, and that they are in constant competition with all other factors of greater or lesser importance to that individual and his society. As Koos has indicated:

> What we can expect a community to provide, and its members to accept, in the way of health activities . . . (and we may add education) . . . must therefore be vested in a framework which is peculiar to that community. This in no way prevents the establishment of uniform goals . . . but it does mean that community efforts . . . are necessarily custom built.[1]

If a man may be regarded correctly as a social being, and if social activities including those concerned with health and education depend upon the interactions among individuals and groups of individuals, some brief consideration of social groupings is indicated. People belong to groups for many reasons. An individual needs the group, but not necessarily only a particular group, or the same group for all needs. While attachments to groups must be strong to be of value, they are not necessarily fixed. They may be and often are broken or transferred, depending upon different purposes to be served. Accordingly, the individual is seldom if ever identified with only a single group. Again, this may be observed even in simple primitive societies, the members of which have multiple group attachments, to family, to a larger kinship group, to a totem group, to a maturation cult or to secret society as well as to the tribe. In our more highly developed or sophisticated society the plurality of group membership is even more marked. In addition to the family one finds the school, the church, the social or recreational groups, the business and professional associations to mention only a few. In most of our communities there are groups concerned with various aspects of health and education,—personal and community, child or adult. It is an interesting phenomenon that man does not always react the same as an individual as he does when a member of a group. Also, as a multiple group member, he is often seen to behave differently in one group than in another.

Since our intention here is a general social analysis for a better understanding of the background and development of community or social organization for the protection and improvement of health, it is important to identify the groups that may be of significance toward those ends. There are three basic identifiable groups of which individuals, including teachers involved with any aspect of community health, must be constantly aware. The first is concerned with ethnic identification. Included are groups based upon religion, language, race or nationality, each with its own prescriptions, prohibitions and ideals, many of which may be of significance to health or sickness. The second relates to ethos identification,—bonds which relate individuals to the same ethical, economic or

[1]Koos, E. L.: New Concepts in Community Organization for Health, Am. J. Publ. Health, *43*:466, 1953.

social group, sometimes a neighborhood in a large city. The economic, educational or moral values of the group may determine attitudes toward health and illness and the extent or manner of participation in efforts to improve the health of the individual or his community. Third and most important of the basic groups is the family. To ignore its predominant position and influence usually guarantees failure. With specific reference to health programs, Koos states:

> We may well question the logic of industry—or school—centered programs that ignore the importance of the family as a "conditioner of attitudes," and which may send the individual back to his family to face conflicting ideologies about health and its values. This is not a plea to abandon school—or industry—centered programs; it is to point out that such programs can work effectively only if they send the individual back to his family prepared to adjust differences that may have engendered; to make him, in effect, a health organizer in his own small family world. If the individual is not so prepared . . . the cost, intentions and frustrations can outweigh any small good the program may have accomplished.[2]

If the life history of the individual is related to the life history of his society, it follows that his behavior and response to matters relating to personal and community health will be determined largely by the culture of his society, transmitted to him through the three basic societal groups—ethnic, ethos and family. It is with this background in mind that a brief review of man's historic struggle with the health hazards of his environment is presented.

A Matter of Definition

There have been a number of attempts to define the terms health, and public or community health. A study of the definitions itself provides a picture of the modern evolution of man's expectations in this field. The best known definition of public or community health is that of Winslow who in 1920 described it as:

> The science and the art of preventing disease, prolonging life, and promoting health and efficiency through organized community effort for the sanitation of the environment, the control of communicable infections, the education of the individual in principles of personal hygiene, the organization of medical and nursing services for the early diagnosis and preventive treatment of disease, and the development of the social machinery which

[2]Koos, ibid.

> will insure to every individual a standard of living adequate for the maintenance of health; so organizing these benefits as to enable every citizen to realize his birthright of health and longevity.[3]

This statement is remarkable in its inclusiveness and modernity. A more recent and increasingly used definition is contained in the Constitution of the World Health Organization:

> Health is a state of complete physical, mental and social well being and not merely the absence of disease or infirmity.

This is of interest in its emphasis on the positive aspects of public health philosophy. In recognition of the place of public health in the total scheme of things, as well as its intent, one of us has defined public health as:

> The social application of the knowledge and techniques of various and varying disciplines to the biological, psychological and sociological advantage of man.[4]

If one approaches definition by way of philosophy or purpose, several other comments may be pertinent here. Over-enthusiastic individuals may propound actions in this field for its own sake. As has been implied earlier in this chapter, it is felt that such reasoning is fallacious. Health in itself has real value only as it promotes efficiency and happiness. It is the quality of life that counts and not the quantity. Either personal or community health, as ends in themselves, is valueless. The only true value of health, therefore, depends upon the activities that may be engaged in by virtue of it. On the other hand, it is important to recognize that public health activities represent part of civilization's struggle for a better life. With civilization and knowledge come an organized conscious opportunity and effort to change man's relation to his physical and social environment. We seek to outwit death for at least a brief span and to protect mankind from illnesses that may cause suffering, unhappiness, inefficiency or premature death. This is accomplished by devising various means of preventing disease from occurring in the first instance, or progressing in the second. Many of these hygienic inventions can be put to use only by means of a broad social movement.

Health and History

In general, the history of man's fight for health begins with what little is known about the millenia during which he was completely at the mercy of nature, and with no effective means of combating its hazards.

[3]Modern Medicine, 2: 186, 1920.
[4]Hanlon, op. cit., p. 23.

The next great period dealt with the appearance and advancement of civilization and the increasing effect of technology on raising standards of living. The most recent period has resulted in a dramatic acceleration in the advancement of the public health. The past hundred years have witnessed the development of an increasing number of techniques based upon new scientific knowledge applied for the development of organized public health programs which have become widespread particularly in Europe and North America. At the moment, knowledge, new discoveries, and techniques have been increasing at a phenomenal rate, and have provided ever more powerful weapons. These in turn give rise to new responsibilities as well as require increased introspection concerning their significance. The extent of this acceleration may be depicted vividly as representing a change from one major medical discovery per century up to 1900, to one per decade between 1900 and 1940, and to one or more per year since 1940. Related to this is the statement commonly made that 90 per cent of all scientists who ever lived are alive today. As indications of the effect of this are the facts that 90 per cent of prescriptions written today are for items that were non-existent a decade ago, and that two-thirds of all the food products now available to the American housewife did not exist 10 years ago.

The Pre-Christian Era

Little is known about either personal or community hygienic measures of prehistoric peoples. The study of the customs of contemporary primitive groups, however, provides some light. It is extremely rare that even the most primitive tribes do not have a certain group hygienic sense. Among tribal rules commonly found are those which prohibit fouling of family or tribal quarters, the use of the downstream side of the campsite or of burial for the disposal of excreta, and the burial or burning of the dead. Pertaining to civilizations for which archeological records exist, it has been learned that the Minoans (about 3000 to 1500 B.C.) had advanced to the construction of elaborate drainage systems, water closets, and even water flushing systems. The dynastic Egyptians (about 3000 to 1000 B.C.) had a marked sense of personal cleanliness, possessed extensive pharmacological resources and constructed earth closets and public drainage systems. The Judaic hygienic code (about 1500 B.C.) as summarized in Leviticus is well known. It dealt with a wide variety of personal and community hygienic responsibilities including the cleanliness of the body, protective measures against the spread of contagious diseases, isolation of lepers, disinfection of dwellings following illness, sanitation of campsites, disposal of excreta and refuse, the choice and protection of water and food supplies, and the hygiene of maternity.

Greece in the time of Pericles is of special interest for two reasons.

Personal hygiene was developed to an extent never previously attained. There was great concern for public cleanliness, exercise and dietetics. The other point of interest was that, in contrast to present day Western humanitarian philosophy, there existed a policy to ignore and even deliberately destroy the weak, ill and crippled. Greece gave way to the Roman Empire which is best known for its administrative and engineering accomplishments. It developed laws for the registration of births and deaths, the prevention of nuisances and foul smells, the destruction of ruinous buildings, of dangerous animals, and of unsound goods, the supervision of weights and measures as they related to food, the registration and supervision of public bars, of taverns and of houses of ill fame, and the regulation of building construction. The government assumed the responsibility for an uninterrupted supply of good and inexpensive grain. Many public sanitary services were provided including paved streets with gutters and drains with provision for their cleaning and repair, the removal of garbage and rubbish, the operation of public baths, and the provision of a notably safe and adequate water supply. In addition, Roman cities were provided with subsurface drains or cloacae for the removal of sewage, many of which are still in use.

Rome to Renaissance

The ascendancy of Christianity saw the development of a reaction against things reminiscent of Rome and its paganism. The attitude was taken that the Roman and Grecian ways of life pampered the body at the expense of the soul. There resulted a belittlement of worldly and physical needs, and the appearance of the concept of "mortification of the flesh." The reaction was so intense that it included attitudes toward personal and community hygiene. It became immoral to see even one's own body. Bathing therefore was infrequent, and clothing undoubtedly dirty. Parenthetically, this is commonly considered to account for the subsequent widespread demand for perfumes. Diets in general were inadequate, consisting of badly prepared or poorly preserved foods. This is said to have given rise to the eventual search for and trade in spices. There was utter disregard for sanitation, and refuse and human waste were allowed to accumulate in and around dwellings. The influence of this period spanned many centuries as is evidenced by descriptions of life in European cities up to the 18th Century, depicted for example in many of Hogarth's prints.

A phenomenon that caused great hygienic problems was the development of extensive movements of large numbers of people for reasons of religion and trade. The known world was expanding, and increasing numbers of ships and caravans plied the seas and the overland trade routes. Christian zeal led to a series of crusades which attracted people from all parts of Europe to Asia Minor and the Holy Land. In addition to this was the development and rapid growth of Islam during the 6th and 7th centuries. It became religious custom to make a pilgrimage to Mecca and Medina, the holy places of Islam. As a result of these several forces, large numbers of individuals who previously had lived their more or less isolated lives without contact with many diseases, criss-crossed their paths and passed their respective ailments on to each other. There resulted a long series of tremendous epidemics and pandemics of bubonic plague, cholera, smallpox, leprosy and many other terrifying diseases. Not only were those involved directly in the population movements affected, but even more serious, when the survivors returned home, the diseases were broadcast throughout the known world.

Leprosy, which is known to have existed in ancient Egypt passed through Asia Minor to Europe whose people had apparently not known it before and were highly susceptible. Under such circumstances it took a very acute and terrifying form. In an attempt to combat this mysterious ailment, laws were passed to regulate the conduct and movement of those afflicted. Lepers were banished from human communities and were often declared officially dead. They had to wear identifying clothes and sound a horn or bell as a warning of their approach. These stringent actions apparently produced some effect by enforced isolation of those infected. It also undoubtedly brought about their relatively rapid death from hunger, exposure and neglect. As a result, by the 16th Century, leprosy was practically eradicated in Europe, but by no means everywhere. There are still millions of people throughout the world afflicted with this dreadful disease, and who are still unfortunately ill-treated.

Meanwhile, an even deadlier menace appeared in the form of bubonic plague. Probably no other single influence, including even the atomic bomb, has or will ever come as close to wiping out the human race as did this one disease. For example, during the 1340's more than 13,000,000 people were thought to have died from it in China. India was practically depopulated. The Middle East was said to have been literally covered by dead bodies. During one of its many upsurges, Cairo lost from 10,000 to 15,000 people daily. In Gaza, 22,000 people and most of the animals were dead within six weeks. A report to Pope Clement VI stated that "half of the population of the known world had died." The important island of Cyprus lost all of its inhabitants, and ships with dead crews drifted aimlessly on the Mediterranean, Baltic and Red Seas, spreading the disease further wherever they were driven ashore. During the single year 1348, Florence lost 60,000, Venice 100,000, Sien 70,000, Paris 50,000, St. Denys 15,000, and Strasbourg 9,000. The port of Marseilles lost 16,000 in one month and in Vienna 1200 perished daily. In much of France not more than one out of every ten people was left alive. In Avignon, the site of the Papal See where about 60,000 died, the Pope consecrated the Rhone River into which large numbers of bodies were thrown because the churchyard could no longer hold them and there were not enough people to dig graves. Everywhere bodies were piled by the thousands in large pits and covered with thin layers of earth. Plague crossed the English Channel and destroyed half the population of Medieval England. London, during just one of its many epidemics, lost 100,000 inhabitants.

In order to appreciate the significance of these figures, it must be realized that the population of the world and its countries and cities was only a small fraction of what it is now. Plague continued to ebb and flow across the known world like a periodic tide sweeping everything before it. This continued until as recently as the 19th Century. Certain desperate groping attempts were made to combat these epidemic disasters. They represent some of the earliest public health actions. In 1348, Venice banned the entrance of infected or suspected ships and travellers. Rogusa, in 1377, ruled that travellers from plague-infected areas must stop outside the port and remain free of disease for two months, later forty days, before being allowed to enter. Thus came about the first quarantine measure. Six years later Marseilles erected the first quarantine station. These are historic landmarks in public health, but unfortunately their effectiveness was limited by communications, ignorance, superstition and the lack of appreciation of the role of vectors such as the rat and its fleas.

Cholera was another of the many diseases which was spread by the mass movement of people. Its historic home has been in the Ganges delta. Repeatedly throughout history it has surged outward and spread around the world. It has continued as a great threat even to the present time. It became one of the most common epidemic diseases of increasingly urbanized Europe and later was rapidly passed on to the American continent by means of the large numbers of settlers and immigrants. It accompanied the '49ers to the gold fields of California and is said to have been the chief cause of death among them. Mention should be made also of syphilis, which was referred to as "the great pox" to distinguish it from the smallpox, which of course is itself considered an extremely dangerous disease. As far as can be determined the early explorers beginning with Columbus' crew exchanged smallpox, measles, and tuberculosis for the syphilis of the American Indian. During the 15th Century, syphilis spread like wildfire throughout Europe in very severe and acute form.

The Age of Enlightenment

Gradually, doubt began to be cast upon the common ideas that diseases were caused by the positions of planets, witchcraft, chance, or vengeful punishment for sin. Those involved in the age of enlightenment and in the budding of scientific thought sought other more rational explanations and ways to control the destiny of man. It should be noted in passing, however, that there persists even today much misconception and superstition about many diseases. One still encounters, for example, individuals who look upon venereal infections and even cancer and tuberculosis as punishment for some sort of sexual misbehavior.

At any rate, the people of Europe slowly emerged from the dreadful and depressing period of Medievalism and cautiously began to open their eyes and to think as free individuals. A number of outstanding philosophers appeared who were to mold the future of mankind. Among these were Descartes, Lyell, Lamarck, Cuvier, Boyle, Adam Smith, Voltaire, and Darwin. Each in his field hammered at the bars which imprisoned the minds and bodies of man. Together they brought about remarkable achievements during the late 18th Century and throughout the 19th Century. The concept of the dignity of man and his right to seek mastery over his fate became established. The search for scientific truth for its own sake was finally advocated.

The 18th and 19th Centuries were not without their unique problems, however. The development of new forms of energy gave rise to the industrial revolution. The struggle for economic power became a dominant factor in the culture of the times with resulting severe abuses of those less educated and the economically less fortunate masses. Slavery reached its peak during this period in order to produce the raw materials for the maws of the industrial centers of Europe. Child labor was an accepted practice, and orphans and abandoned children were in effect purchased from workhouses and foundling homes by factory owners who sometimes literally chained the children to machines. Understandably malnutrition, tuberculosis and many other diseases ran rampant. As a result, by the middle of the 19th Century, the average age at death among the working classes in London was 22 years as compared with 44 for the gentry and professional persons. Abuses became so flagrant that reaction was bound to set in. Charles Dickens, Jonathan Swift, Charles Reade, Jeremy Bentham, Victor Hugo, Harriet Beecher Stowe and others focussed attention upon the many social problems of the time by means of their widely read writings. In terms of hygienic reform, Edwin Chadwick's momentous "Report on an Inquiry into the Sanitary Condition of the Laboring Population of Great Britain" was especially significant and led to the establishment in 1848 of a General Board of Health for England. In the same year, Sir John Simon was appointed the first Medical Officer of Health for London. Seven years later he assumed the same office for Great Britain as a whole, and improvements in public health followed rapidly.

Public Health in the New World

Meanwhile, the new North American colonies were developing their own health problems. Many of the early settlements were seriously threatened and sometimes obliterated by epidemic diseases, most notably smallpox. Ironically, the diseases the colonists brought aided them unwittingly in the establishment of their footholds. The natives, who had had no previous contact with many diseases, such as tuberculosis, measles and smallpox, died in large numbers, and were less able to resist the settlement and expansion of migrants from Europe. It is estimated that during this period the Indian population was decimated by diseases introduced by the settlers.

Very early, the settlements along the eastern seaboard instituted certain measures that may be regarded as of a public health nature. Laws were passed as early as 1639 in the Massachusetts Colony for the registration of births and deaths. Other legislation dealt with the prevention of the pollution of harbors, the control of nuisances and offensive trades, the isolation of cases of smallpox, and the quarantine of ships. The increasing threat from various diseases, especially yellow fever, about the time of the American Revolution led to a widespread interest in the development of Boards of Health. Permissive legislation for this purpose was passed in 1797 by New York and Massachusetts and in 1805 by Connecticut. There is some question as to which city had the first permanent Board of Health. Boston is commonly considered to have organized the first in 1799 with Paul Revere as its chairman. Priority has also been claimed by Petersburg, Virginia (1780), Baltimore (1793), Philadelphia (1794) and New York (1796).

In 1798, the recently formed American Congress created a Marine Hospital Service in order to provide for sick and disabled merchant seamen. This is significant for three reasons: first, it was the origin of what eventually became the U.S. Public Health Service, second, it provided an organization for effecting a national and interstate quarantine, and third, it represents probably the first instance of prepaid medical insurance. For 20 cents per month deducted from his pay (later replaced by a tonnage tax) each merchant seaman was assured medical and hospital care. By 1800 the merchant marine had grown to such an extent that it became practical to construct in Norfolk, Virginia the first of many hospitals which are still administered by the U.S. Public Health Service.

Between 1800 and 1850 the nation expanded rapidly in size and population, but public health activities remained stationary. Problems, however, kept pace with national development. Many epidemics especially of smallpox, yellow fever, cholera, typhoid and typhus rapidly entered and swept over the land. Tuberculosis and malaria reached very high levels of prevalence. For example, in Massachusetts, for which good records exist, the tuberculosis death rate in 1850 was over 300 per 100,000 population per year. The infant mortality was about 200 per 1000 live births, and smallpox, scarlet fever and typhoid fever were high on the list of leading causes of death. As a result, at that time, the average length of life in Boston and most of the other older cities in America was even less than that in London, which was itself the object of widespread criticism. The American social scene also became the subject of scathing comments by visitors from abroad who left with the impression of cruelty and barbarism of life in the United States, as well as of the generally unkempt appearance of its communities.

An important indication of inadequacy was the low quality of medical care. Professional teaching facilities were few and inadequate. A large proportion of the "physicians" were self-designated and itinerant. Professional licensure was non-existent. A wide spectrum of healing philosophies and cults arose, many of them based upon weird and mystical concepts. Treatment consisted of generally crude and far from sterile emergency surgery, and of empirical remedies brought over from Europe. These were augmented by newly discovered "remedies" borrowed from the native American aborigines. This state of therapeutic evil led Oliver Wendell Holmes to remark that, "If the whole materia medica as now used could be sunk to the bottom of the sea, it would be all the better for mankind, and all the worse for the fishes."

Boards of Health, to the extent that they existed, tended to be temporary makeshift organizations which consisted of a group of physicians and other citizens who were called together to meet emergency situations as they occurred. Gradually it was realized in some places that some measure of permanency in hygienic affairs was desirable and practical. This led to the formation of permanent local health departments in an ever increasing number of urban centers: Baltimore (1798), Charlestown, South Carolina (1815), Philadelphia (1818), Providence (1832), Cambridge (1846), New York City (1866), Chicago (1867), Louisville (1870), Indianapolis (1872), and Boston (1873). As might be expected, their activities were determined by current theories about the causation of disease, and placed emphasis upon the elimination of insanitary nuisances. Thus, in mid 19th century New York City, with a population of 300,000, the community health program was concerned with crowded living conditions, dirty streets, and the regulation of public baths, slaughter houses, and pigsties.

The most notable document in public health history in the United States appeared about this time. Lemuel Shattuck (1793-1859) produced his extraordinary "Report of the Sanitary Commission of Massachusetts." Shattuck was a remarkable individual who led the diversified life of teacher, historian, bookdealer, sociologist, statistician and eventually a legislator in the State Assembly. Although a layman, he had a keen and vocal interest in sanitary reform which led to his appointment as chairman of a legislative committee to study the health problems of the Commonwealth of Massachusetts. The resulting report, released in 1850, was remarkable since it related to existing and future public health needs not only of Massachusetts, but also of the nation as a whole. In some respects, even now more than a century later, it would be considered ahead of its time. In order to evaluate the report properly, it must be remembered that when it was written there were no national or state public health programs, and such local health agencies as had been organized were still embryonic and as has been mentioned, operated almost entirely on the basis of fallacious theory. Medical practice was far from scientific and in a confused state, the training of nurses was non-existent, and almost another half century was to pass before the spectacular era of Pasteur, Koch, and the other contributors to the golden age of bacteriology.

Among the many recommendations in the report were those for the establishment of permanent state and local Boards of Health and operating health organizations, a regular system of sanitary inspection, the state and nationwide collection and analysis of vital statistics with a routine system for the exchange of data and information, sanitary programs for towns and buildings, studies of and programs dealing with the health of school children, studies of tuberculosis, alcoholism and mental diseases, the sanitary supervision and study of the problems of immigrants, the erection of model tenements, public bath houses and wash houses, the control of smoke nuisances, the control of food adulteration, the exposure of quacks and nostrums, the preaching of health from pulpits, the establishment of nurses training schools, the teaching of sanitary science in medical schools, and the inclusion of preventive medicine in clinical practice with routine physical examinations and family records of illness. Unfortunately this report which appeared in 1850 fell on sterile soil and was allowed to lie unappreciated for about two decades. Finally, in 1869 the first permanent State Board of Health was established in Massachusetts as had been recommended by Shattuck. The second, incidentally, was organized on the opposite side of the continent in the new state of California in 1870. By the close of the century, 37 other states had followed suit. Eventually, as a result of action by Texas in 1909 and by New Mexico in 1919, every state in the union had a board of health and a permanent operating department of public health.

To return to the national level, more and more the expanding United States Public Health Service fulfilled the function of a federal public health agency. The national government accepted responsibility for certain other groups in addition to the merchant marine. In time, it became practical for the Public Health Service to develop a full-time career staff of commissioned officers. Responsibility for interstate and federal quarantine, and the supervision of interstate carriers were added to its responsibilities. This led naturally to investigation of the epidemiology of various diseases which in turn gave rise in 1901 to the establishment of the National Hygienic Laboratory. In subsequent years this expanded into the vast research complex of the National Institutes of

Health and the National Clinical Center in Bethesda, Maryland, the Center for Disease Control in Atlanta, Georgia, and the National Institute of Environmental Health Science near Durham, N. C. These carry out or underwrite a major part of the medical and public health research in the nation. In recognition of its expanding function, the name of the agency was changed in 1902 to the Public Health and Marine Hospital Service under the direction of a Surgeon General. In 1912 it was reorganized further and received its present name, the United States Public Health Service.

By now, the basic framework for official health activities in the United States had been established, except for one notable gap. On the national level there existed the Public Health Service. All but one state had organized boards and departments of health. On the local level, most of the larger cities and towns had set up permanent public health agencies, and an increasing number of smaller communities were doing likewise. However, in 1910, less than one-half of the population lived in urban circumstances, in contrast with about 80 per cent now. Furthermore, in 1910, two in three of the rural population lived and worked on farms as compared with only 5 per cent at present. The remainder of the non-urban dwellers do not live or work as farmers. In fact, the majority live relatively close to cities. Accordingly, even if the communities of all of the urban dwellers in 1910 had had public health programs, which of course they didn't, there still would have been more than one-half of the population, those in the rural areas, left unserved and unprotected.

Meanwhile, two sets of circumstances were at work to change this situation. As the rural population grew in numbers, it began to experience an increasing number of individual and group health problems. This was all the more serious because the growing urban population depended upon them for food, and could be infected by it. One place where this was true was in Yakima County, Washington, where a series of epidemics of typhoid fever had occurred. In the year 1910-11, the situation became particularly serious and the local and state authorities requested the assistance of the Public Health Service. After bringing the immediate situation under control, it was strongly recommended that the county establish a small, full-time resident staff of professional workers to deal with all public health matters. During the same period, the Rockefeller Sanitary Commission (later to become the Rockefeller Foundation) was working on the serious problem of hookworm disease in the southeastern United States. After several years of effort, it concluded that no single disease or public health problem could be successfully attacked by itself. For permanent effect, all phases of public health had to be dealt with. Therefore, quite independently, they recommended the establishment of county health departments with full-time qualified staffs. The coincidental result was the simultaneous establishment of the first two county health departments, Guilford County, North Carolina in June, 1911, and Yakima County, Washington, in July, 1911. As a result of these various events and approaches, by now almost all of the nation's population is served by local public health services.

The period around 1912 was of significance to the public health movement for still another reason. As the women of America became more powerful and vocal, it was natural that one of their dominant interests was the welfare of children. Infant mortality was very high, about 5 times the present rate. Malnutrition was common as were all of the communicable diseases of childhood. Furthermore, there were still few restraints to the employment of children in industry. Considerable pressure was brought to bear first upon President Theodore Roosevelt and subsequently upon President Taft, largely by organized groups of women, to act in the situation. As a result, on April 9, 1912, an act was passed which established a federal Children's Bureau. Organizationally it was placed in the Department of Labor where it remained until 1946 when it was transferred to the Federal Security Agency which in 1953 became the U.S. Department of Health, Education and Welfare. Subsequently, in 1963, soon after its 50th anniversary, the Children's Bureau was placed in a new Welfare Administration, and more recently in August 1967 became part of a major unit in the Department. This unit, The Social and Rehabilitation Service, also includes the other functions of the former Welfare Administration, the Vocational Rehabilitation Administration, the Administration on Aging, and The Mental Retardation Division of The Public Health Service. This larger agency is designed to join and coordinate under single leadership the programs for those in need and the social service and rehabilitation programs that many individuals and families require.

The original act which established the Children's Bureau directed "That said Bureau shall investigate and report . . . upon all matters pertaining to the welfare of children and child life, among all classes of people, and shall especially investigate the questions of infant mortality, the birth rate, orphanages, juvenile courts, desertions, dangerous occupations, accidents and diseases of children, employment, legislation affecting children in the several states and territories." Over the years, by staff action and by subsequent legislation the Children's Bureau has contributed greatly to the definition, understanding, and solution of a large number of the health and other problems of the children and youth of America.

Arising out of many factors, not the least of which was the economic depression of the time, the Congress in 1935 passed the Social Security Act. Among other effects, this legislation was significant in terms of the role of the Public Health Service. Among other things, it provided for assistance to state and local jurisdictions in the establishment and maintenance of public health programs, the construction and equipment of needed physical facilities, and for the training of various categories of professional personnel. Since then, substantial amounts of federal grants-in-aid have been made available through the Public Health Service. In general, these subsidies to states, and through them to localities, have been made on the basis of four factors; (1) population (2) public health problems (3) economic need and (4) professional personnel training needs. There is no question but that the provisions of this act, and numerous subsequent related acts, and its praiseworthy administration have played dominant roles in the effective development of state and local health programs throughout the nation.

In 1939, President Franklin Roosevelt established the Federal Security Administration which brought together many of the federal governmental units concerned with health, education and welfare. One result was a closer relationship between the Office of Education and the Public Health Service. Further reorganization occurred in 1946 when the National Office of Vital Statistics was transferred from the Department of Commerce to the Public Health Service, and the Children's Bureau of the Department of Labor and the Food and Drug Administration of the Department of Agriculture were transferred to become components of the Federal Security Administration. Finally, in 1953, a federal Department of Health, Education and Welfare, under a Secretary with cabinet rank was created to replace the makeshift Federal Security Administration. Since that time there have been numerous reorganizations and internal realignments as well as many new programs resulting from much new legislation. The result is that by now, the Department of Health, Education and Welfare is the second largest unit of the Federal government with a current budget (1970) of over 52 billions of dollars. This compares with the largest, the Department of Defense which has a current budget of about 78 billions of dollars. The organization and activities of the Department of Health, Education and Welfare are discussed in the following chapter.

Education in the New World

Their fervid desire for freedom to live and worship as they pleased prompted the early colonists to crowd into sailing vessels and to brave the terrors of the Atlantic and the dangers of the wilderness. These dauntless people brought with them to the New World an ethical and cultural heritage which helped to determine the form and direction of education in the colonies and to shape the governmental structure of the emerging nation toward democracy.

From the dynamics of the Renaissance in Europe stemmed the rise of the spirit of scientific inquiry, and experimentation in the application of scientific principles which changed man's thinking and many of the conditions surrounding his life. This period was marked by the development of great universities with their emphasis upon Latin, Greek and the humanities—les artes liberales. The years which followed brought a manifestation of the spirit of inquiry as applied to religion and philosophy. The teachings of the great religious philosophers channeled thinking toward the recognition of man as a self, the consideration of the value and dignity of man, and the right of each individual to shape his own life toward ultimate transcendence to a higher future life. A significant outcome of the Age of Enlightenment was the rise of the vernacular school as the means of permitting each person to work out his own destiny. By the time the colonists came to America, elementary schools for children of freemen had been established in practically all large towns of the Western European countries. Thus, the colonists brought with them a concept of education at two different levels but with little in common. It follows logically that this concept should have been reflected in the early educational pattern in the New World.

Early Efforts

The colonists who settled in the New England area, did not delay in turning their thoughts toward schools for their children. The Boston Latin School, established in 1635, set a pattern for secondary education in other colonies. Harvard College, founded in 1642, stressed admission requirements which called for sound proficiency in the classics. The Massachusetts Law of 1647 required that a teacher be appointed in every township of fifty or more householders and that every town of more than one hundred householders should establish a grammar school. Through the mechanism of the town-meeting, a close but informal relationship existed between these early tax-supported schools and the church. In Virginia, few parish schools were established. Here the tutorial system prevailed, influenced not only by Locke's philosophy, but also by the great distances between large plantations.

It is interesting that the leaders in government were also deeply concerned with education as well as with health matters. Both Thomas Jefferson and Benjamin Franklin stressed the importance of schools for all, and higher education for the preparation of leaders so sorely needed in the new and struggling democracy. At the higher level, Jefferson strongly favored selective education for those qualified, with emphasis upon the classics, but Franklin pointed out the additional need for practical education in preparation for different kinds of tasks. He advocated the inclusion of English, foreign languages, and mathematics.

Nineteenth Century Developments

During the 19th century, many problems which deeply affected education faced the developing nation: the expansion of the nation's land area, the tremendous influx of immigrants from many countries and with vastly different heritages some of which were not as advanced as those of the early settlers, the War Between the States with its aftermath of complex socio-economic problems, the change from an agrarian to an industrial nation, the shift from rural to urban living, the great technical development which accompanied the rise of industry, the changing economy, and the phenomenally rapid rise of the young nation to a position of great power and wealth. Concurrently, there appeared to occur a decline in the importance of the church and an increased materialism in the lives of the people.

The increase in the population, the gradual enactment of compulsory attendance laws, and the provision of state support of education caused the enrollment in elementary schools to multiply. According to Monroe, in the middle of the 19th century the average elementary school curriculum "included only reading, spelling, and English grammar, while those of a superior sort included writing, arithmetic, geography, and history."[5] By the close of the 19th century practically all children of school age were enrolled in elementary school but only 7 per cent of those of high school age were attending secondary school.[6]

The great national changes naturally precipitated cultural changes. There seemed to be a growing awareness of the need for a re-examination of the purpose and direction of education. The writings of Locke, Pestalozzi, Froebel, and Herbart had left their mark on American education. Society was at last aware that children were more than family pets or expendable commodities. During the last quarter of the century, the dual system of education established by the early colonists was superseded by a single system of universal, tax-supported public schools.

The Twentieth Century

The problem of the individual in society now became the center of attention. The concept of the development of each individual to his highest potentialities reflected the new emphasis upon psychology. Scientific and industrial training were introduced into the secondary school, but at the same time these subjects were supposed to be taught in such manner as to contribute to preparation for citizenship. The emphasis upon science, sociology, and psychology turned attention to consideration of educational purpose, methods, and the processes of learning and teaching as well as to the selection of subject matter.

In 1918, the Report on the Cardinal Principles of Education offered the following re-definition of education:

> The purpose of democracy is to organize society that each member may develop his personality primarily through activities

[5]Monroe, Paul: *A Textbook in the History of Education.* New York, The Macmillan Company, 1957, p. 701.

[6]Annual Report, 1952. Washington, D.C.: Office of Education, Federal Security Agency. p. 14.

> designed for the well-being of his fellow-members and society as a whole . . .
>
> Consequently, education in a democracy, both within and without the school, should develop in each individual the knowledge, interests, ideals, habits, and powers whereby he will find his place and use that place to shape himself and society toward ever noble goals.[7]

The Report stipulated that in order to achieve these goals, the pupil should be inculcated along the lines of what were termed the seven cardinal principles stated in this order: (1) health, (2) command of fundamental processes, (3) worthy home membership, (4) vocational training, (5) citizenship, (6) worthy use of leisure, and (7) ethical character. The position of health in this list is significant. This marked a shift of emphasis from the mere scholarly purpose of education in the high school to a concern for daily living, the development of character and other phases formerly considered to be the duty of the family and the church. This thinking also moved high schools toward meeting the needs of the student through a wider diversification.

In 1938, the cardinal principles were re-grouped in a report issued by the Education Policies Commission as (1) self-realization, (2) human relationships, (3) economic efficiency, and (4) civic responsibility.[8] Health is implicitly fundamental to all of these. This quadrad, in the years that followed, served as the basis for curriculum construction throughout the nation.

About the beginning of the 20th century, along with the increased consideration for the child, came a new approach to learning which left its imprint upon education. This movement, known as progressive education, advocated an approach to learning through an appeal to the child's interests. When thus aroused, it was hoped that the child would be moved to greater efforts. So much misunderstanding attended the implementation of this philosophy that eventually it fell into disrepute. Before this happened, however, many of its basic concepts had been implemented by educators and formed the basis of many useful methods and procedures in the schools today.

The entrance into the atomic era, the dramatic recent adjustments in international relationships, and the reality of exploration of extraterrestrial space have spurred serious revaluation of education in the nation. More acutely than ever before, our people have come to realize that the public school, as a core social institution, has proved its worth

[7]*Cardinal Principles of Secondary Education.* Report of the Commission on the Reorganization of Secondary Education, Washington, D.C.: U. S. Bureau of Education, 1918, p. 9.

[8]Educational Policies Commission, *The Purpose of Education in American Democracy.* Washington, D.C.: National Education Association of the United States and the American Association of School Administrators: 1201 Sixteenth Street, N.W., p. 47.

as one of the nation's greatest forces for stability and character building, and that therein lies the hope of the future of our nation and for the free world.

With this brief view of education as a base, the evolution of school health which it nurtured should now be examined, with particular reference to total community health with which it is so inseparably enmeshed.

The Evolution of School Health

A generation inured to the phenomenon of social planning so common to the second half of the 20th century, may find it difficult to realize that no such comprehensive planning preceded the introduction of health and health education into the public schools. Indeed, so gradual was its inception that decades sometimes elapsed between the recognition of a health need and any actual ameliorative action. For the most part, the school health program developed inconspicuously, feature by feature, usually at the behest of some persistent health-minded individual or an enthusiastic vocal group. Nevertheless, note should be taken of certain milestones along the way, keys to the understanding and full appreciation of the how's and why's of today's school health program.

Early in the 19th century there appeared in various parts of Europe evidence of awakening interest in the health and welfare of children. As mentioned, Rousseau, Locke, and others had aroused a consciousness of the real nature of the child and the scope of his needs including those commonly related to health, such as poverty, over-work, poor nutrition. In the struggling American colonies, the major health concern had centered upon the communicable diseases which from time to time ravaged whole segments of the population and increased in magnitude and frequency with the growth of towns and schools. During the first half of the 19th century, the pioneer educator, Horace Mann, earnestly voiced the need for schools to give some attention to the health of children and to plan for the training of teachers who would be able to develop in children an awareness of health with emphasis upon prevention of disease. As a result, the teaching of hygiene and physiology followed mathematics as the second subject of a scientific nature to be introduced into the elementary school curriculum in this country.

In 1850, Lemuel Shattuck, in his famous Report to the Sanitary Commission in Boston, to which earlier reference has been made, is credited with pointing out the health needs of children and with offering practical suggestions to teachers on such matters as daily health inspection and the importance of teaching health and hygiene.

> Every child should be taught, early in life, that to preserve his own life and his own health and the lives and health of others, is one of his most important and constantly abiding duties. Some

> measure is needed which shall compel children to make a sanitary examination of themselves and their associates, and thus elicit a practical application of the lessons of sanitary science in the everyday duties of life. The recommendation now under consideration is designed to furnish this measure. It is to be carried into operation in the use of a blank schedule, which is to be printed on a letter sheet, in the form of a prescribed appendix, and furnished to the teacher of each school. He is to appoint a sanitary committee of the scholars, at the commencement of school, and on the first day of each month, to fill it out under his superintendence. . . . Such a measure is simple, would take but a few minutes each day, and cannot operate otherwise than usefully upon the children, in forming habits of exact observation, and in making a personal application of the laws of health and life to themselves. This is education of an eminently practical character, and of the highest importance.[9]

In the years which followed, a few States introduced the teaching of hygiene. However, most attempts at systematic teaching of health or hygiene consisted mainly of memorizing the facts of anatomy or physiology.

The initial steps leading to specific legislative action came during the period from 1880 to 1890 mainly through the zealous efforts of temperance organizations deeply concerned with the problems of alcohol and tobacco. Through the influence of these organizations during the next decade every State in the nation passed laws requiring its public schools to include the teaching of the undesirable effects of alcohol and tobacco. Some States required that these be taught along with hygiene. In many instances these laws still stand, and units in present day courses of study in health may be found marked "mandatory by the State."

During the last quarter of the century there appeared in many communities a growing interest in the introduction of physical education in the public schools. Sporadic interest had been shown principally in sections of the country where Scandinavian or German groups had settled and perpetuated their old-country interest in physical culture, particularly formal gymnastics. In 1882, Ohio became the first state to require physical education in its first and second class cities, and in 1890 North Dakota took the lead in requiring it in all common schools. Health and physical education, although closely related, were introduced into the public schools during the same decade but as two separate entities.

With communicable diseases of childhood a paramount problem, it was logical that the medical profession should turn its attention to the

[9] Shattuck, Lemuel. *Report of the Sanitary Commission of Massachusetts, 1850.* Facsimile edition. Cambridge, Mass., Harvard University Press, 1948. p. 178-179.

schools. Boston was the first city to introduce medical inspection in its public schools in the year 1894. During the next four years, Chicago, New York, and Philadelphia followed suit. In 1905 the New York schools began to examine each child for physical defects. In 1906, Massachusetts legislation required medical inspection in its public schools. By 1910, medical inspection was quite firmly established in most large cities in the United States of America. For a number of years, the term medical inspection provided an accurate description of the program. Defects disclosed by the inspection were charted but there was scant time or attention devoted to the follow-up and corrective procedures which forward-looking communities today regard as a basic part of school health services. In far too many schools and communities, the means, *i.e.* medical inspection, was considered in effect as an end in itself. Unfortunately, this is sometimes true even today.

Another milestone along the road to school health was the appointment in 1902 in New York City of the nation's first public school nurse. Her appointment by the Board of Education was preceded by a month's demonstration arranged by Lillian D. Wald, the famous Director of the Henry Street Settlement. Contacts with settlement children had furnished moving evidence of the enormity of their existing health needs. The demonstration of what one nurse could accomplish during one month was sufficiently convincing to result in the official appointment of 24 nurses during that same school year. The first public school dentist was appointed in Reading, Pennsylvania in 1903, and in 1914 the first school dental hygienists were appointed in Bridgeport, Connecticut. The following year the State of Vermont introduced compulsory eye, ear, nose and throat examinations.

With the involvement of our nation in World War I, the general public became truly aroused by the great number of draft rejections for physical reasons. As a result, intensive post-war emphasis was given to health and welfare, particularly among children from infancy to fourteen years of age.

A generation later, with the advent of World War II, the people learned to their consternation that the percentage of draft rejections was practically no better than it had been at the time of World War I. Health efforts since World War I had been concentrated mainly upon young children and college students, but the junior and senior high school years had been largely neglected. This realization led to immediate increased efforts with the health concerns of children and youth from grades 7 through 12 and with school health in general.

The White House Conferences

Of great importance in giving impetus to interest in child health have been the White House Conferences on Children and Youth, the first of which was called by Theodore Roosevelt in 1909. The announcement of the Golden Anniversary White House Conference on Children and Youth in 1960 included the following brief reviews concerning the main outcomes of each of the preceding decennial conferences:

> This first Conference (in 1909) gave impetus to the establishment of the United States Children's Bureau in 1912, the enactment of child labor laws, and the organization of the first national voluntary agency concerned with the welfare of children. In each decade that followed, a White House Conference called by the President left its mark—
>
> 1919—Established national responsibility in setting minimum health and welfare standards for mothers and children
>
> 1930—Produced the most comprehensive collection of data on health and welfare of children ever assembled, including the Children's Charter
>
> 1940—Led to strengthening of personnel and training standards in equipping American children for the successful practice of democracy
>
> 1950—Endorsed a platform for meeting the problems which prevent young people from achieving healthy personalities; developed machinery for continuing activity during the time between conferences.[10]

Each conference had far-reaching effects upon school health developments. Moreover, through the publicity attending the conferences, school personnel and the general public were kept informed about trends and needs. The 1919 Conference stressed the importance of health services and minimum standards for healthful living. Some of the rights of children as set forth in the Children's Charter[11] at the 1930 Conference were directly concerned with the three main phases of school health (see page 243). A continuation of these emphases characterized the 1940 Conference. The Mid-Century Conference centered around mental, emotional, and spiritual qualities essential to individual happiness and responsible citizenship. The need for health education to be integrated throughout the entire school experience was given special emphasis.

The Golden Anniversary White House Conference for Children and Youth held in 1960 announced:

> Its Purpose—to promote opportunities for children and youth to realize their full potential for a creative life in freedom and dignity.
>
> Its Focus— on the effects of our rapidly changing world on the

[10] *Golden Anniversary Conference on Children and Youth.* Washington 25, D.C.: Golden Anniversary Conference on Children and Youth, 330 Independence Avenue S.W., 1960. A folder.

[11] *The White House Conference,* 1930, New York, The Century Co., 1931, p. 45.

> development of our young . . . on appraising and reappraising the values and ideals we live by . . . on studying the factors that influence individual fulfillment—family, religion, education, health, community life.[12]

The custom of holding local meetings prior to each decennial conference was inaugurated with the 1919 Conference. Scores of regional preconference meetings serve the useful purpose of familiarizing people, including parents and school personnel, with the problems to be discussed. Each succeeding conference has involved more people in preliminary preparation. Preparation for the Golden Anniversary Conference in 1960 and for the 1970 Conference involved thousands of people in local communities throughout the entire nation in discussions of assigned topics leading to the definition of needs and the framing of recommendations. By now, a major portion of the values of the conferences lies in these preliminary local study groups which concentrate upon grass roots versions of the problems to be considered later on a national scale. The broad involvement of many types of organizations and agencies interested in some aspect of child health and welfare, and the development of strenuous follow-up efforts for the implementation of the conference recommendations tend to make these conferences a truly continuing influence. The responsibility for the follow-up of the Golden Anniversary Conference was centered in the National Committee on Children and Youth with headquarters in Washington, D.C. This committee stimulated interchange of experiences and the holding of interim conferences on State and Regional bases, with special emphasis upon the formation of a permanent Governor's Committee in each state.

The following excerpt from the 1960 State Report indicates the direction of future emphasis:

> "The priorities which the States see for the sixties all add up to the major goal of equalizing opportunities for all children and youth, urban and rural, white and non-white of whatever economic and social group, in whatever state or region.
>
> These are the priorities: a major upgrading of the quality of education, with much greater attention to special needs; an enlargement of opportunities for youth, with better preparation for employment; an enlargement of opportunities for the constructive use of leisure; a concentrated effort to improve the physical and especially the mental health of our children and youth; and a concentrated effort to strengthen family life."[13]

[12]op. cit.

[13]The State Report on Children and Youth, Golden Anniversary White House Conference on Children and Youth, National Council of State Committees for Children and Youth. Printed in US of America, National Committee, Mrs. Rollin Brown, Chairman.

Voluntary Health Agencies and the School Child

In a pioneer country where people were peculiarly dependent upon each other, the spontaneous rise and growth of the voluntary health agency seemed a natural expression of this sense of responsibility for one's less fortunate neighbor. It is logical that such organizations should have played key roles in the development of the school health program, sometimes even blazing a trail by calling attention to a special existing problem which needed consideration. Particularly noteworthy among such organizations was the National Tuberculosis Association (now the National Tuberculosis and Respiratory Disease Association) which in 1915 began a movement known as the Modern Health Crusade which promoted programs stressing desirable health habits in children. Later, the Association promoted tuberculin testing, x-raying, the provision of consultant services, pilot demonstrations, and in-service education of teachers.

The American Child Health Association, which existed from 1922 to 1935, greatly influenced the trends and direction of school health. Through its conferences it stimulated interest in various problems and encouraged practical self-study and analysis, surveys, demonstrations, and research. Many other non-official agencies contributed to school health but space prevents their mention.

Professional Organizations and the School Child

Professional organizations have given continuous support and stimulation to the various phases of the school child's health. Particularly noteworthy in this respect have been the American School Health Association, the American Public Health Association especially through its School Health Section, the American Association for Health, Physical Education and Recreation, the National Education Association, and the American Medical Association. A notable attempt at a unified approach to school health was made in 1911 when a Committee of the National Education Association and the Committee of the Council on Health and Public Instruction of the American Medical Association met together to consider the child health program in schools. This led to the establishment of the Joint Committee on Health Problems in Education of the National Education Association and the American Medical Association whose authoritative publications have contributed immeasurably to the school health program of today.

International Agencies and the School Child

The United States of America has joined whole-heartedly in the international efforts of the United Nations in its attempt to raise the general level of child health throughout the world. It has done this by extensive support of the work of the United Nations International Children's Emergency Fund (UNICEF) and the World Health Organization (WHO). Every health educator and teacher should regard as part of her professional preparation, cultural background and fundamental philosophy, familiarity with the Declaration of the Rights of the Child which was adopted at the General Assembly of the United Nations on November 20, 1959.

The International Council of Health, Physical Education and Recreation holds its conferences in relation with the World Confederation of Organizations of the Teaching Profession. In addition to these conferences, the ICHPER stimulates regional workshops for member groups and research studies. Its offices are located at the headquarters of the National Education Association in Washington, D.C.

Professional Preparation in Health Education

The professional preparation of classroom teachers and specialists in health education has long been the concern of the various professional organizations centered upon health. With specific regard to the specialty of health education, the American Public Health Association published first in 1948, and subsequently revised a listing of suggested qualifications and functions.[14] It is recommended that those interested in a career in this specialized field attend one of the accredited Graduate Schools of Public Health and obtain the degree of Master of Public Health. Many fellowships are available for this purpose and information concerning them may be obtained readily by contacting one's state health department.

During recent years, teacher preparation in health education has been the focus of numerous conferences participated in by members of all the professional organizations most concerned. Various reports, prepared under the leadership of the American Association for Health, Physical Education and Recreation have served as guidelines in raising the general professional level. Current emphasis upon unity in terminology, goals, and purposes points toward future progress in school health.

Research in School Health

Recent years have witnessed some excellent research which has helped to chart sound progress in health and health education in schools. The famous studies in Malden, Massachusetts and elsewhere have demonstrated that health education can be effective in changing health habits. Grants from various foundations and organizations have been largely responsible for many projects with the leadership and guidance supplied by professional groups.

[14]Educational Qualifications of Health Educators. New York, American Public Health Association.

The American School Health Association, mainly through its numerous study committees which focus upon special problems or specific areas or phases of the school health program, and its many publications, has contributed consistently and invaluably to the improvement of the school health program and to the increased public recognition of its importance.

The year 1961 marked the beginning of a noteworthy, comprehensive School Health Education Study (referred to by the acronym SHES) with promising implications. With the aid of the American Association for Health, Physical Education, and Recreation and a grant from the Samuel Bronfman Foundation of New York City, this study was preceded by a preliminary survey[15] of on-going health education in a nation-wide random sampling of grades 6 through 11, and the assembly and publication of a synthesis of completed, independent, voluntary research studies on related phases of school health.[16] Under dedicated professional leadership and with the cooperation of many skilled professionals there resulted from these coordinated efforts a curriculum guide and corresponding teaching materials for kindergarten through Grade 12 designed to aid local curriculum planners in meeting more effectively the health education needs of children and youth. Nation-wide application and implementation of these study results could have far-reaching effects upon the future quality and directions of health instruction in the United States. (SHES is described in detail in Chapter 14.)[17]

Special mention should be given to the increased amount of research by graduate students and teachers under the aegis of various colleges and universities throughout the nation, dealing with or related to various phases of the school health program. The exchange of findings and results is encouraged by research sections or councils within the professional organizations and their publications and periodicals.

Although such research studies and pilot demonstrations have reached into many phases of school health, what has been accomplished is slight in comparison with the existing need.

Questions for Discussion

1. What are the implications for the teacher of the several definitions of health presented in this chapter?
2. What do the words "health" and "illness" really mean in practice to various people? Ask a sample of your acquaintances which conditions they consider illnesses and which they do not. Where does health stop and illness begin?

[15]Sliepcevich, Elena M.: *School Health Education Study: A Summary Report.* Washington, D.C., School Health Education Study, 1964.

[16]Veenker, C. Harold (ed.): *Synthesis of Research in Selected Areas of Health Instruction.* Washington, D.C.: School Health Education Study, 1963.

[17]School Health Education Study: *Health Education: A Conceptual Approach to Curriculum Design.* St. Paul, Minnesota: Minnesota Mining and Manufacturing Company, 1967.

3. What statements can you find in our Constitution which give sanction to activity in public health?
4. Have there been individuals in your community who have contributed notably to the development of medicine, nursing, or the promotion of public health and social welfare?
5. From your readings, can you think of instances in which the course of history has been determined or affected by disease?
6. Do you know of any well known works of art in which obvious signs of disease can be identified? (ex., cretinism in some of Velasquez's paintings.)
7. Can you name some individuals notable in the history of literature, art and music who suffered from various diseases that may have affected their work and the course of their lives? (ex., Beethoven's deafness)

Suggested Reading

1. Butts, R. Freeman: *A Cultural History of Western Civilization,* New York, McGraw-Hill Book Co., 1955.
2. Hanlon, J. J., Rogers, F. B., and Rosen, G.: A Bookshelf on the History and Philosophy of Public Health, Am. J. Pub. Health, *50*:445, 1960.
3. Winslow, C.-E. A.: *The Evolution and Significance of the Modern Public Health Campaign,* New Haven, Yale University Press, 1923.
4. Rosen, George: *A History of Public Health,* New York, M. D. Publications, 1958.
5. Sigerist, Henry E.: *Civilization and Disease,* Ithaca, Cornell University Press, 1943.
6. Galdston, Iago (Ed.): *The Epidemiology of Health,* New York, Health Education Council, 1953.
7. Rogers, Edward G.: *Human Ecology and Health,* New York, The Macmillan Co., 1960.
8. Ulich, Robert: *The Education of Nations,* Cambridge, Harvard University Press, 1961.
9. Monroe, Paul: *A Textbook in the History of Education,* New York, The Macmillan Co., 1957.
10. Bruner, Jerome S.: *The Process of Education,* Cambridge, Mass., Harvard Univ. Press, 1963.
11. Means, Richard K.: *A History of Health Education in the United States,* Philadelphia, Lea & Febiger, 1962.

Chapter 3

Social Organization for Health

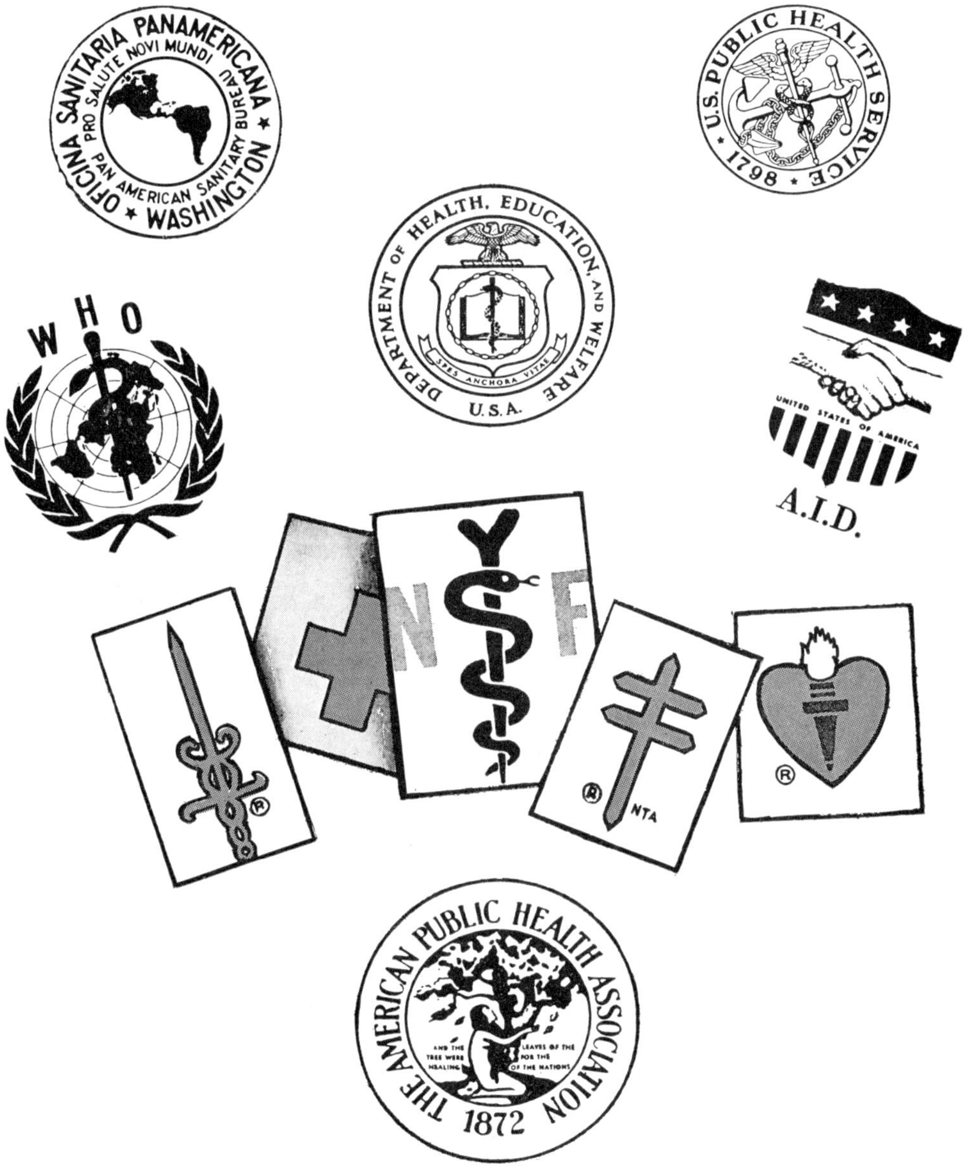

FIG. 5. "And the leaves of the tree were for the healing of the nations" (Revelation 22:2).

Introduction

In the United States of America, the protection of the health of the public is very much a shared responsibility. This is in contrast with the situation in many other countries where all health care, protection as well as treatment, is provided by a strongly centralized national government, either because of a poor economy and low standard of living, or because of a broad program of social insurance. Without question, the approach in this country is the most complex in the world. It involves the participation of a large number of interested individuals and organizations. Until recently, in the United States, health has been regarded essentially as a private and individual responsibility. Accordingly, the private practitioner of medicine, his ancillary co-workers in related professions, and privately operated hospitals traditionally have been regarded as forming the basic structure of our system of medical and health care. As time has gone on, however, this concept has tended to become more and more diluted by the increasing involvement in health matters not only of government, but also of groups such as private industry, unions, and many citizen groups. The result is that by now the average person in this country obtains his personal and community health protection and care not from one, but from a broad spectrum of sources. A partial listing of these would include, in addition to self-treatment, various types of private practitioners of medicine, psychiatric and behavioral counsellors, a wide variety of ancillary or para-medical personnel, private hospitals and out-patient clinics, local, state and federal government hospitals and clinics, an increasing number of industrial, business and labor-union in- and out-patient health facilities, many types of medical and hospital insurance programs sponsored either by government or private auspices, official community or public health programs, school health programs, and a large number of citizen sponsored and supported voluntary health agencies established for a wide assortment of special interests and problems. The mere listing of part of this confusing array of sources of health protection makes necessary a consideration of the differences among therapeutic medicine, preventive medicine and community or public health.

Traditionally, the private practitioner of medicine, and the ancillary personnel and institutions that assist him are concerned essentially with therapy or the repair of damage already done. For the most part, individuals still seek the services of private physicians primarily for diagnosis and care of some malady, the repair of a broken limb, the healing or removal of a diseased organ, or the amelioration of mental stress. Necessarily, both the relationship and the services are highly individualized and personal. Preventive medicine involves a concept which goes beyond therapy by attempting to prevent either the development of a physical or mental ailment, or its progression to more severe or irremediable proportions. In this sense, it is more concerned with causes than with effects. Ideally, of course, and with increasing frequency, private practitioners of medicine combine therapeutic and preventive medicine in their services to individuals. The unique characteristic or distinction of community or public health is that it regards an entire community or society as the patient, and recognizes that health protection and promotion may and indeed must be applied to the total community, as well as to the individual. It recognizes also that, in order to accomplish this, many different kinds of people and professions have both separate and collective contributions to make. Thus, in addition to physicians with post-graduate training in public health or in one of a variety of pertinent clinical specialties, there are needed on the community health team dentists, veterinarians, nurses, engineers, sanitarians, laboratorians, statisticians, social scientists, health educators, and many others. They must all work in coordination with each other and with the personnel of all other community organizations and groups concerned in any way with health. Important among these are teachers and institutions whose primary responsibility is the education of young people.

The foregoing discussion which attempts to distinguish among the various participants in community health work should not be interpreted as indicating areas of real or potential conflict, although unfortunately there have been occasional instances where shortsighted private physicians, public health workers, school officials or others have made this appear to be so. Dr. Franklin D. Murphy, speaking as President of the University of Kansas, when asked whether health was a public or private matter answered "It is neither and it is both." He argued that the effective resolution of the many complex health and medical problems that challenge us "will be hastened as we blend public and private effort on the basis of logic and need," concluding appropriately that "there may be times when we can afford the luxury of foolish unproductive in-fighting, but this is not one of them."[1]

The Scope of Community Health

What is the scope of activity in community or public health? Generally speaking, community or public health activities may be considered to fall into five categories, individual components of which may or may not be observed in a given situation depending upon circumstances.

1. Fields in which activity must of necessity be on a community basis:
   a. Supervision of the food, water, and milk supplies
   b. Insect control
   c. Prevention of atmospheric and stream pollution
   d. Supervision of consumer products potentially hazardous to health and safety
   e. Supervision of the manner of disposal of wastes

[1]Murphy, F. D.: Health—Public or Private? Am. J. Publ. Health, *46*:15, 1956.

2. Fields which deal with preventable illnesses, disabilities, or premature deaths:
   a. Communicable diseases, including infestations
   b. Dietary deficiencies
   c. Addiction- or habituation-producing drugs and narcotics
   d. Allergic conditions and their sources
   e. Mental, personality, and behavior disorders
   f. Conditions related to occupational illness and injury
   g. Cancer (prevention where possible, or arrest of progression)
   h. Cardiovascular diseases (prevention where possible, otherwise arrest of progression)
   i. Conditions associated with the risks of maternity, growth, and development
   j. Certain genetic or hereditary conditions
   k. Home, community, and industrial accidents
   l. Rehabilitation of victims of injuries and disease
   m. Dental caries

3. Fields of medical care which need organized official leadership:
   a. Facilitation of pregraduate and postgraduate education
   b. Promotion of equitable distribution of personnel and facilities

4. School and community health education

5. Research and evaluation—no health agency can ignore professional and scientific investigation and evaluation and remain progressive

Organization for Community Health

The complexity of the situation as it exists in the United States, makes it necessary to consider organization for community health in at least two dimensions, the various levels of government on the one hand, and the various auspices, official and nonofficial, on the other. The respective inter-relationships are shown in simplified form in the several accompanying illustrations which depict health organization as if it were a three storied physical structure (Fig. 6). On the street level, closest to the citizens and their problems, are the various local resources. Figure 7 presents in the form of a theoretical floor plan some of these local resources as they are usually found. They fall into three general categories, official agencies of local government concerned in any way in health matters, voluntary or citizen sponsored agencies interested in various aspects of health, and the private physicians and dentists and their auxiliary personnel who practice their professions in the community. In terms of individual health, as has been pointed out, this last group of private practitioners is the most important. From the standpoint of responsibility for over-all community health, however, the most important is the official health department which does or should occupy the

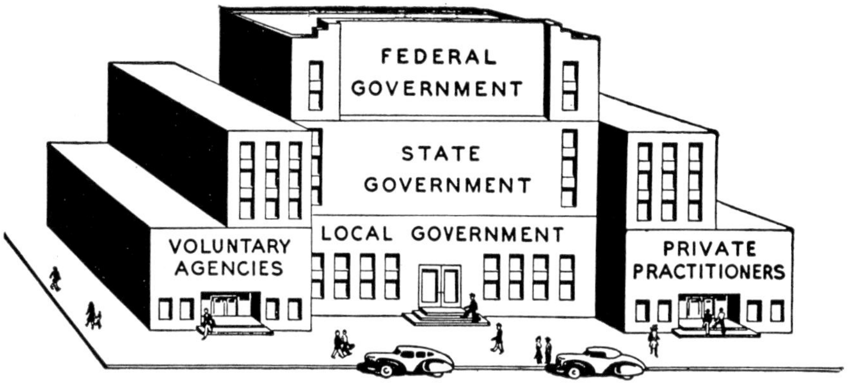

FIG. 6. The structure of community health organization.

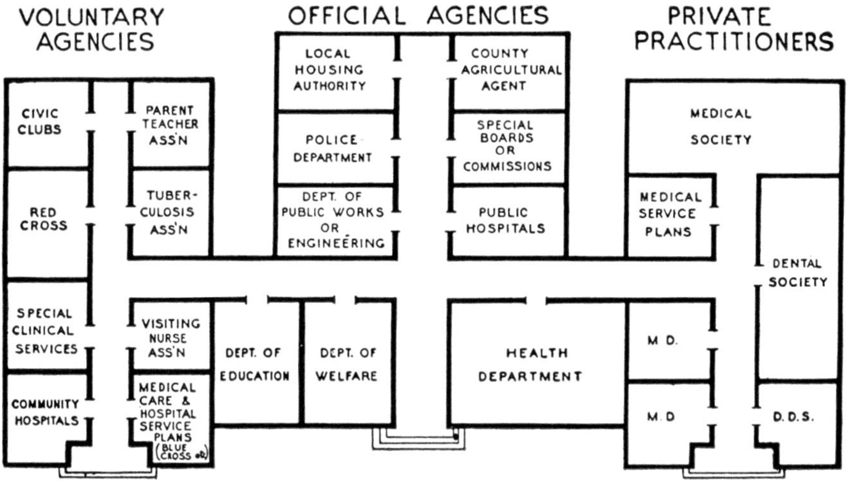

FIG. 7. Health organization on the local level.

pivotal catalytic and coordinating position. Numerous other official agencies share concern and responsibility for certain special aspects of the well-being of the community. For example, the police department is concerned with accidents, one of the leading causes of disability and deaths; the local housing authority is concerned with the hygiene of housing; the department of public works is commonly responsible for the production and distribution of an adequate supply of safe water and usually for the disposal of sewage, refuse, and garbage; the department of welfare makes available to the indigent and other disadvantaged persons certain of the necessities of life and health such as food, clothing, and shelter, while public hospitals and clinics provide for their medical care.

One of the most important of the local official agencies is the department of education in that it has under its direct supervision and influence for a significant part of their time a complete cross-section of the community between certain age limits. The group for which the schools and their teachers are responsible is of particular significance from the standpoint of health for two special reasons: first, students are in a period of life when they should be learning about personal and community health, and second, they are in the age span when certain health problems are particularly common and where the seeds of many future health problems may be planted and progress. The organization of school health programs will be dealt with in more detail later.

Local Health Organization: Official

Because of its position of primary responsibility for community health matters, the organization and function of the official local health agency merits special consideration. Local government in the United States takes many forms: municipalities, towns, townships, counties, and a wide variety of districts organized for special purposes. Accordingly, a number of different approaches to local health organization may be observed. Every progressive urban center has its own health department. As one approaches the more rural situation, however, certain practical factors must be taken into consideration, especially the number of people and the size of an area adequate to produce sufficient tax funds to support at least a minimum staff of qualified public health workers. It is usually recommended that an area should contain at least 50,000 people before it considers an independent health unit. Exceptions may occur, of course, on the basis of wealth, density of population, special health programs will be dealt with in more detail later.

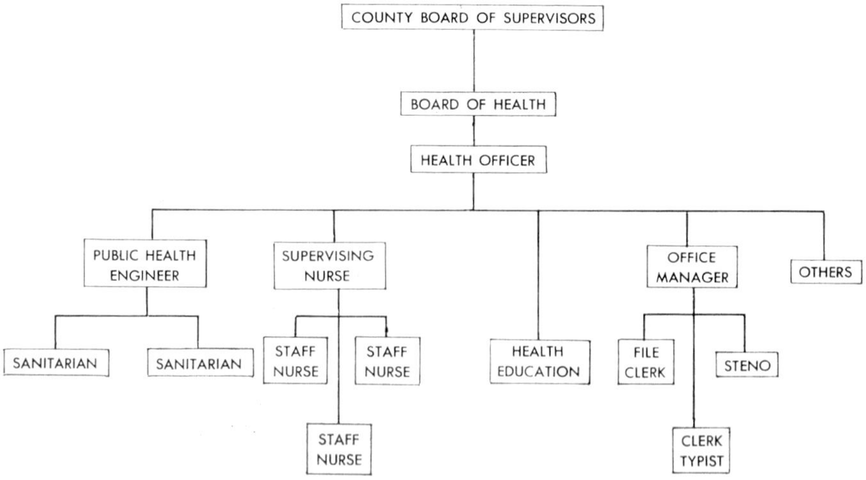

FIG. 8. Typical organization of a small County Health Department.

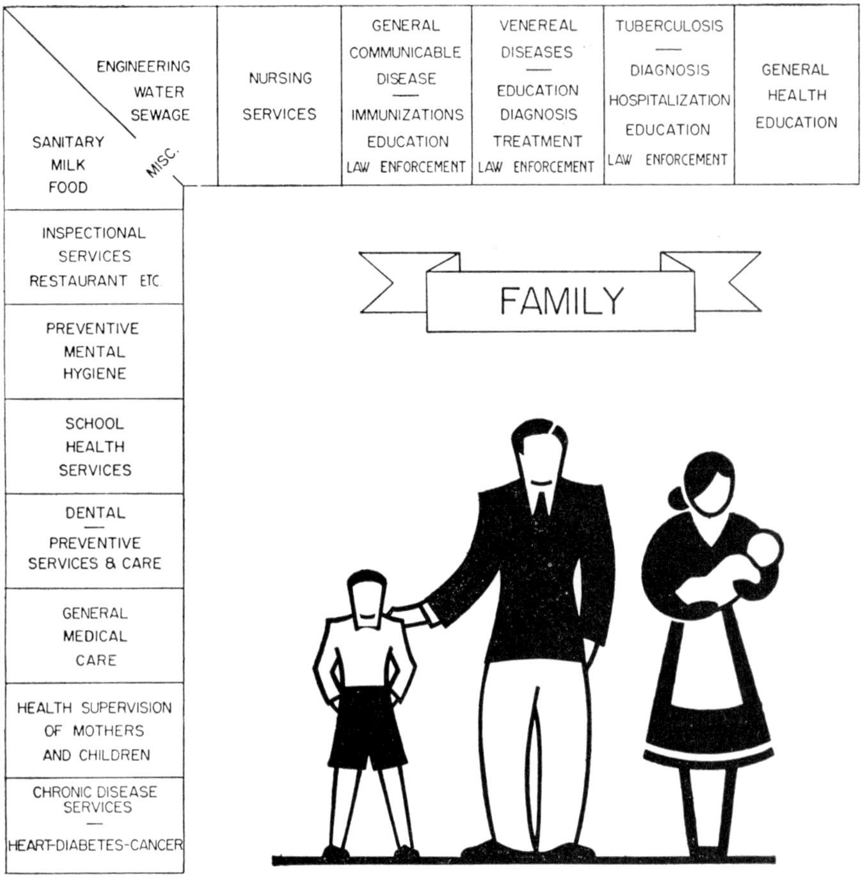

FIG. 9. **Services and activities of a local Health Department.**

tion have improved, the small inefficient and inadequate village and township health departments have been replaced for the most part with much more satisfactory county-wide health departments which include all towns or cities within their area. (Fig. 8). Sometimes, even an entire county cannot support a health department. In such instances there are two recourses: the joining with one or two other counties to form a multi-county health unit, or the establishment of state health districts consisting of several counties with the program determined and the budget and staff provided by the State Department of Health. In certain circumstances this is most practical. Such state health districts must be regarded as a last resort since the personnel, hence the services, are inevitably minimal. By now, there are about 1600 full-time local health departments of one type or another, serving almost 2500 counties, including more than 300 cities. They protect the health of a combined population of almost 180,000,000 people. This represents about nine-tenths of the population of the nation.

While local health departments are involved in a wide variety of services and activities, as illustrated in Figure 9, their basic functions should include at least the following: (1) vital statistics, (2) environmental health, (3) maternal and child health, including family planning, (4) communicable disease control, (5) chronic disease control, (6) mental health, including addictive disease programs, (7) promotion of adult health, (8) laboratory services, and (9) health education. According to the American Public Health Association, as presented in an official policy statement, in order to achieve an effective community program the local health department should provide the following services:

1. Recording and analysis of health data
   a. Recording and analysis of reports of births, deaths, marriages, divorces, and notifiable diseases
   b. Maintenance of registers of individuals known to have certain specific long-term diseases and impairments
   c. Conduct of special surveys to determine the prevalence and resultant disability from various diseases
   d. Collection and interpretation of morbidity data from such sources as clinics, hospitals, organized nursing services, prepayment plans, industry, and workmen's compensation and disability insurance programs
   e. Maintenance of continuing records on the number and qualifications of all types of health personnel, the quantitative and qualitative resources of available facilities, and the types and extent of health services provided through various voluntary and public programs
   f. Periodic evaluation of community health needs and services, both personal and environmental.

2. Health education and information
   a. Stimulation of the general public, government and the professions to recognize health problems that exist, to study the resources available for meeting the problems, and to develop and put into action programs designed to solve them
   b. Cooperation with and assistance of official and voluntary organizations such as departments of education, and civic, youth, and other community groups in the development of their health programs
   c. Provision of individual instruction by public health nurses and other personnel, of women attending pre- or postnatal or child health clinics, of families in which communicable or certain chronic non-communicable diseases exist, and of patients who are required by their personal physician to follow certain regimens

d. Organization of lectures, classes, and courses for parents, food handlers, teachers, police, diabetics, and community groups

e. Use of mass educational and informational media such as newspapers, magazines, pamphlets, movies, radio and television

f. Development of a well-rounded program of professional education, designed to assist the health professions to maintain and improve the quality of their service

3. Supervision and regulation

a. Assurance of sanitary food, water, and milk supplies

b. Assurance of the safety and salubrity of various products and equipment used in the household

c. Control of nuisances, sanitary disposal of wastes and control of water and air pollution

d. Prevention of occupational diseases and accidents

e. Control of human and animal sources of infection

f. Regulation of housing

g. Inspection of hospitals, nursing homes, and other health facilities by means of:

i. Public education and individual instruction

ii. Issuance of regulations

iii. Laboratory control

iv. Inspection and licensure

v. Revocation of permits and, as a last resort, court action

4. Provision of environmental health services (as necessary)

a. Construction of pit privies

b. Drainage and larvicidal treatment of mosquito breeding areas, residual spraying of homes for insect control

c. Rat proofing of buildings, and other insect and rodent control measures

5. Administration of personal health services

a. Immunization against infectious diseases and other preventive measures such as the application of fluoride to children's teeth

b. Advisory health maintenance service, as in child health conferences, prenatal clinics, parents' classes and public health nursing visits

c. Case finding surveys of the general population, such as chest x-ray surveys, serological tests for syphilis, cancer detection programs, and school health examinations. Adult health inventories and "multiphasic" surveys for the detection of various groups of diseases may also be included

d. Provision of diagnostic aids to private physicians, such as laboratory services and diagnostic and consultation clinics for crippled children, cancer, cardiac, and other conditions as circumstances indicate

e. Provision of diagnostic and treatment services for specific diseases such as syphilis, tuberculosis, dental defects in children and expectant mothers, and orthopedic, cardiac, and other crippling impairments in children

6. Operation of health facilities
   a. Operation of neighborhood health centers and clinics
   b. Operation of general or special hospitals (as necessary)
7. Coordination of activities and resources
   a. Provision of effective leadership to meet community health needs
   b. Encouragement of coordination of various official and voluntary agencies to avoid duplication and overlapping and to assure efficient and economical administration
   c. Participation on interdepartmental or regional boards dealing with public water supplies, sewage and refuse disposal, control of atmospheric pollution, housing, city planning, hospital planning, zoning regulation, development of recreational areas and other public programs which have significant implications for community health

To perform the foregoing activities and services, a basic multi-disciplinary professional staff is necessary. Current standards suggest the employment of the following types and numbers of professional personnel in order to provide the minimum desirable services to a community:

Medical personnel–1 per 50,000 population (the best qualified to serve as health officer, the others preferably to direct the school health program, the maternal and child health program, and the epidemiology program)

Sanitary personnel—1 per 15,000 population (one preferably a public health engineer)

Staff nursing personnel–1 per 5,000 population (one per 2,500 population if bedside nursing of the sick is included)

Supervisory nursing personnel–1 per 6 to 8 staff nurses

Office personnel–1 per 15,000 population

Other specialized personnel–as problems demand and funds make possible

The health organizations of larger communities, because of their more complex and specialized types of problems, necessarily require more extensive personnel and organization. Figure 10 presents as an example the organization of the official community health agency of one of the largest cities in the nation. Its staff includes physicians of various

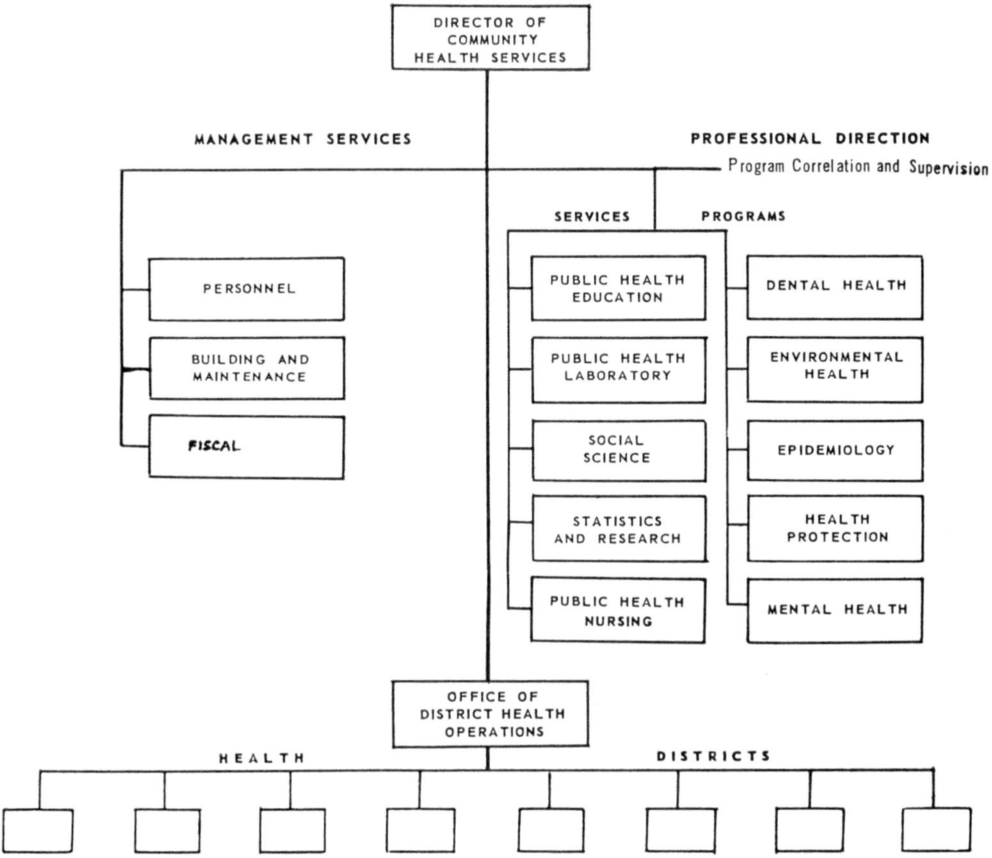

FIG. 10. Example of a decentralized large City Health Department.

specialties, dentists, veterinarians, experts in radiation and air pollution, physicists, laboratory workers, health educators, statisticians, social scientists, and many other categories of professional personnel.

Legal responsibility for the protection and promotion of the health of the community is usually placed in a local board of health. Ordinarily, such a board consists of five or seven individuals, professional and lay, appointed from the community by the elected executive of the community, the mayor in cities or the board of supervisors in counties. Typically, appointments are overlapping and compensation, if any, is nominal. The Board of Health usually selects and appoints the Health Officer, Health Commissioner, or Director of Public Health, the title depending upon local custom. Appointment is frequently subject to approval by either or both the local legislative body, and/or the state health department. Fortunately, it has been possible for most state health departments to obtain the establishment of high standards and qualifications for appointments to local public health positions as a condition for eligibility of the community for state aid. Increasingly, all personnel other than the Health Officer are included in civil service systems.

Voluntary Health Agencies

Another factor of considerable importance in the pattern of efforts to improve community health should be mentioned. Its development was peculiarly American in nature, and consisted of the formation of a large number of citizen conceived, sponsored, financed, and operated agencies concerned with various types of health problems. This voluntary health agency movement began with the Anti-Tuberculosis Society of Philadelphia in 1892. From this beginning the movement has grown to include more than 20,000 voluntary health agencies which are concerned with all types of health and disease problems. Some are concerned exclusively with specific diseases such as cancer, tuberculosis or diabetes, some with conditions of certain organs or parts of the body such as blindness, hearing or crippling, some with specific groups such as mothers or children, and some with certain broad phases of community health such as safety or sanitation. (Appendix B provides a listing of some of the more important of these voluntary health agencies.)

These agencies typically are financed by public solicitations, the sale of special stamps or seals, or as part of Red Feather, Community Chest, or United Fund drives. They have played a valuable role in augmenting the efforts of the official local health agencies. In general, their purposes are to fill existing gaps and to lead the way. An extensive study and analysis of them has described eight basic functions of voluntary agencies which may be summarized as follows.[2]

1. Pioneering—exploring or surveying unserved needs, and trial of new methods of dealing with recognized needs.
2. Demonstration—adopting or subsidizing experimental projects to demonstrate practical methods for community health improvement, or for the wide application of proven methods. Examples have been the demonstration of the value of full-time local health departments, home delivery services, visiting nursing services, nutrition programs, and community disease registries.
3. Education—this is probably the single most important function of voluntary health agencies. While primarily concerned with public education, many voluntary agencies have assisted in professional training by means of fellowships, in-service training courses, and the subsidization of field training areas.

[2]Gunn, S. M. and Platt, P. S.: *Voluntary Health Agencies,* New York, The Ronald Press, 1946.

4. Supplementation of official activities—often official health agencies cannot enter new fields of service and activity because of political or appropriation restrictions or because of public reservation. In many such instances, voluntary agencies have played a most important role by filling the gap between currently accepted public practice and more advanced scientific knowledge. Usually, this is done with the expectation that within a reasonable period of time the official health agency will be able to carry on.

5. Guarding citizen interests in health matters—because of their nature, representation, and support, voluntary health agencies are important in guarding the public interest, not only by promoting the official health program, but also, by defending it against political and other interference. Occasionally, they serve the public interest by studying and criticizing the official health agencies' programs and officials.

6. Promotion of health legislation—it is the primary responsibility of the health officer to provide leadership in the field of community health legislation. Usually, he cannot do this entirely alone. One of his greatest sources of strength and support in this regard is the group of cooperative voluntary health agencies that exist in his community. Through their informed membership they are usually able to bring the weight of intelligent public opinion to bear upon proposed or existing legislation.

7. Group planning and coordination—with the development of many agencies, both official and voluntary, interested in the health needs of a community, there is a potential of duplication or conflict which can be avoided only by means of careful planning and coordination. This has become one of the chief concerns and contributions of community health federations or health divisions of councils of social agencies.

8. Development of balanced community health programs—this is really the total cumulative result of all of the foregoing purposes and functions of voluntary health agencies. By protecting and promoting official health programs, by increasing the hygienic consciousness of the community through public education, and by providing funds, facilities or personnel where substantive gaps exist, voluntary health agencies may make the difference between a mediocre community health program and one that is truly effective.

In addition to voluntary health agencies, there exist a large number of philanthropic foundations, professional associations and community health councils that have played very significant roles in the development of community or public health progress. (See Appendix B)

Special reference should be made to one particular type of non-official health agency, the Visiting Nurse Society. It apparently began with the Woman's Branch of the New York City Mission which was organized in 1877 to teach hygiene in the homes of the underprivileged. In 1886 the first agency specifically designated as a Visiting Nursing Society was established in Philadelphia. Since then, many others have been established in communities throughout the nation. These excellent agencies have performed invaluable service, not only by augmenting the efforts of public health nurses in official health agencies, but also by providing bedside nursing care of the sick, follow-up on request of instructions to patients of private physicians, public education, and professional field training. In recent years there has been a trend in many places to merge or at least more effectively to coordinate the work of the private visiting nursing societies and of the nurses in official health agencies. Properly effectuated, this can lead to much greater efficiency and more service to more individuals.

State Health Organization

The pattern of public health organization on the state level is more complex and varied than on the local level. In all fifty states, as well as in the several territories, more than one agency has significant responsibilities in the field of health. A study by the United States Public Health Service showed that over-all there were about sixty different types of state agencies involved in public health activities. A consolidated tabulation of these is as follows:

- Department of health
- Department of welfare, social security, emergency relief, general assistance, *etc.*
- Department of agriculture
- Department of labor, labor and industry, labor and immigration, *etc.*
- Department of education, public instruction, *etc.*
- Special boards, commissions, or independent offices established specifically for the activity indicated (tuberculosis board or commission, cancer commission, workmen's compensation commission or bureau, industrial accident board, dairy and food commission, hotel commission, livestock sanitary board, water resources board, commission for the blind, crippled children's commission, mental disease commission or department, state toxicologist, state veterinarian, *etc.*)

Board of control of affairs, department of state institutions, *etc.*
Independent state hospital, independent state laboratory
Department of conservation
State university or college
Department of mines and minerals, or of natural resources
Department of engineering, department of public utilities
State experiment station
Independent licensing and examining boards
Department of motor vehicles, department of public safety
Department of civil service and registration, department of registration and education
Other departments or offices of state government

The number of agencies that may be involved in some type of health activity in specific states may range from ten to thirty-two. Furthermore, very often within a given state, a number of different agencies may be found active in the same field. For example, in one state, thirteen separate agencies are engaged in various aspects of accident prevention work, while in another, twelve agencies participate in some way in health education. The chief reason for these variations is the complexity of state government and the fact that the United States of America is exactly what the title indicates, a union of essentially independent governmental units each of which has the inherent power to organize itself and to conduct its affairs essentially however it wishes.

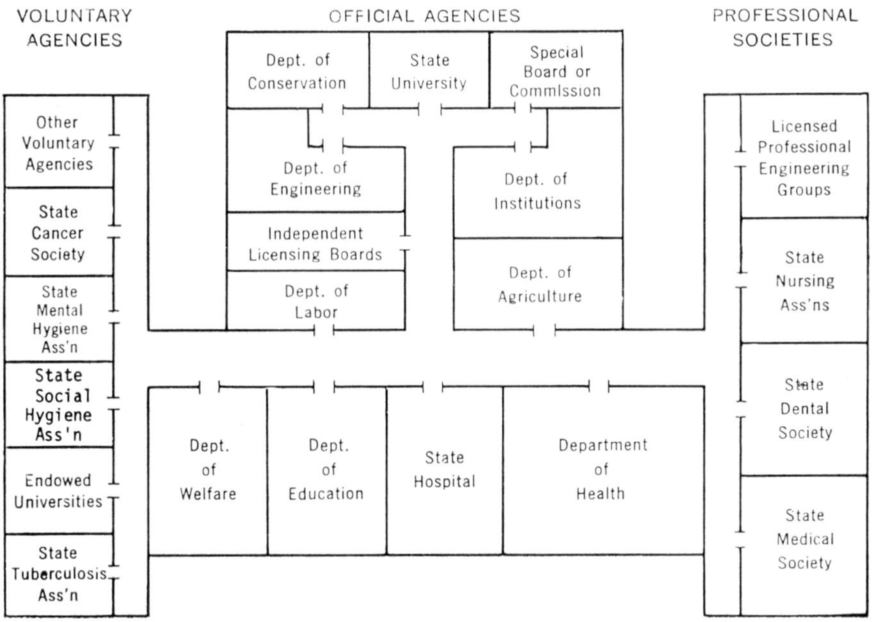

FIG. 11. Health organization on the state level.

Despite this, every state without exception has one particular agency which is given primary responsibility for the protection and promotion of the health of the public. As on the local level, the state health department is expected to provide leadership in health matters on its level, all other agencies serving in effect in a contributory, auxiliary or specialized manner. The relationship of a state department of public health with other agencies on its governmental level is illustrated in Figure 11 which presents the second floor plan of our structure for health.

In contrast with local community health activities, the direct personal service activities of state health agencies are typically few and limited. More or less typically, their functions may be considered to consist of the following:

1. To represent the public health interests and goals of the state to the elected governing body of the state
2. To promulgate and enforce public health rules and regulations applicable throughout the state
3. To determine state public health policy and to provide a state-wide coordinated public health program with clear objectives for the guidance of local health departments
4. To promote the establishment of full-time local health units
5. To develop an appropriate plan for the coordination of local health services with related hospital and medical programs which may be developed on a regional basis
6. To provide financial assistance to supplement the resources of local health departments
7. To make selected consultation and other special services available throughout the state.
8. To assist localities to set up demonstrations on a temporary basis.
9. To establish minimum and stimulate optimum standards of performance
10. To develop a recruitment and training program for local health department personnel
11. To delegate certain legal responsibilities of the state health agency, insofar as feasible and practical, to well-organized and adequately staffed local health departments
12. To carry on all relationships with local citizens and groups through or in cooperation with the local health departments
13. To carry on a state-wide program of health education
14. To evaluate existing state and local programs

15. To represent the interest of the state in interstate health relations
16. To represent the interests of the state in state-federal health relations

The foregoing may be condensed into the four functional categories of: (1) state-wide planning and policy making, (2) inter-state health relations, (3) state-federal relations, and (4) encouragement of the development and maintenance of local health programs. While the first three of these are obviously of great importance, perhaps the best single measure of the effectiveness of a state health department is the extent to which it succeeds in stimulating the formation of local health departments, and helps them in turn to do an effective job of direct service to and protection of the public.

The spectrum of specific professional activities in which the personnel of state health agencies may be involved is indicated by the following which is relatively inclusive:

Vital statistics collection, recording, analysis and preservation
Leadership in comprehensive state health planning
Maternal and child health services
School health services
Crippled children's services
Communicable disease prevention and control
Chronic disease prevention, early diagnosis and treatment
Mental health and mental retardation programs
Dental health programs
Speech, vision and hearing programs
General medical care of the needy
Health services for migratory labor
Physical and vocational rehabilitation
Public health nursing services
Nutrition education and services
Social services related to health and illness
Surveillance of sanitation of water, sewage, and solid wastes
Supervision of sanitation of dairy products, foods and food service
Supervision of drugs and pharmaceuticals
Rodent and insect vector control
Supervision of plumbing, housing, hotels, motels and camps
Air pollution control
Surveillance and control of sources of radiation
Occupational health and safety programs
Workman's compensation
Public and professional health education
Consumer protection and education
Professional licensure
Laboratory services
Research activities

Each state organizes its public health agency to suit its own wishes and situation. As time has gone by, however, certain general similarities have developed. Figure 12 presents the organizational structure of the official health agency of one of the more typical states.

State Responsibility for School Health

The allocation of responsibility for the health of the school child follows different patterns according to the organizational structure of the particular state or local government. The state constitutes the legal power in

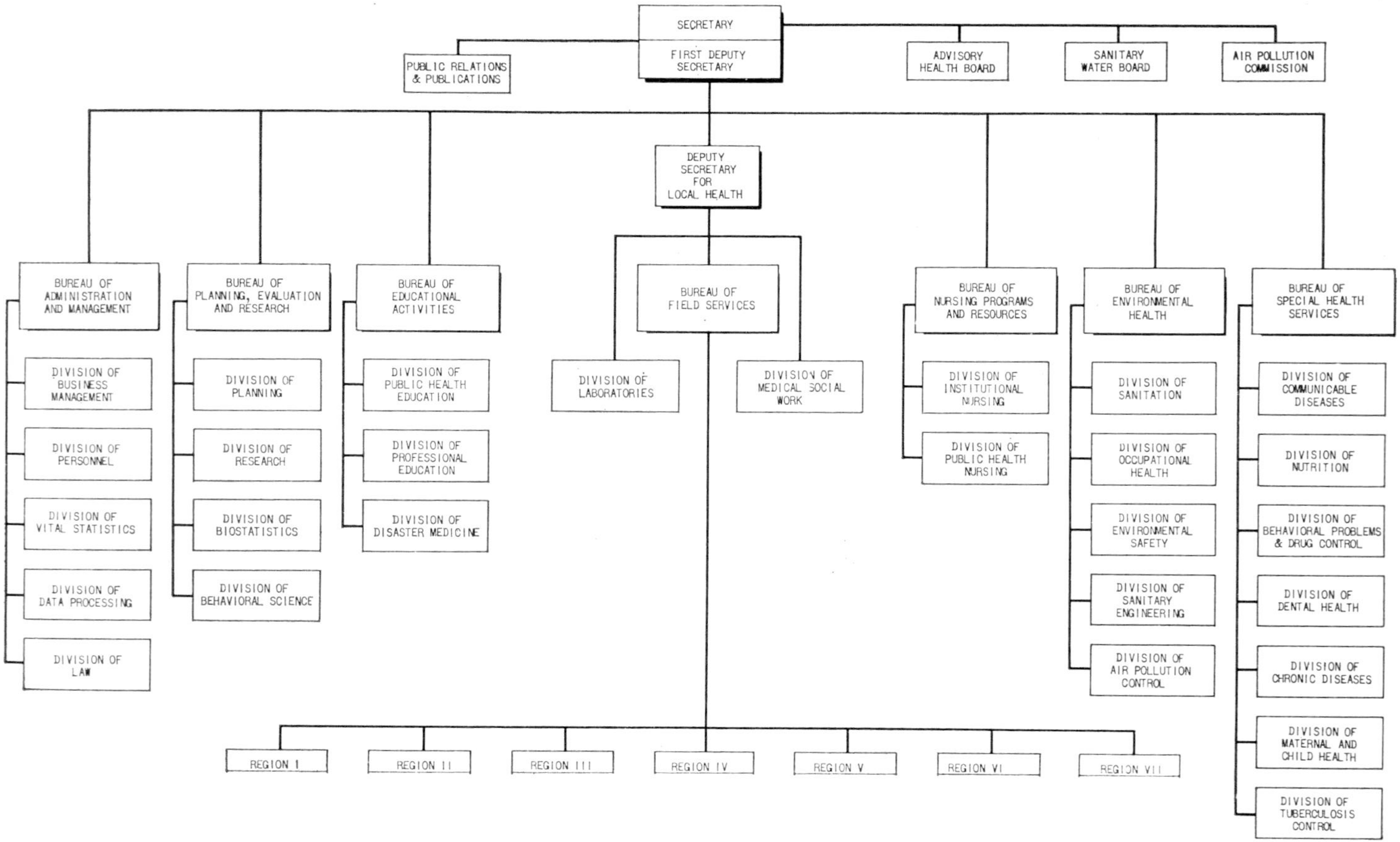

FIG. 12. Organization of a State Department of Health.

public education but the long-time insistence of the people of this democracy that the public school is the prerogative of the local community is reflected in the policy of all states to establish minimum requirements and recommendations concerning education, thereby permitting the local school district considerable latitude in determining the details of its own school program.

In some states and localities, the major responsibility for the school health program rests with the department of health; in others, with the board of education or department of public instruction. In still others, it is divided between the two, with the health department carrying the major responsibility for matters pertaining to school health services and healthful school living, and the department of education focusing upon health instruction and certification regulations. Today, in most instances, regardless of the officially designated pattern, the two departments appear to work together in the adoption of common policies, joint planning and administration, with the implementation procedures clearly defined and carefully allocated.

The head of the Department of Education, known as the Secretary (or in some states as the Commissioner or State Superintendent of Schools) is usually appointed by the Governor. The Secretary, assisted by an advisory board, is responsible for the quality of education in the state. This includes the establishment of certification regulations pertaining to pre-school, elementary, and secondary school teachers, supervisors, administrators, and certification in special subjects including, in some states, health education. The certification of all school health workers might also fall in this domain.

The Secretary of Education or his deputy would apportion the administrative tasks by establishing various divisions as needed, each with its own administrative head or adviser. Included might be a Division of Health, Physical Education, and Recreation. Today in many states this is likely to be sub-divided into three divisions each with its own director or adviser: (1) health and safety education, (2) physical education, and (3) recreation and outdoor education. The main responsibilities of the director of health and safety education would be the implementation and maintenance of quality health instruction throughout the state at all levels, including teacher education in state colleges and universities. His duties include the following:

(1) advisory and consultative services to school districts
(2) provision of minimum curriculum guides or courses of study at all levels
(3) leadership in the preparation of guides in health instruction
(4) leadership in surveys, evaluative procedures, investigations, curriculum studies, research projects
(5) provision for resource materials available to schools

(6) cooperation with health-related departments, agencies, and professional organizations within the state
(7) compilation of reports as requested by the Secretary of Education or the Governor

If, as sometimes is the case, the health department is called upon to carry full responsibility for the total school health program, the staff of its division of health education must be expanded to include consultants in health instruction. If, on the other hand, the entire responsibility for school health is centered in the department of public instruction, its division of health and safety would have to include personnel specially qualified in medicine, nursing, dentistry, sanitation, and numerous other related professional fields.

Regardless of the pattern followed, the success of the school health program will depend upon the establishment of sound policies, a well-coordinated approach, the clarity with which the role of each department is stated, understood and observed by their respective staffs, and the willingness of the members of the health team to work together.

In some states and localities, the plan of having a state health council or advisory health committee composed of representatives of various official and voluntary agencies, schools and universities, has been found effective in the identification and solution of problems and the efficient integration of activities.

A number of jurisdictions have achieved highly successful results in increasing general interest in the school health program, and in raising its general level, by means of establishment of an Inter-agency Planning Committee. Included in the membership of such committees are representatives of various official and voluntary health agencies and of professional groups. By pooling their services, finances, and resources, many worthwhile projects have been possible. With the cooperation of colleges and universities, summer workshops in school-community health have been made possible for school and public health personnel through the establishment of scholarships and the integrated use of the personnel and other resources of all pertinent agencies. Special workshops for school administrators, college health conferences, demonstrations, and research studies have similarly contributed to the total improvement of the health of the school population.

Federal Health Organization

Because of the manner in which federal interests in health matters originated and developed, there exists a confusing maze of departments, bureaus, offices, agencies, commissions, services, and authorities, each responsible for one or several health functions. As discussed briefly in the preceding chapter, part of the confusion was mitigated by the establishment in 1953 of a federal Department of Health, Education, and Welfare. Despite this, federal health interests are still scattered throughout a considerable number of other government agencies. They run the gamut from some very logical responsibilities of the Department of Agriculture to such fascinating anachronisms as the responsibility of the Fish and Wild Life Service of the Department of the Interior for the medical and health services for the inhabitants of the Pribiloff Islands off mainland Alaska.

Federal agencies concerned with public health fall into four general categories. The first is concerned with broad general health interests and includes only one agency, the United States Public Health Service. The second category is concerned with the well being of special population groups and includes such agencies as the Department of Labor, Children's Bureau, the Women's Bureau, the Farm Security Administration, the Agricultural Extension Service, the Office of Indian Affairs, the medical divisions of the Armed Forces, and the Veterans Administration. The third category includes agencies concerned with special problems or programs such as the Office of Education, the Office of Vocational Rehabilitation, the Food and Drug Administration, the Federal Trade Commission, the Bureau of Mines, the Division of Labor Standards, and the Bureau of Labor Statistics in the Department of Labor, various bureaus within the Department of Agriculture concerned with plants, animals, human nutrition, the Maritime Commission, the Atomic Energy Commission, and the Tennessee Valley Authority. The Social Security Administration and the Bureau of Employees Compensation may be included here since they provide medical care to special groups. The fourth category consists of certain quasi-independent institutions such as the St. Elizabeth's Hospital and the Freedman's Hospital. In addition, one might add a fifth category of agencies concerned with the international health interests of the United States Government. The two significant partners here are the U.S. Public Health Service and the Agency for International Development of the Department of State.

For practical reasons detailed consideration will be limited to the few agencies which are most significantly concerned with health. As has been indicated the majority of these are now located within the Public Health Service of the Department of Health, Education and Welfare.

The Public Health Service

The principal federal health organization is the United States Public Health Service, the history of which was presented briefly in the preceding chapter. It is directed by a Surgeon General who is appointed by the President, but who reports to the Secretary of Health, Education, and Welfare, through the Assistant Secretary for Health and Scientific Affairs. The Service is organized into five administrative units: the

Office of the Surgeon General, the Health Services and Mental Health Administration, the Environmental Health Service, the Food and Drug Administration, and the National Institutes of Health. Included also is the National Library of Medicine which is supervised by a board of regents and administered by an executive director who reports to the Surgeon General. For purposes of operational convenience, many of the activities of the Service are conducted through ten regional offices located in Boston, New York, Philadelphia, Chicago, Atlanta, Kansas City, Dallas, Denver, San Francisco, and Seattle. Through the years, the responsibilities of the Public Health Service have been increased tremendously. This is emphasized by the fact that the total funds available to the Public Health Service amounts to about $3.5 billions, four-fifths from appropriations and authorizations and one-fifth from repayments from other agencies and unobligated balances. It is notable that about one half of the funds available were devoted to grants and research contracts to state and local agencies, private institutions, universities, hospitals, and individuals outside the federal government. In personnel, the Service has a staff of almost 45,000 of which about 7 percent are active regular Commissioned Corps Officers and the remainder are civil service personnel. In addition there are about 8000 inactive Reserve officers.

The present functions of the Public Health Service may be summarized as follows:

1. Study of the causes and means of propagation and spread of the diseases of mankind, and the development of methods of prevention and control. In this work the Public Health Service maintains a number of world renowned research laboratories, chief among which are those of the National Institutes of Health, Bethesda, Maryland;* the National Institute of Environmental Health Sciences near Durham, N.C.; the Center for Disease Control at Atlanta, Ga.; the Arctic Health Research Center at Fairbanks, Alaska; and the Appalachian Center at Morgantown, W. Va. In addition to investigations carried on at these Institutes and centers, financial assistance is given through research grants to a large number of universities, professional and technical schools, laboratories, and other public and private institutions for research projects, upon the recommendation of professional advisory councils. Funds are also available for research fellowships, both in the Institutes and in various educational institutions.

*The National Institutes of Health now include a spectrum of research institutes concerned with cancer, heart and lung diseases, arthritis and metabolic diseases, neurological diseases and stroke, allergy and infectious diseases, eye, dental, general medical services, child health and human development and environmental health sciences (the last located near Durham, N.C.)

2. Maritime quarantine and the inspection of passengers and crews of vessels and airplanes arriving from foreign ports, for the protection of the country from the importation of quarantinable diseases from other countries. Examination of immigrants for detection and isolation of persons suffering from mandatorily excludable disease. Medical inspection of aliens is performed in collaboration with the Immigration and Naturalization Service of the Department of Justice.

3. Interstate quarantine for the prevention of the spread of diseases from one state to another. The Service prescribes the conditions under which persons and things may move in interstate commerce. It assists states in controlling epidemics, and may on request take complete charge of serious outbreaks. Regulation of conditions existing within the boundaries of a particular state is a duty that remains under state jurisdiction.

4. Dissemination of public health information, including the collection and publication of reports of disease prevalence in the United States and foreign countries, and other pertinent information regarding conservation of the public health.

5. Assistance, through grants to states, counties, cities, and health districts, in establishing and maintaining proper sanitation facilities, general public health services—including industrial hygiene, mental hygiene, and cancer control—and special programs for the control of venereal diseases and tuberculosis. Grants made under this authority represent an actual transfer of funds from federal to state treasuries for the employment and training of personnel for state and local health work, the purchase of supplies and equipment, the provision of appropriate facilities for care and treatment of designated illnesses, and the payment of general operating expenses. Services include the loan of personnel for temporary duty, and the provision of consultation and advice to state and local health departments. Assistance is also furnished states in the development of hospitalization plans and the construction of hospital and allied health facilities.

6. Supervisory control and licensure of the manufacturers of biological products—vaccines, serums, toxins, antitoxins, arsenicals, and similar preparations— used in the prevention and treatment of diseases. This control has been established to insure safe and standard products.

7. Study of mental diseases and drug addiction and investigation of legitimate needs for narcotic drugs.

8. Provision of hospitalization, general medical and dental care, and preventive health services for American merchant seamen, members of the United States Coast Guard and the Coast and Geodetic Survey, and for other legal beneficiaries of the Service. In this connection, the Service operates a number of hospitals and out-patients clinics, and contracts for service in over 100 other places not served by Public Health Service facilities. It assigns medical and dental officers to ship duty to provide medical and dental care at sea for the Coast Guard and Coast and Geodetic Survey. The Public Health Service in cooperation with the Bureau of Prisons, maintains a medical and health program in Federal prisons. The Public Health Service also is responsible for the provision of medical care and public health services to American Indians, Eskimos and Aleuts.

9. Operation of special hospitals—these include the National Leprosarium at Carville, Louisiana, the two hospitals for the care of persons addicted to narcotics at Lexington, Kentucky, and Fort Worth, Texas, St. Elizabeth's Hospital for mentally ill civilian beneficiaries of the Federal Government in Washington, D.C., and Freedman's Hospital associated with Howard University, also in Washington, D.C.

10. Cooperation with other Federal agencies in discharging their various health functions, through assignment of personnel for assistance.

11. Collaboration with and participation in the functioning of international health organizations. In carrying out this service, particular attention is given to the provision of consultation and training, the direction of programs, and the exchange of international health and related personnel.

12. Collection and publication of data on vital statistics, which are basic materials for public health programs and give valuable information concerning public health trends. Through measurements of death rates from different causes, the progress of health programs directed toward reduction of particular diseases or conditions can be evaluated.

In summary, the activities of the U.S. Public Health Service may be said to be in the areas of: (1) research, (2) demonstration, (3) inter-state and international quarantine, (4) advice on technical matters to the other federal agencies as well as to state and local governments and perhaps most significantly, (5) financial grants-in-aid to state and territorial health agencies for the expansion and improvement of their programs and those of the local jurisdictions they include. As only one of many possible examples of the efficency of the Public Health Service, it can be pointed out that, as a result of the efforts of its Division of Foreign Quarantine, there has been no outbreak of a quarantinable disease introduced from abroad for almost a quarter of a century.

The Children's Bureau

Another unit within the Department of Health, Education and Welfare which has played a significant role in the improvement of the health of the American people is the Children's Bureau. As indicated previously, since 1967 it has been part of the Social and Rehabilitation Service of the Department of Health, Education and Welfare. Its existence apart from the Public Health Service, although somewhat illogical, came about largely on the basis of the argument that the needs of children should be considered as a whole, and that since they were unable to organize and speak for themselves, there was a need for some agency in the government constantly to look after their interests. One of the chief functions of the Children's Bureau, has been to encourage and enable each state to establish and extend direct health services for mothers and children. Through the years this has been accomplished by means of financial and expert assistance to the states in the support of the development of prenatal, postnatal and well-child clinics, of demonstrations of adequate delivery services, and of public health nursing services for maternal and child health supervision. It was largely through the persistent efforts of the Children's Bureau that all state health departments eventually established divisions of maternal and child health. Another important activity of the Bureau is in the field of a wide variety of services for crippled children. It conducts many surveys and studies on the nature and extent of all types of problems that affect the welfare of children including health problems, and produces many analyses, reports and statistics relating to these problems. In addition to relating operationally with other official agencies, the Children's Bureau cooperates with many national, state and local non-official or voluntary organizations and institutions, and stimulates interest, participation and coordination of resources and services on the part of educational, social and welfare agencies.

The Food and Drug Administration

The Food and Drug Administration, since 1968 a part of the Public Health Service of the Department of Health, Education and Welfare, is the federal agency concerned with the quality of foods and drugs. It promotes the purity, safety, standard potency, and accurate labeling of the many and rapidly increasing numbers of substances within its legal jurisdiction including foods, drugs, cosmetics, certain milk products, and poisons. In addition it has responsibilities in relation to therapeutic devices, flammable fabrics, dangerous toys and a variety of other items that may be hazardous to health and safety. Its inspectors maintain inter-state and international surveillance over such materials, and serve as consultants to state and local public health and food and drug officials.

The Office of Education

On the federal level, the principal resource for school health education is centered in the United States Office of Education. Its staff includes specialists in health education, safety education, and physical education on the elementary, secondary and higher education levels and in teacher education. The contribution of this office to health education includes leadership in the form of advisory and consultation services, research, conferences, investigations, publications, the dissemination of information concerning statistics, data and progress. It cooperates actively with various professional organizations concerned with raising the level of school health and health programs. In cooperation with the Department of Agriculture, it promotes school lunch programs and administers a grant-in-aid program for vocational education in health.

The Department of Agriculture

The Department of Agriculture with separate Cabinet status is involved in a wide variety of activities of considerable public health concern. Its Agricultural Research Service conducts research on human and animal nutrition and on consumer food use as well as on the control and eradication of pests and plant and animal diseases, some of which may affect man. The Department administers the federal meat inspection program and carries out investigations and education relating to the sanitary production and handling of milk and milk products. Its Consumer and Marketing Service is responsible for several programs of particular importance to schools and school children. Among these are (a) The National School Lunch Program (b) The Pilot School Breakfast Program (c) The Special Milk Program for Children and (d) The Equipment Program for initiation or expansion of school food service. In addition, this service administers the Food Stamp Program for assistance to needy families. In cooperation with state land-grant universities and state Departments of Agriculture, much is done to improve rural health and nutrition through emphasis upon family life and education by the stimulation of improved services.

The International Scene

Recent history has truly made this "One World" from a health standpoint. No longer are seas and mountains barriers to invading disease any more than they are to attack by military forces. The chapter which dealt with history indicated a few very early concerns with this problem, which led most notably to the concept of quarantine. In the larger and more effective sense, it is necessary to jump to the twentieth century wherein there have been developed a series of organizations and programs designed to cope with health problems on a global scale.

The first truly international health organization, and the longest-lived up to the present, resulted from an Inter-American Health Conference which was held in Mexico City in 1902. At that conference there was established a permanent *Pan-American Sanitary Bureau,* recently renamed the Pan-American Health Organization. It has headquarters in Washington, D.C., and it is governed by an elected Directing Council and a Director General and is supported by annual financial quotas contributed by each of the American Republics. It serves as the center of coordination of international action and information on health matters in the Western Hemisphere; provides technical aid, consultation, and guidance upon request; promotes professional and public education in health; and conducts an annual conference which is attended by delegates from all member nations. When the World Health Organization became a reality in 1946, as described subsequently, the P.A.H.O. was designated as its regional representative in the Western Hemisphere.

By 1907, growing recognition of the need for some type of world-wide center and forum for health affairs, led to the establishment of an *International Office of Public Health.* The movement was relatively ineffective because of lack of genuine international interest, inadequate financial support, and questions of international law and relationships. When the League of Nations was formed at the close of World War I, the International Office of Public Health was absorbed into the newly organized *Health Organization of the League of Nations.* The function was still limited largely to epidemiological intelligence and the holding of international health conferences. During World War II, the League of Nations fell apart. The Health Organization, however, continued to receive international support and to function.

Even before the war was over, however, the allied nations recognized not only the necessity of continuing an international health agency but the importance of expanding its functions. As a result, a constitution for a *World Health Organization* was signed in New York City in 1946 by sixty-one nations. Its existence became official on September 1, 1948. Transferred to it were the duties and powers of the Health Organization of the League of Nations, and the health functions of the temporary United Nations Relief and Rehabilitation Administration (UNRRA). The World Health Organization, while one of the specialized agencies related to the United Nations, has its separate and independent existence in terms of constitution, powers, membership and financing. It is the largest of the international specialized agencies with a membership of over 120 nations.

The World Health Organization has its headquarters in Geneva, Switzerland, with regional offices as follows: Washington, for the Americas (Pan-American Health Organization); Copenhagen, for Europe; Alexandria, for the Eastern Mediterranean; Brazzaville, for Africa—South of the Sahara; New Delhi, for South-East Asia; and Manila for the Western Pacific. Its activities are financed by pro-rated quotas and special contributions from its member nations and from the United Nations Technical Assistance Board. Each year, usually in May, a World Health Assembly (Fig. 13) convenes as a legislative body to determine international health policy and programs. Each member nation is allowed three delegates (plus advisors) but only one delegate may vote. An Executive Board, elected at the Assembly, is responsible for putting the decisions and policies of the Assembly into effect, and to deal with emergencies in the name of the Assembly. This board of eighteen health experts ordinarily meets twice a year. The day-to-day work of the WHO is conducted by a secreteriat of technical and administrative personnel under a Director-General. Each geographic region has a representative committee to formulate regional policies and to supervise the activities of the regional office. The WHO also appoints a number of expert panels and technical committees to advise it on various aspects of its responsibilities and work.

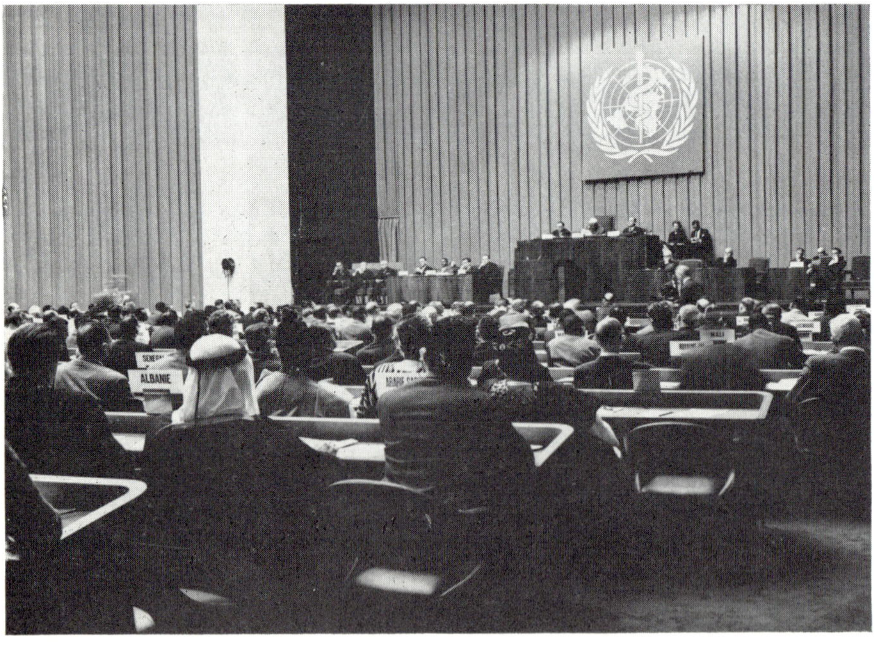

FIG. 13. The World Health Assembly in session, Geneva, Switzerland.

The functions of the World Health Organization have been summarized as follows:

1. It is the one directing and coordinating authority on international health work. It is not a supra-national ministry of health, but rather a world-wide cooperative through which the nations help each other to help themselves in raising health standards.

2. It provides to member countries various central technical services, *i.e.*, epidemiology, statistics, standardization of drugs and procedures, a wide range of technical publications, *etc.*

3. Its most important function is to help countries to strengthen and improve their own health services. Upon request it provides advisory and consulting services through public health experts, demonstration teams for disease control, visiting specialists, *etc.*

The Constitution of the World Health Organization has been referred to appropriately as the Magna Carta of health because of its affirmation that health is "one of the fundamental rights of every human being, without distinction of race, religion, political belief, economic or social condition" and because of its recognition that "the health of all peoples is fundamental to the attainment of peace and security."

At the end of World War II there was great concern over the plight of large numbers of children in the war-torn areas of the world. When the United Nations Relief and Rehabilitation Administration brought its activities to a close, certain of its resources were transferred to a newly

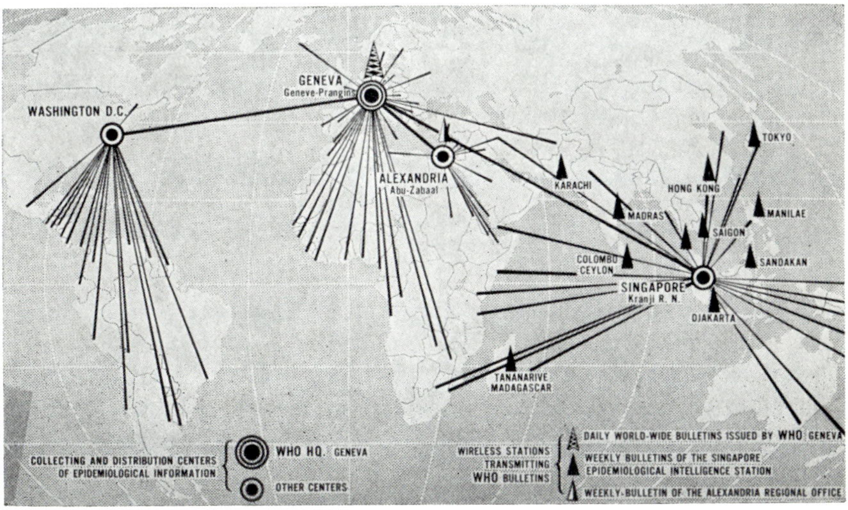

Fig. 14. World-wide Epidemiological Intelligence System of WHO.

formed organization called the *United Nations International Children's Emergency Fund* (UNICEF) in order to continue the much needed assistance to and care of children. As an emergency agency, it provided large amounts of food, powdered milk and supplies for child and maternal welfare activities in many parts of the world. In doing so, its attention was called to many continuing problems which affected children, not only in countries devastated by the war but also in the so-called under-developed areas of the world. As a result, it was allowed to reorganize into the *United Nations Children's Fund* and has expanded its activities in certain special problem directions, notably nutrition, maternal care, B.C.G., tuberculosis vaccination, and demonstrations of the control of certain diseases such as yaws and malaria. It conducts its activities in close partnership with the World Health Organization.

One of the great responsibilities which the United States of America bears as a result of being the most affluent and one of the technically most advanced nations in the world is to share its knowledge and resources with areas of the world which for various reasons have not been in the main stream of progress. Actually, we became involved in this by necessity when we were forced to enter World War II. The early and rapid successes of the Nazis, Facists, and Japanese militarists cut off the Allies from much needed natural resources. In January 1942, the Conference of Foreign Ministers of the American Republics became concerned with the necessity of joint effort for common good and survival. As a result, they recommended the establishment by the United States of an Office of the Coordinator of Inter-American Affairs. Shortly this became a government corporation named the *Institute of Inter-American Affairs.* Its function was to provide technical assistance leading to the more adequate development of the much needed resources of Central and South America, by means of bi-laterally conceived, financed and conducted programs. At once it was recognized that the single most important resource was the human factor. As a result, the first international agreement for technical assistance by the United States was with Ecuador in the field of health. From this, the program spread rapidly to involve cooperative developmental activities in many countries and in many substantive areas other than health, most notably education and agriculture.

When World War II was over, this type of activity was spread to certain countries in Europe and the Middle East, and subsequently to some of the countries in the Western Pacific and South Asia. Unfortunately, this much needed and fruitful program of technical assistance to under-developed areas has suffered by its eventual organizational relationship with programs of military and economic assistance and by repeated reorganizations and changes of names. For a number of years it was well known as the *International Cooperation Administration* (ICA). Its present name is the *Agency for International Development*

(A.I.D.). The programs of technical assistance in health matters of the A.I.D. work in close cooperation with the United States Public Health Service, the United States Peace Corps, the World Health Organization, and the Pan-American Health Organization.

In addition to the foregoing international health activities of an official or governmental nature, mention should be made of the many notable contributions made over the years by certain religious groups and philanthropic foundations. Outstanding have been the activities of the American Friends Service Committee, the Unitarian Service Committee, certain foreign mission programs of the Roman Catholic, Seventh Day Adventist, Baptist, Methodist, and Lutheran Churches as well as the Church of the Latter Day Saints, the American Bureau for Medical Aid to China (no longer active on the mainland), the Near East Relief Agency, and many others. The representatives of these groups have done notable service in the improvement of health and health knowledge, working quietly and effectively, hand in hand with people in villages and on farms throughout the world.

Several of the large philanthropic foundations, especially the Rockefeller Foundation and the Kellogg Foundation, have made truly remarkable contributions not only in the widespread control of certain devastating diseases such as yellow fever, malaria, hookworm and plague, but perhaps more significantly in the training and education of large numbers of health workers of all types and in the establishment of professional schools of high standards.

Questions for Discussion

1. What is the general death rate of your community? How does it compare with that of the state? With that of the nation?
2. Does your community have a health department? When was it organized and under what circumstances? Does it have a full-time staff? What professional disciplines are represented? What are their qualifications? How are they selected? In what activities does your health department engage? How much per capita does your community spend for public health work?
3. What efforts have been made, and by whom, to assess or evaluate the health situation in your community and the programs of its health department?
4. What are some examples of personal health problems that may become community health problems?
5. What voluntary or non-official health agencies exist in your community and what are their activities? How do they relate to the activities of the official health department?
6. What services does your community receive from the State Health Department? From the United States Public Health Service or the Children's Bureau?
7. In what ways can your community be affected by health conditions in another country?

8. What are some specific ways in which the Pan-American Health Organization and the World Health Organization help the people of underdeveloped areas?

Suggested Reading

1. Hanlon, John J.: *Principles of Public Health Administration,* 5th ed., St. Louis, C. V. Mosby Co., 1969.
2. Mustard, Harry S.: *Government in Public Health,* New York, Commonwealth Fund, 1945.
3. *Health is a Community Affair,* Ntl. Comm. on Community Health Services, Cambridge, Mass., Harvard Univ. Press, 1966.
4. *Health Administration and Organization in The Decade Ahead,* Ntl. Comm. on Community Health Services, Washington, D.C., Public Affairs Press, 1967.
5. Confrey, Eugene A. (Ed.): *Administration of Community Health Services,* Chicago, Intern. City Managers Assn., 1961.
6. Mattison, B. F. and Richman, T. L.: *Community Health Services,* Public Affairs Pamphlet No. 180-S, New York, 1962.
7. Winslow, C.-E. A.: *A City Set on a Hill,* New York, Doubleday, Doran, 1934.
8. *The City Scene, a symposium*: Pub. Health Repts., *77*:376, May 1962.
9. *United States Public Health Service,* Washington D. C., 1963, Govt. Printing Office.
10. *Children's Bureau: Five Decades of Action for Children,* Washington, Supt. of Documents, 1962.
11. *World Health Organization, what it is, what it does, how it works.* Geneva, 1965, World Health Organization.
12. Hanlon, John J.: *Bookshelf on International Health,* Am. J. Publ. Health, *48*:413, 1958.
13. Galdston, Iago (Ed.): *Voluntary Action and the State,* New York, International Univ. Press, 1961.
14. Carter, Richard: *The Gentle Legions,* New York, Doubleday, 1961.
15. Sills, David L.: *The Volunteers,* Glencoe, Ill., The Free Press, 1957.

PART II
The Play: Problems

The play, in which each of us participates, consists of a myriad of experiences fraught with many problems. Some of the most crucial of them relate to the health and well-being of the individual on the one hand and of the social complex on the other. They are by no means mutually exclusive. To the contrary, each affects and in fact determines the other. A broad spectrum of factors has the potential of influencing health directly or indirectly. Many things may go awry as one moves through life, hence many types of health problems may appear. Perhaps the single most important concept to bear in mind in this respect is that man does not stand alone. He is an intimate part of an extensive ecological system. He has an impact upon all other creatures and upon all aspects of his environment. They in turn may and often do have an adverse effect upon him. Health problems may be categorized therefore into several broad areas: those which arise from the environment, those which result from encounters with other biological organisms, those which stem from certain intrinsic physical or mental mishaps, and difficulties that may be encountered in attempts to remedy the foregoing. This then constitutes the play,—the genesis, development and solution of health problems.

Chapter 4

Man vs. Disease—Epidemiology

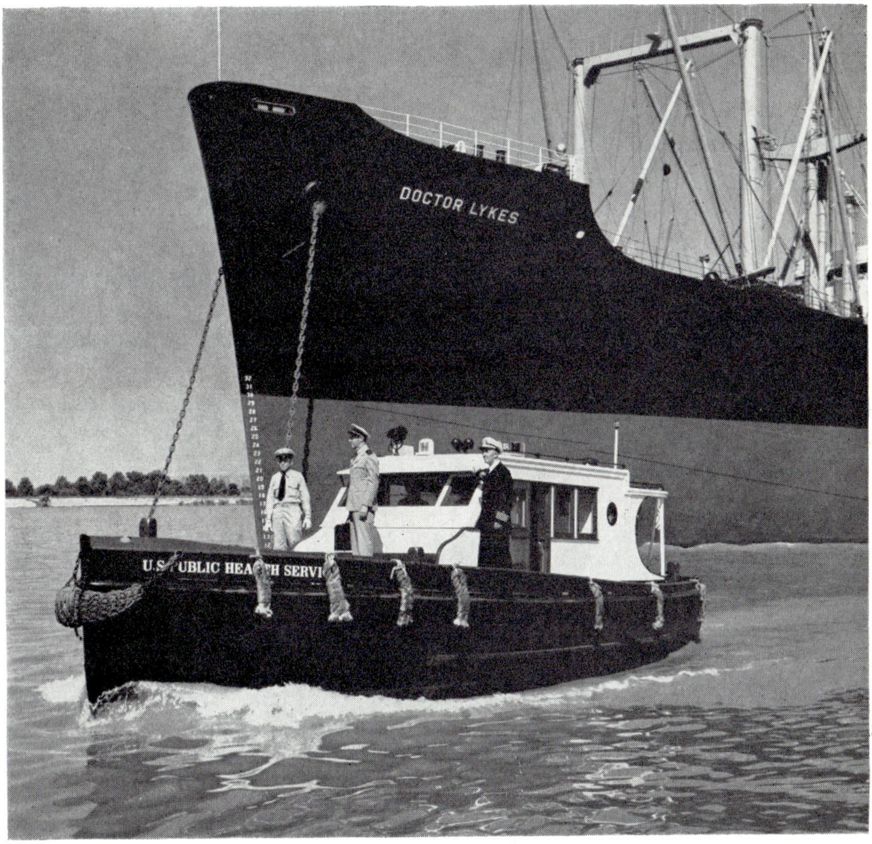

FIG. 15. A quarantine boat.

Introduction, The Meaning of Epidemiology

One of the many problems which confronts all teachers is the actual or potential presence of disease among his or her pupils. The primary school teacher has particular need to be concerned, especially with regard to certain acute communicable diseases which are most apt to occur in the age group with which the teacher has most frequent contact. It is the purpose of this chapter to provide a general background on the subject of disease and its control in order to assist the teacher in understanding his or her role, and in passing on to pupils certain fundamentals of the subject. An attempt is made to present the subject in broad general terms rather than by means of an encyclopedic description of a long series of disease entities.[1] This approach is used in the belief that memorized details tend to fade through time, while broad fundamental concepts tend to grow.

We are concerned here with the field of epidemiology. Originally, the term arose in relation to the study of epidemic disease, such as cholera or measles. Through the years, however, it has come to be applied in a much broader, biologically universal sense, so that now one speaks not only of the epidemiology of a communicable ailment such as influenza, but also of the epidemiology of a non-communicable condition such as heart disease, the epidemiology of physical hazards such as home accidents, the epidemiology of congenital conditions such as birth defects, and even the epidemiology of group effects such as births or infant deaths. The science of epidemiology deals essentially with the ecology of disease—"The circumstances under which diseases occur, where diseases tend to flourish, and where they do not."[2] Since the approach is ecological, it may be concerned with the widest possible spectrum of factors; biological, physical, genetic, environmental, social, economic, religious, political or whatever. The following may be helpful as a workable and descriptive definition:

> Epidemiology is the study of the natural history of disease or injury with reference to their cause and the factors influencing their occurrence. It (1) provides a picture of the extent, distribution and type of disease or injury at different times and in different places, and (2) relates these phenomena to the external conditions which surround the individual and determine his mode of life.

[1]The reader is urged to obtain a copy of *Control of Communicable Diseases in Man,* 11th Ed., 1970, American Public Health Association, 1740 Broadway, New York 19, New York, pp. 234 (price $1.75). This invaluable, authoritative and convenient handbook, which provides practical summaries of each disease, is widely used throughout the world.

[2]Paul, John R.: *Clinical Epidemiology,* University of Chicago Press, 1958, p. 9.

In considering epidemiology in its more traditional concern with the control of communicable disease, it is important first of all to regard the situation from nature's viewpoint. In the past, epidemiology has been considered almost exclusively from the point of view of only one of the myriad of factors—man, whose involvement in many instances is quite incidental or accidental. It is appropriate and useful to reorient our thinking and to consider epidemiology in an ecological sense wherein the phenomena of health, illness, or injury are seen as no more than selected instances among the many results of the total interaction between man and his environment. In this sense, communicable disease in man does not represent an independent or unique relationship set apart from all the other life processes, nor do its problems constitute a law unto themselves. Through time, many kinds of living things have been created or evolved. We, the members of the human species, Homo sapiens, represent only one of these types of biological creations out of an unknown number of other different types. Nature, of necessity, is concerned with the immediate and long-range needs and interests of all living things. Nature plays no favorites. As a result, we share with all other living things, plant as well as animal, certain fundamental needs, desires or drives:

(1) The need for food and shelter.
(2) The desire for personal survival.
(3) The drive for perpetuation of our kind.

Man and Microorganism

Because of the complexity of nature, the great variety of living things, and the tendency for the physical environment to become overcrowded by them, it is inevitable that some biological creations impinge upon others. As a matter of fact, this is probably a universal rule and a good one, since it provides the constant competition which determines which are most fit to survive and carry on nature's work. As far as nature is concerned, man is but one of many involved. From this point of view. then, it must be recognized that the various microorganisms in nature have no innate malevolence toward man. For that matter, man could not exist without them since many of them assist in his function and survival: the normal bacteria of the intestinal tract that help digest our food; the organisms in the preparation of many foods such as vinegar, wine, sauerkraut, and bread; those that play a role in industrial processes such as tanning; and those that produce some of the most valuable gifts to man such as penicillin, streptomycin, and other antibiotics.

Actually, only a very small proportion of all the many kinds of microorganisms are pathogenic, or disease-causing, in man. In such situations, the so-called pathogen has merely found in man a convenient steppingstone or way-station in its own attempt to survive. From the standpoint of nature and the pathogen or parasite, the most desirable or practical situation is one in which they and man find it possible to live in non-fatal harmony, symbiosis or joint survival. In a sense, an organism which kills its host, especially rapidly, represents a biological failure. This is why a disease such as anthrax is uncommon. For one thing, the disease, which is primarily an infection of farm animals, rapidly makes the individual quite ill, thereby taking him out of circulation. More than that, the organism which enters through a cut or other lesions in the skin multiplies rapidly in tremendous numbers in the blood stream and glands. Essentially, it has locked itself in since direct contact with infected tissues is necessary for its transmission. As a result, its rare occurrence is limited to industrial workers with contaminated hides, hair and wool, and occasionally agricultural workers and veterinarians. By way of contrast, consider the tuberculosis bacterium which quietly settles itself into a group or perhaps joins a family. It grows slowly and is in a position to cause a long term infection which provides more than ample time not only for its own growth but also for repeated passage on to others.

In consideration of the individuals who nature places in the path of infection, it is no accident that certain types are much more significant than others in terms of successful serial passage, and therefore, survival of the microorganism. Thus, the typhoid germ which infects a food-handler finds itself in an extremely advantageous biological position. On the other hand, consider the gonococcus which finds itself in the eyes of a newborn baby. True, it can cause much harm to the child it has infected, but it has reached a dead end. In contrast is another more usual gonococcus which acclimates itself to the genital glands of a promiscuous person. It is in an ideal situation for its survival and transmission. The first key, then, to understanding what is involved in disease, is an appreciation of what nature is trying to do for all of its creatures.

Disease, A Dynamic System

In recognizing disease in man as the result of ecological forces, it becomes evident that we are dealing with a dynamic system which consists of three primary factors; (1) an agent of disease or injury, (2) a recipient or host, and (3) a common environment. Each of these is made up of a varying number of subfactors, some interrelated and some not.

The Agent

The agent of disease or injury may be practically anything in nature. As far as communicable ailments are concerned, the agent is, of course, biological in character: viruses, rickettsia, bacteria, protozoa, molds or fungi, or certain segmented worms called helminths. Then there are physical agents which may be harmful to man under certain circumstances. Excessive exposure to heat, cold, and radiation fall into this category. In addition to harmful biological and physical agents are chemical agents. Curiously, chemical agents of disease may cause harm either by their presence or by their absence. If certain substances, such as vitamins, essential minerals, or proteins are inadequate in the diet, specific medical syndromes or illnesses will result—scurvy, goiter, or kwashiorkor as examples. On the other hand, there are the rapidly increasing numbers of toxic chemicals to which we are being exposed via air, water, food and otherwise, in our western industrialized culture: lead, various hydrocarbons, corrosives, detergents and many others.

The Host

There are many characteristics of the host that play a role in determining whether or not he succumbs to the influences of an agent of disease or injury. To begin with, anatomic structure can be important. Thus, infection of the inner ear is more common in young children, because of the shortness and straightness of the ear canal in early life. One's general physiological state obviously plays a role: nutrition, muscle tone, energy reserve, vital capacity and the like. Easily overlooked is the psychic constitution. High-strung, nervous individuals are more subject to certain skin conditions and gastrointestinal illnesses. The various intrinsic personal factors such as age, sex, and race may be critical. Some conditions are quite selective on either the basis of opportunity for infection or for biological reasons. Thus, race or nationality differcences may be observed. Among others, Negros, Eskimos and Irish

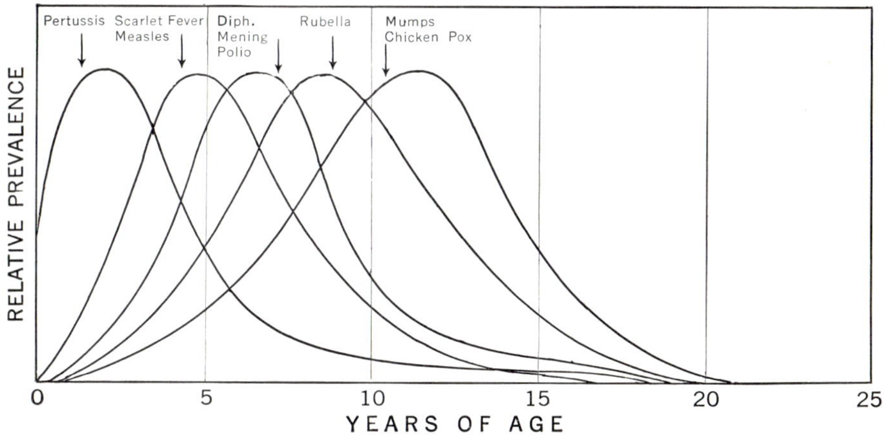

FIG. 16. Relative prevalence by age of acute communicable respiratory diseases.

appear to be more susceptible to tuberculosis than the average. Similarly, Jews appear to be more subject to stomach or gastric ulcers than non-Jews. Measles and many other acute diseases affect primarily young children (Fig. 16), and tuberculosis is most prevalent among young adults. Some diseases favor one sex over the other for various reasons. Thus, histoplasmosis is about 7 times as common in males as in females. In the cases of certain diseases, genetic resistance or susceptibility may exist. An example of the latter is sickle cell anemia which is limited to members of the Bantu tribe.

Finally, there is the possibility of *acquired resistance or immunity.* This may be natural immunity as a result of long-term group exposure with selective survival. Thus, Negros are much more resistant to yellow fever than are members of the white race, and Jews are more resistant to tuberculosis than most non-Jews. *Artificial acquired immunity* may be either active or passive. The former, *active immunity,* results when an antigen, in the form of a vaccine consisting of live or killed organisms or their byproducts, is inoculated or injected into a susceptible person. The antigen stimulates the cells of the person inoculated to produce or generate substances called antibodies which act against or *anti* the material injected so that exposure to larger amounts of more virulent material later is neutralized. The effect might almost be regarded as a physiological conditioned reflex. Effective antigenic agents or vaccines now exist against a large and increasing number of infectious agents including smallpox, yellow fever, plague, cholera, rabies, typhus fever, typhoid and paratyphoid fever, diphtheria, measles, rubella or German measles, tetanus, pertussis or whooping cough, poliomyelitis, many strains of influenza, to mention only the more important.

One problem is that the development of active immunity takes time, a number of weeks at least. Sometimes circumstances arise where an individual is known to have been exposed to a disease to which he is known to be susceptible and there is insufficient time to develop active immunity before the incubation period of the disease is passed. With some diseases one can resort to *passive immunity* by injecting blood or blood serum from an animal which has been actively immunized against the specific disease or from a human who is known to have had the disease. For example, the danger from tetanus (lockjaw) and diphtheria is largely from the toxin or poison which the bacteria produce. Animals such as horses may easily be injected with tetanus toxin or diphtheria toxin as an active immunizing antigen. The animal produces huge amounts of antitoxin, which circulates in its blood serum. Blood can be drawn in controlled amounts, the antitoxin-bearing serum separated, sterilized, put in vials and stored for use in emergencies such as mentioned above. In such cases, the exposed susceptible person borrows or uses antibodies (in these examples antitoxin) which the horse's body has manufactured at leisure. The pooled mixed blood of adult humans who through the process of maturing have been exposed to various microorganisms also contains significant amounts of antibodies that are effective against certain infections. The antibodies which are concentrated in the so-called gamma portion of the globulin of the blood plasma of human volunteers may also be available for emergency use in case of exposure to infectious hepatitis or exposure of a pregnant woman to German measles. In the latter case, if the disease is allowed to develop, the infant is very apt to be born with a congenital defect, especially, cataract, imperfect formation of the heart, or deaf mutism.

The Common Environment

The third primary factor involved in the existence and continuation of a communicable disease is the common environment, which contains within it elements of various types conducive to the epidemiologically effective bringing together of the agent of disease and the potential host. Much more is involved than the mere coexistence of the two. For each disease, a certain naturally prescribed set of circumstances is necessary. In some cases, it is relatively simple. Thus, an individual who has never had measles (a susceptible) need only be relatively casually exposed to the virus (the agent) in the droplets from the nose and throat of an infected person (a case) in order to allow successful transmission. The disease is so communicable that talking or laughing in the same room may be sufficient. By contrast, ankylostomiasis or hookworm disease requires a case or carrier with poor hygienic habits and facilities who deposits infected feces upon a certain type of surface, warm moist sandy soil, which allows the eggs of the hookworms to develop into larvae. Then there is necessary a relatively simple rural socio-economic circumstance which provides new potential hosts in bare feet to pick up the larvae which pass through the skin and enter the circulation. Even then, if the general state of health and nutrition is high, the developing worms will be cast off in the intestinal tract of the host.

The latter example indicates that the common environment itself is made up of three components, all of which are important and any one of which may be causal or critical in the transmission of the infection. The first of these consists of certain physical factors: weather, climate, season (Fig. 17), soil, terrain, sunlight, and the like. As examples, one may point to the high incidence and death rate from pneumonia in the cold thin air of the high Andes, and the large numbers of mosquitoes and possibly much malaria in marshy areas. The second is the biological component such as the presence of infected animal hosts, such as the pig in trichinosis; of vectors or living transmitters, such as the mosquito in malaria; of type and adequacy of the food supply, *i.e.*, nutrition; and competition among species. The third component is concerned with social factors and includes consideration of a great many things such

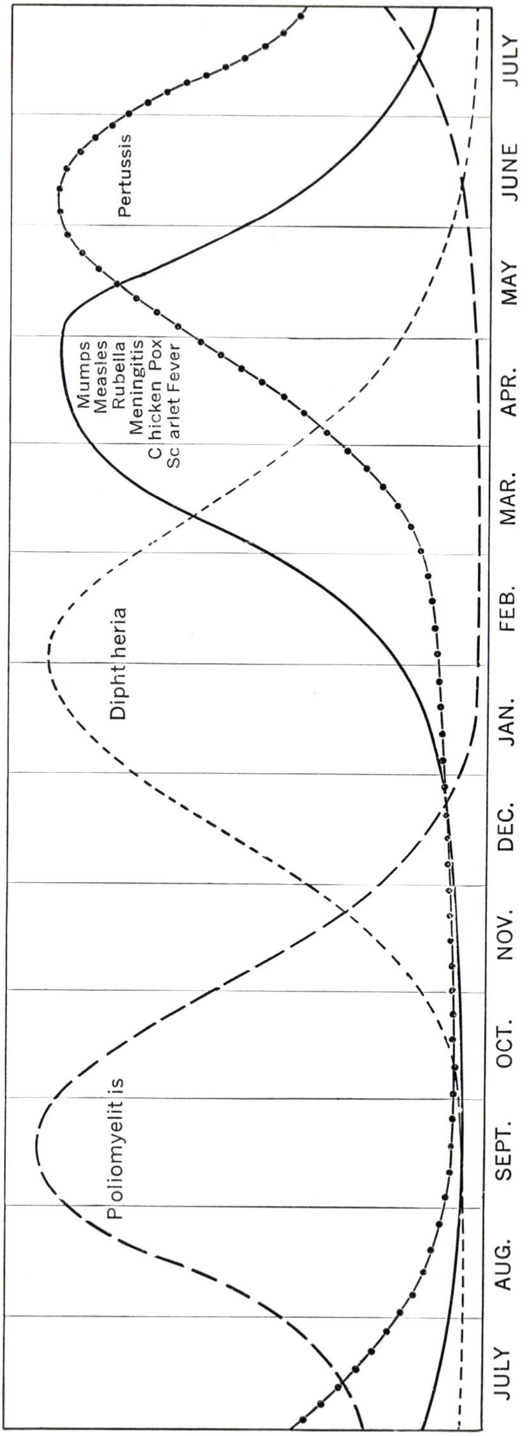

FIG. 17. Seasonal prevalence of acute communicable respiratory diseases (northern hemisphere).

as amount, density, and rate of increase and movement of population; frequency and extent of congregation at school, church, work, recreation; mode and extent of use of transportation; housing and clothing; economic pressures and potentials; social motivations, habits, customs and traditions; quantity and quality of general and professional education; existence of social welfare programs; availability of medical services for diagnosis, treatment and prevention; and psychological motivations and reactions, both individual and mass.

Steps in the Spread of Disease

In order to proceed with a consideration of steps involved in the transmission of communicable disease it is necessary to define several terms, a few of which have already been used. Necessarily, the definitions presented are designed on the basis of the use of the terms in epidemiology.

Agent refers to a material of a biological, physical or chemical nature which has the potential of causing disease or injury to man (or other animals).

Case refers to a person who has been affected by an agent in a way and to an extent that specific clinical signs and/or symptoms appear.

Carrier refers to a person who has been infected by a biological agent, continues to carry and disseminate it, but does not himself develop into a clinical case.

Reservoir refers to animals, plants, soil or inanimate organic matter on which a biological agent depends primarily for survival, and in which it reproduces itself so it can be transmitted to a susceptible host.

Host refers to a human or other living animal into which an agent can gain entry and find adequate sustenance for its multiplication.

Vector refers to insects which transmit agents of infection from a case, carrier, or reservoir to a host. They may do so by inoculation into or through the skin in the process of biting, or by deposit onto the surface of the skin, food or other objects with which the host subsequently comes into effective relationship. A vector may be infected itself (ex. mosquito) or may serve merely in a mechanical transporting sense (ex. housefly).

Fomite refers to an inanimate object or material which becomes infected with an agent and from which a host through effective relationship may acquire the agent (ex. soiled clothing, food, milk, *etc.*).

Contact refers to a person or animal known to have been in such relationship with a source of an infectious agent as to have had sufficient opportunity to acquire the infection.

Immune refers to a person who possesses specific antibodies, as a result of either previous infection or artificial immunization, sufficient to protect him against most exposures to the corresponding infectious agent. Immunity is relative and may be overwhelmed by a massive exposure or an unusual mode of entry of the agent.

Susceptible refers to a person or animal presumably not possessing resistance against a particular disease-causing agent, and is thereby liable to contract the disease if exposed to its specific agent.

Incubation Period refers to the time interval which usually transpires between effective exposure of a susceptible host to an agent, and the appearance of signs or symptoms of the specific disease.

Epidemiologically Effective Contact refers to a type and extent of exposure, of a person or animal to an agent of disease or injury, that if susceptible, the disease or injury will occur.

It is obvious that as long as a biological agent of disease is completely contained within an infected source, it cannot constitute a threat to other potential hosts. A series of steps indicated in Figure 18 are necessary before such a threat can become a reality. First, the agent must find a way to get out of the infested host. Any method will not suffice. It must be biologically possible and epidemiologically suitable. That is, it must fit in with the chain of events necessary to provide an opportunity for eventual infection of a new host. Each biological agent, and the disease it causes, has its own characteristics in this regard. The spirochete of syphilis provides a good example. It is an exceedingly frail organism and can exist only within narrow temperature limits and dies quickly when exposed to drying or light. It is not surprising, therefore, that it passes from one host to another almost exclusively by means of the most intimate, interpersonal relationships which preclude its exposure to these hazards. Other organisms prefer exit through other natural openings of the body. Some find more than one exit possible. On getting out of the infected host, the agent must now find a suitable mode of transmission to the new or potential host. Again, the factor of specific selectivity of method is involved. Some agents are carried mechanically by means of infected hands or a variety of inanimate objects. Those included in the category of acute respiratory diseases travel on tiny droplets which are thrown out into the atmosphere in the process of speaking, sneezing, coughing and the like. Because of their almost microscopic size, these droplets may remain suspended in the air for considerable periods of time.

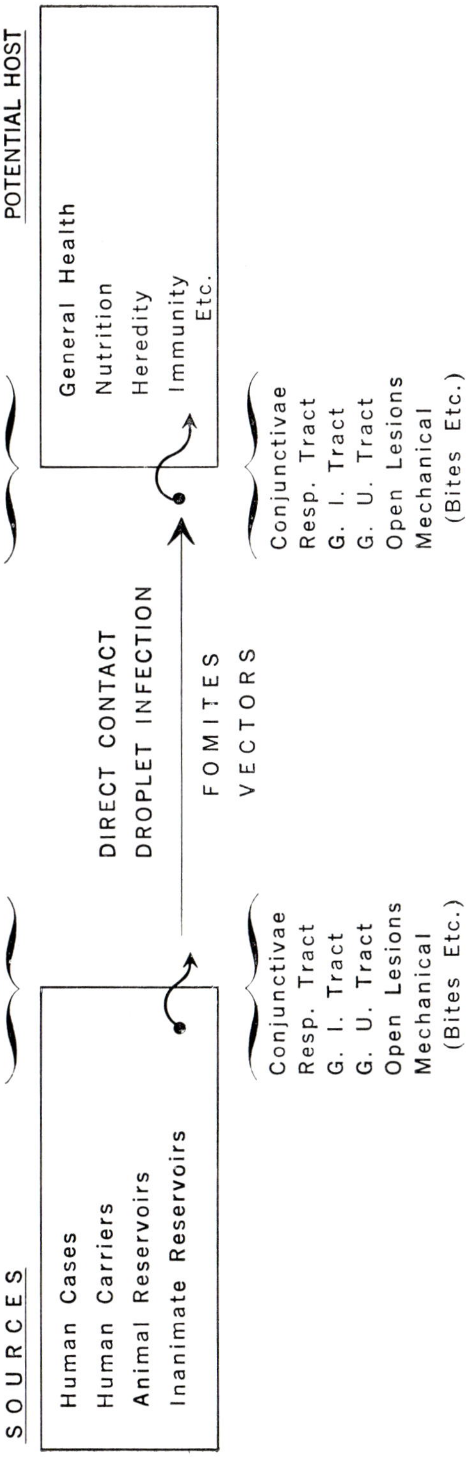

FIG. 18. Sequence of events in transmission of diseases.

Certain other agents travel by means of other animal species, predominantly insects. Some insects carry the agent in a purely mechanical sense as in the case of the housefly which picks up infected material on the surface of its body. Others, like the mosquito, are actually involved in the life cycle of the biological agent of disease. In such instances the agent escapes as a result of the insect biting the infected host, following which part of the agent's development occurs within the insect and eventually passes from the insect to a new host by means of another biting episode. On reaching the new host, therefore, the agent of disease

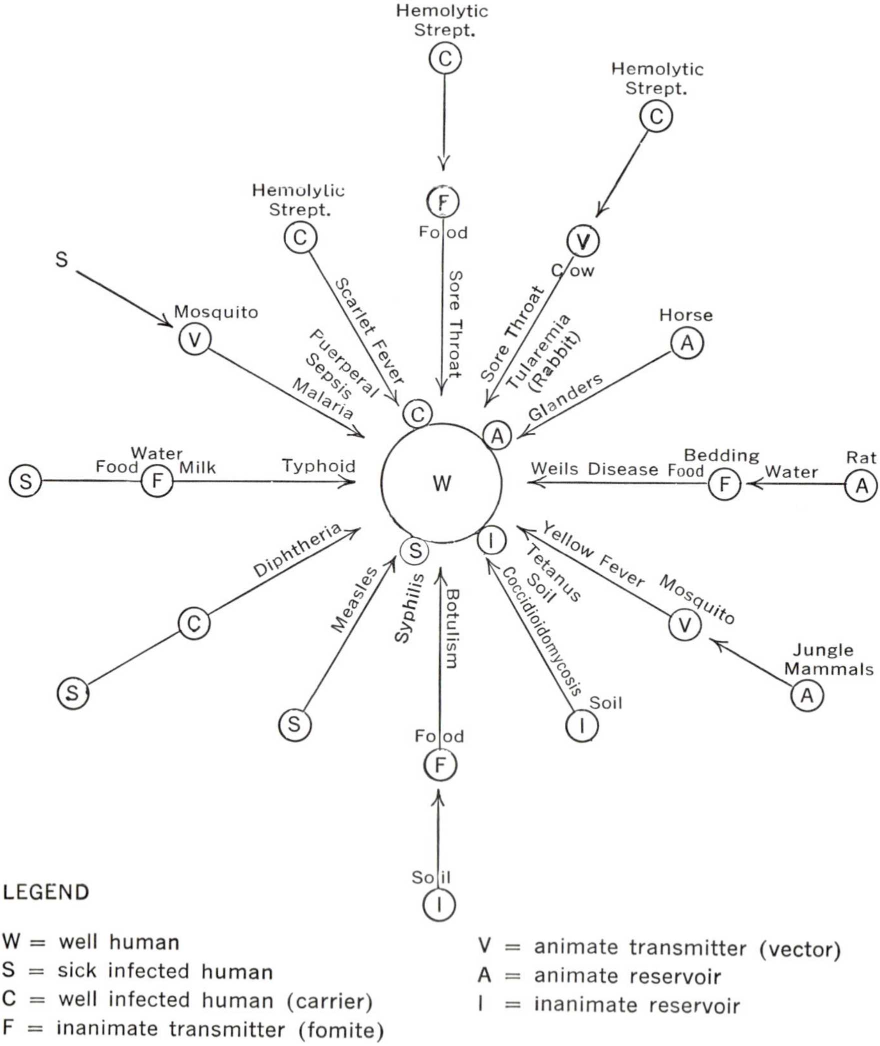

FIG. 19. Modes of spread of communicable disease.

must find a biologically suitable method of entrance. Generally speaking, the choice of mode of entrance parallels that of the mode of exit, agents which escape through the nasopharynx, for example, entering a new host through its nasopharynx. Even when the agent has succeeded in entering the new potential host, the agent may not survive and disease may not result. This may be attributable to a number of factors among which are the general or specific state of immunity, nutrition, general health, the presence or absence of anomalies, and the like.

Each of the steps in the foregoing chain of events is necessary for the perpetuation of an agent and its disease. Each step also represents a potential place for the application of control measures. As the adage states, "The chain is only as strong as its weakest link." A successful attack on any single link in this chain can lead to the control or even eradication of certain diseases.

Figure 19 presents this from a slightly different point of view. The well person (W) may be affected by outside biological agents of disease in a wide variety of ways. There are in his environment a number of factors which may threaten him: clinically ill infected humans (S), apparently well but infected human carriers (C), animate non-human reservoirs of disease in the form of lower animals (A), inanimate reservoirs of disease such as soil (I), animate transmitters or vectors (V), and inanimate transmitters of disease or fomites (F). As indicated, the well person may be infected by any one or a combination of these factors, depending upon his own habits and activities, and the biologically adapted habits and activities of the various factors in the environment that may potentially affect him. In some cases, such as the venereal diseases, direct and intimate contact must occur between the well and the infected human. This is shown as (S)(W). With some other diseases such as measles and smallpox, the well person may be infected across a certain distance by means of droplets from an infected human in a non-intimate relationship (S)→(W). In some instances an apparently healthy human carrier may be interposed, as occurs sometimes with diphtheria where an individual may acquire the organism from a clinically ill person and transmit it in turn to a healthy person who becomes ill, without the carrier himself showing signs of clinical diphtheria (S)→(C)→(W). Sometimes, as usually occurs with typhoid, the intervening factor may be an inanimate transmitter or fomite such as food, milk, or water (S)→(F)→(W). With many diseases the intervening factor is an animate vector such as a mosquito, louse or other biting insect (S)→(V)→(W). Sometimes well individuals are infected by intimate contact with healthy carriers. An example of this is the transfer of hemolytic streptococci from the hands of an accoucheur to the tissues of a woman in labor, thereby causing puerperal sepsis (C)(W). In other cases, organisms may be transferred over a distance, as with droplets infected with hemolytic streptococci passing from the nose or throat of a carrier to a well person (C)→(W). This type of situation may be further complicated by the interposition of an inanimate fomite, such as food infected by a carrier, and later consumed by the well person (C)→(F)→(W). Again using the hemolytic streptococci as an example, the apparently healthy human character may infect an animate transmitter such as a cow, which, developing mastitis, infects its milk, which is consumed by a well person, who may develop septic sore throat. The resulting pattern in such a case would be (C)→(V)→(F)→(W). Animate, but non-human reservoirs of disease may threaten the well person in a number of similar ways. Sometimes intimate contact is necessary between the animate reservoir and the potential human host. Among examples that may be mentioned are the handling of the carcass of an infected rabbit resulting in tularemia in man, and the transmission of rabies by the bites of rabid dogs (A)(W). Some animal diseases, such as glanders in horses, may be transmitted over a distance in a manner similar to measles (A)→(W). Sometimes an inanimate transmitter or fomite is involved as in the case of the contamination of bedding or food by discharges of rats carrying the agent of infectious jaundice (A)→(F)→(W). Certain diseases affect primarily lower animals, but man may occasionally get in the way. An important example is jungle yellow fever which is sometimes transferred by mosquitos from small jungle mammals to man (A)→(V)→(W). Even the inanimate environment may sometimes be a source of infection either by direct contact as with tetanus acquired from the soil (I)(W), or over a distance as may possibly be the case in the transmission of the pathogenic fungus, coccidioides immitis (I)→(W).

The foregoing scheme and distribution is by no means all inclusive. When protozoan parasites are involved, the pattern of transmission becomes much more complex, since their life cycles typically involve a number of steps and a number of hosts. For example, the large tape worm *Diphyllobothrium latum* infests man in the following way:

dog		water		crustacea		fish		human
(A)	→	(I)	→	(A)	→	(A)	→	(W)

For an even more complicated picture, that of infestation by the liver fluke is presented:

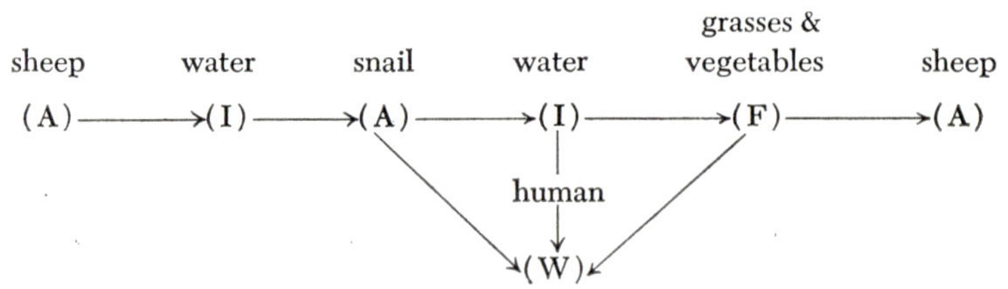

Epidemics Can Be Different

Although each disease tends to have its own characteristics to a remarkable degree, it is interesting to observe the extent to which they may be influenced by the foregoing factors. Thus, certain diseases may increase for any of a number of different reasons. While it is recognized that the school teacher in the United States is not apt to have contact with malaria, it does provide a convenient means of illustrating, by means of a number of actual examples, these points which are in effect basic epidemiological principles or phenomena.

(1) *Increase due to a new species of mosquito vector.* For an historically long time, tertian malaria has existed in certain parts of Rumania but not in the delta of the Danube River. During World War I, Bulgarian and Turkish troops brought with them a new mosquito species, with breeding habits that enabled it to thrive in the delta. As a result, severe malaria spread rapidly through the area.

(2) *Increase due to the introduction of new hosts.* At the end of World War I, many Greek villages, whose inhabitants over generations had reached an endemic-epidemic balance with regard to malaria, received large numbers of displaced refugees. Malaria suddenly became epidemic due to this upset in the ratio of susceptible newcomers to resistant inhabitants.

(3) *Increase due to altered social environment.* During World War II, Greece which had done much to control malaria suffered much physical destruction and displacement of people. Food and drugs were lacking for continued suppression of the disease. This combined with increased breeding of the mosquito vector in the debris allowed the disease to flourish epidemically, even in places like Athens where it had long since been eliminated.

(4) *Increase due to altered physical environment.* One of the great accomplishments of Mussolini early in his regime was the draining of the Pontine marshes around Rome, thereby eliminating an historic hotbed of malaria. Toward the end of World War II when the Nazis retreated up the Italian peninsula, they deliberately reflooded the area in order to delay the allied troops. This flooding also allowed malaria-transmitting mosquitoes to breed rapidly, and malaria again became a problem until the Pontine marshes were redrained.

(5) *Increase due to change in climate.* The spread of malaria depends upon certain species of mosquitos, which breed best in warm moist circumstances. In 1961, the spring rains in the East African highlands were unusually heavy and there was much flooding. There resulted a marked increase in mosquito breeding and in the incidence of malaria.

(6) *Increase due to change in economy.* Malaria may be controlled by the widespread use of suppressive drugs and by means of spraying and dusting with various insecticides. If, as has happened in a number of places, the economic situation precludes the purchase of these materials, malaria can soon spread from those individuals who have remained infected.

(7) *Increase due to change in agriculture.* On several occasions we have seen valleys in South America, previously planted in grain and fruit then changed over to vineyards for more profitable wine manufacture. This necessitated irrigation which allowed the breeding of an efficient mosquito-transmitter of a particularly severe type of malaria brought into the area by new workers. The situation became so dangerous that these fertile valleys had to be completely abandoned.

(8) *Increase due to changes in communications and travel.* The world has become remarkably small, relative to the modern speed of travel. This has very serious epidemic implications. Before and during World War II, Brazil had achieved great success in the control of malaria. Then a new and especially dangerous mosquito, *Anopheles gambiae,* was accidentally introduced apparently by a plane from Dakar in West Africa to Natal in eastern Brazil. Strenuous efforts eventually brought the resultant flare-up of malaria under control but only after the death of many people.

As has been indicated earlier, some diseases may be spread in more than one way. When this is true, what happens in a particular episode depends upon the method of spread involved. A good example is typhoid fever which may be transmitted by a carrier (an apparently well but infected person), or by contaminated water, food or milk. If it is a carrier, spread is dependent upon personal contact which tends to result in a long drawn-out epidemic involving perhaps only a few people at a time, and limited to ages characteristic of those contacted (Fig. 20).

If contaminated water is the mode of spread of typhoid a definite epidemic curve results. However the epidemic tends to be a little slow in building up and is often preceded by a primary epidemic of milder

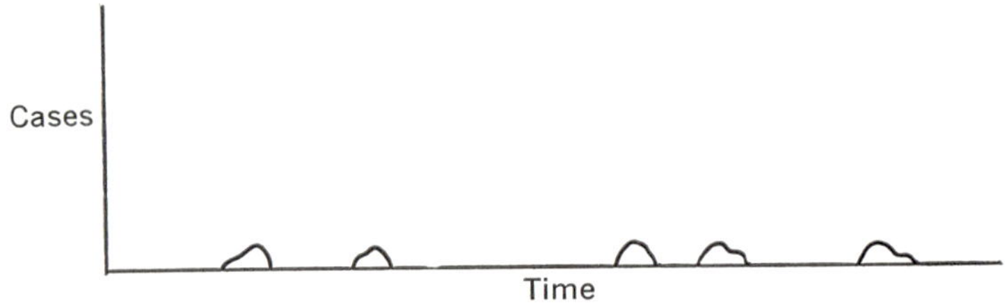

FIG. 20. Carrier-contact borne typhoid.

diarrhea or dysentery due to other and more acute contaminating organisms. The initial outbreak of typhoid fever then occurs followed after a short interval by a series of secondary cases who acquire the disease by contact with those infected early. In this type of epidemic, the disease tends to be relatively mild and all ages are affected (Fig. 21).

If contaminated food is involved, the typhoid organism will usually have had some time to incubate and multiply. Furthermore, exposure through eating is usually a one-time event. As a result, food-borne epidemics are much more sudden in nature, the disease tends to be more severe since more organisms are ingested, and usually all ages tend to be involved, depending of course on the circumstances of the meal (Fig. 22).

When milk is infected with typhoid bacteria, a splendid culture

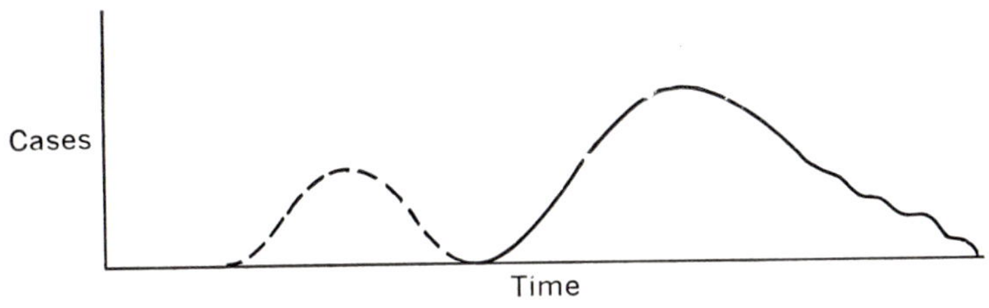

FIG. 21. Water borne typhoid epidemic.

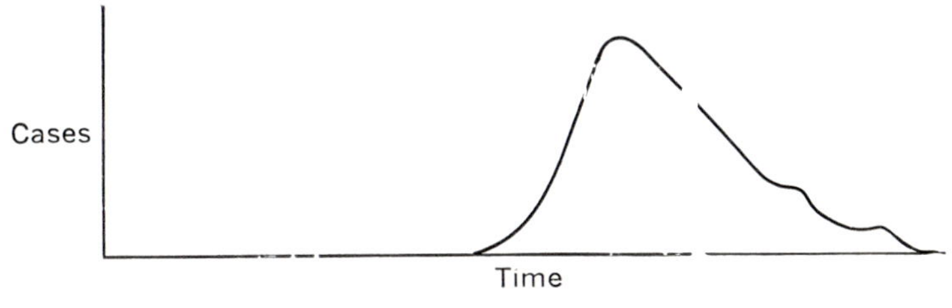

FIG. 22. Food borne typhoid epidemic.

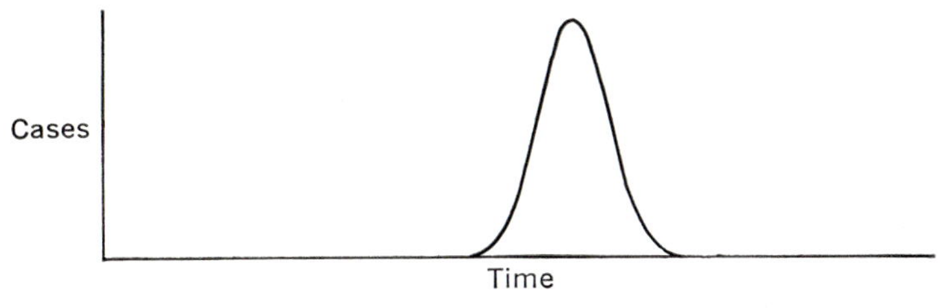

FIG. 23. Milk borne typhoid epidemic.

medium is provided. There is usually a rapid and extensive increase in the number of organisms. Because of this and the limited time period over which the contaminated milk is consumed there results an extremely explosive epidemic. Cases tend to be severely ill with a higher death rate and younger persons are especially affected because they consume more milk (Fig. 23).

Measures for Control of Communicable Disease

Man's attempts to exercise some control over the hazard of communicable disease go far back into history. Primitive people, both in ancient times and at present, have used noise, smoke, frightful masks, charms and incantations, in the belief that these diseases were caused by evil spirits. Even modern man has resorted to such procedures. As recent as the end of the 19th century, some American communities shot off cannon and burned barrels of pitch in the streets in an attempt to combat yellow fever and other pestilences. Sulphur candles may still be purchased, hence continue to be used by some in the belief that they "kill germs," and some individuals rely on asafoetida bags, good-luck charms and amulets of various types in the belief or hope that they protect against disease.

From what has been presented with regard to the various factors involved in the development and spread of disease, it may be correctly surmised that the methods to be followed for the effective control of communicable disease depend to a considerable extent upon the ecology of that particular disease. In other words, an approach which may prevent or control one disease, may be worthless in the case of another. The various approaches to control, therefore, may be considered in somewhat the same manner as were the steps involved in the spread of disease. For convenience, the spectrum of possible control measures is presented in semi-outline form.

I. Prevention of the Spread of Disease

A. *Measures Aimed at the Microorganism*

1. Fumigation, the exposure of infected material to toxic gases or fumes such as burning sulphur. This procedure originated with the miasmatic theory of disease and is long since outmoded. It has no practical effect upon microorganisms.
2. Disinfection, the direct application of physical or chemical agents to infected material. This is of value in the destruction of certain pathogenic agents under particular circumstances. Examples are the chlorination of drinking water,

the pasteurization of milk, and the exposure of various fomites to heat, drying and sunlight.

3. Sterilization, the complete destruction of all living contaminants by the direct application of physical or chemical agents. When this can be done, it is of course most effective. Several examples that might be cited are the treatment with strong chemicals of stools from patients with typhoid fever, the burning of sputum from persons afflicted with tuberculosis, the cooking of pork to destroy the larvae of trichinosis, and the use of drops of a silver salt solution in the eyes of the newborn in order to destroy any gonococci that might be present.

B. *Measures Aimed at the Reservoir*

1. Eradication of the reservoir. If an animal serves as a natural reservoir for a microorganism, the complete elimination of the reservoir would be very effective. Sometimes this is actually possible and practical. Examples are the seeking out, slaughtering and destruction of cattle or goats infected with undulant fever; of rabbits with tularemia; of dogs, foxes, bats, *etc.* with rabies; parrots and related birds with psittacosis; and of squirrels, rats and other rodents infected with plague, typhus and various other diseases. Partial eradication of a human reservoir may be considered to be represented by the surgical removal of a chronically infected gall bladder from a chronic typhoid carrier, or of chronically infected tonsils from chronic carriers of hemolytic streptococci or diphtheria organisms.

2. Reduction of the communicability of reservoirs. If, as is the case with humans, it is not practical or possible to eradicate disease reservoirs, their communicability may be reduced or eliminated by other means.

   (*a*) Discovery of reservoirs. It is obvious that before anything definitive can be done about reservoirs or sources of infection, they must be located to as complete a degree and as early as possible. This requires the cooperative activity of many individuals and groups, parents, private physicians, hospitals, schools, and the official health department, to mention only the most important. With respect to the child population, in a true sense, the ultimate responsibility lies with the parents. It is to be expected logically that they are in the best position to observe or hear of any deviation from normal health and well being in their children. This being so places the initiative for action in their hands. The initiative should take the form of keeping the school child home, of notifying the school, and preferably of obtaining medical guidance. If circumstances indicate and make it possible, a school nurse may visit the home. If the school nurse suspects that the child is suffering from a communicable disease, she should urge medical attention and report her findings to the public health authorities.

Similarly, it is incumbent upon attending physicians or hospitals to report such information to the health department. It is then the responsibility of the health department to carry out whatever investigations may be indicated in order to locate the source from which the patient received the infection, and those contacts to whom the patient may have passed it on. A properly functioning health department also is on a constant lookout for possible sources of infection by the routine checking of death certificates, burial permits, hospital records, and requests for certain diagnostic kits and materials for treatment. It may also conduct certain community diagnostic programs involving the widespread application of tests for tuberculosis, intestinal parasites, infections of the nose and throat such as diphtheria, venereal diseases, and other conditions. Frequently activities such as these are carried out in intimate partnership with teachers and school authorities.

A few words of description of death certificates is appropriate here. The death certificates of the fifty states are more or less standard in form in conformance with suggestions of the National Office of Vital Statistics of the United States Public Health Services. A typical example is shown in figure 24. They consist essentially of three parts, (*a*) certain sociological data which may be obtained or provided by a relative, acquaintance or non-medical attendant, (*b*) medical certification of the cause of death which must be filled in and signed by the medical attendant, a medical examiner or a coroner, and (*c*) certification of registration of death and burial by the local registrar of vital statistics and the funeral director. The immediate and contributing causes of death must conform with the terminology in the "International List of Diseases, Injuries and Causes of Death" in order to ensure, inasmuch as possible, accuracy and uniformity. Accurate death certificates are of great value to public health agencies in indicat-

HVS-20143 REV. 11/59

LOCAL REG. NO...

PRIMARY
DIST. NO...

COMMONWEALTH OF PENNSYLVANIA
DEPARTMENT OF HEALTH
VITAL STATISTICS

CERTIFICATE OF DEATH

1. DEATH OCCURRED IN: a. County b. City or borough
c. If death did not occur in City or borough, give name of township (Do not use R. D. or Box Number)
d. Full Name of Hospital or institution (if not in hospital, give street address)

2. DECEASED'S MAILING ADDRESS a. Street address, R. D., or Box Number
b. Post Office, Zone, and State

3. VETERAN Yes ☐ NO ☐
a. Which War.......................... b. Serial No.......................

4. NAME OF DECEASED (Type or print) a. (First) b. (Middle) c. (Last)

5. DATE OF DEATH (Month) (Day) (Year)

6. WHERE DID DECEASED ACTUALLY LIVE? a. State.................................... b. County....................................
c. Did deceased live in a township?
☐ Yes, deceased lived in....................................township.
☐ No, deceased lived within actual limits of....................................city or borough.

7. SEX | 8. COLOR OR RACE | 9. MARRIED ☐ NEVER MARRIED ☐ WIDOWED ☐ DIVORCED ☐ | 10. DATE OF BIRTH | 11. AGE (in years last birthday) | If under 1 year: Months, Days | If under 24 hours: Hours, Min.

12. USUAL OCCUPATION (even if retired) | 13. SOCIAL SECURITY NO. | 14. BIRTHPLACE (State or foreign country) | 15. CITIZEN OF WHAT COUNTRY?

16. FULL NAME OF SPOUSE | 17. MOTHER'S MAIDEN NAME

18. FATHER'S NAME | 19. INFORMANT'S NAME AND ADDRESS

MEDICAL CERTIFICATE (Items 20 through 23 must be completed by physician only)

20. CAUSE OF DEATH: Enter only one cause per line for (a), (b) & (c).

INTERVAL BETWEEN ONSET AND DEATH

PART 1. Death was caused by:
IMMEDIATE CAUSE (a) ....
Conditions, if any, which gave rise to above cause (a) stating the underlying cause last.
DUE TO (b) ....
DUE TO (c) ....

PART II. OTHER SIGNIFICANT CONDITIONS: contributing to death but not related to the immediate cause given in Part I (a)

21. WAS AUTOPSY PERFORMED? Yes ☐ No ☐

22. a. ACCIDENT Yes ☐ No ☐ | 22. b. DESCRIBE HOW ACCIDENT OCCURRED | 22. c. TIME OF ACCIDENT Hour m E.S.T. Month Day Year

22. d. ACCIDENT OCCURRED While at work ☐ Not while at work ☐ | 22. e. PLACE OF ACCIDENT (e.g., home, farm, street, etc.) | 22. f. CITY, BOROUGH, TOWNSHIP COUNTY STATE

23. I hereby certify that I attended the above named deceased and that death occurred from the causes and on the date stated above at m., E.S.T.
a. Signature M. D. or D. O. b. Address c. Date signed

24. a. BURIAL ☐ CREMATION ☐ REMOVAL ☐ | 24. b. DATE | 24. c. NAME OF CEMETERY OR CREMATORY | 24. d. LOCATION (City, Boro., Twp., & County) (State)

25. DATE REC'D BY REG. | 26. REGISTRAR'S SIGNATURE | 27. SIGNATURE AND ADDRESS OF FUNERAL DIRECTOR

FIG. 24. Example of a Death Certificate.

ing problems, evaluating progress and in planning programs. They also are a deterrent to homicide, and provide much needed legal data and documentation in order to inherit, claim life insurance and pensions, and the like. They also are useful for genealogical purposes. The responsibility for filing a death certificate rests with the individual who inters the body. The certificate is checked by the local registrar who, after abstracting certain locally essential or useful information, forwards it to the state registrar of vital statistics. The state is responsible for compiling, analyzing, tabulating, and interpreting the data provided by the accumulated certificates on a weekly, monthly and annual basis. The state is also responsible for the permanent preservation of the original certificates in fireproof vaults as part of the state's archives.

(*b*) Treatment of reservoirs. When sources of infection are discovered, it is most important from their own standpoint that they be treated as promptly and as thoroughly as possible. This is also of great concern to the community since it assures the most prompt rendering of the patient non-infectious. This is particularly true of certain chronic communicable diseases such as tuberculosis and syphilis. With the former, prompt collapse of the infected lung combined with certain antibiotics, tends to reduce greatly the infectiousness of the patient. In the case of infectious syphilis, the prompt administration of penicillin or a related antibiotic renders the patient noninfectious to others. In all cases, it must be remembered that complete treatment is necessary, else the patient will not achieve ultimate recovery and may lapse back to the infectious state.

(*c*) Isolation. This is the separation, for the period of communicability, of infected persons from others, so as to prevent the direct or indirect spread of the infectious agent. Strict isolation is important with certain few diseases such as smallpox, typhoid, or plague. It is not a practical procedure with most common diseases, especially the so-called acute communicable diseases of childhood. With these, there are many missed or hidden cases, and the period of greatest infectiousness precedes the appearance of clinical signs and symptoms upon which a diagnosis may be based. Often, however, an attending physician may isolate such patients, not so much for the protection of the community as for the protection of the patient against secondary infections that might be acquired from well meaning visitors and other persons. Except under most unusual circumstances, the placarding of premises is no longer considered socially or epidemiologically practical.

(*d*) Quarantine. This is the limitation of movement of well persons, who have been exposed to a communicable disease, for a period of time equal to the longest usual incubation period of the disease, in order to protect those who have not been exposed. For a long time, great reliance was placed upon quarantine, not only of ships, households, and institutions, but even of entire ports and cities. As with isolation, recent years have brought a recognition of its limitations, and as a result quarantine restrictions have been greatly modified. Selective quarantine is frequently used. Examples which depend upon the disease and circumstance, are the exemption of immune persons or of wage earners except those who work as food handlers, the limitation of movement of military populations, and the exclusion of exposed children from school.

The latter leads to consideration of a problem which often confronts the teacher and the school administrator. Frequently, when epidemic disease exists or threatens, there arises a public clamor to close the schools. On the surface this may appear logical on the basis of limiting contact among the school age population. However, the closing of schools usually results in greater and more intimate contact among children since they tend to play unrestricted and unsupervised in their neighborhoods, and circulate freely among groups and crowds rather than to remain at home. Therefore, in communities with well organized and efficient school health and public health services, epidemics can best be controlled if the schools remain open and the children are engaged in controlled activities under intelligent surveillance.

In considering this subject, the National Committee on School Health Policies has suggested that each locality decide for itself on the basis of the answers to two questions: (1) Are nurses and medical staffs so adequate and so alert that the inspection, observation and supervision of students will keep sick students out of school? (2) If a school is closed, will students be kept at home and away from other students so that its closing will not increase opportunities for contact with possible sources of infection?

Generally speaking, if the first question can be answered affirmatively, or the second question answered negatively, schools should be kept open in the face of an epidemic. This is usually the case in large public schools and in thickly settled communities. Schools should be closed when the first question is answered negatively or the second question affirmatively. In smaller communities with scattered houses, where opportunities for personal contact are limited, this is frequently the situation. In rural areas, especially where pupils are transported in buses thereby increasing intimate contact, it may also be advisable, under certain circumstances, to close the schools.

To summarize the issue of quarantine and isolation, the following statement of current policies of the health department of a large city is presented. It illustrates the trend toward more reasonable and practical controls of communicable disease cases and contacts.

Quarantine of Contacts

chickenpox–none
measles–none
mumps–none
*poliomyelitis–none
*scarlet fever–none
*diphtheria–yes, pending negative nose and throat cultures
pertussis (whooping cough) non-immune child contacts excluded from school and public gatherings for 14 days after last exposure
smallpox–16 days from last exposure unless successfully vaccinated
typhoid and paratyphoid fevers–no quarantine, but household contacts cannot act as food handlers
*(With poliomyelitis, scarlet fever and diphtheria, wage earners permitted to enter and leave premises if they have no contact with patient, with children or with food for public consumption.)

Isolation of Cases

Until recovery—erysipelas, influenza, meningococcic meningitis, mumps, septic sore throat, typhus.
For specific periods–
chickenpox–until skin entirely clear.
smallpox–until skin clear of crusts
diphtheria–until 2 successive negative nose and throat cultures, 24 hours apart, otherwise 14 days.
measles–7 days from rash minimum.
pertussis–3 weeks minimum.
poliomyelitis–7 days minimum from onset
scarlet fever–7 days minimum in uncomplicated cases, otherwise until recovery.
typhoid and paratyphoid–until 3 consecutive negative stool cultures at least 24 hours apart.

Excluded from school, public gatherings, or work until recovery–impetigo, epidemic kerato-conjunctivitis (pink eye), scabies, trachoma.

Excluded from intimate contact (not merely sexual)–syphilis, gonorrhea, chanchroid, yaws, granuloma inguinale, lymphogranuloma venereum.

Isolation not required but desirable–common cold, dysenteries, pneumonia, tuberculosis (preferably in hospital or sanatorium).

Separation from pregnant women–rubella (German measles), mumps.

C. *Measures Aimed at Vectors*

1. Fumigation, disinfection and direct killing. With certain diseases, if it is impossible or impractical to attack the microorganism itself or the reservoir of infection, successful control may sometimes be achieved through measures aimed at vectors. Included here are such activities as destruction of lice and fleas with insecticidal sprays and powders, the direct killing of flies and mosquitoes, and the dipping of cattle to eliminate ticks.
2. Prevention of breeding. This carries control measures back still one more step. For example, the oiling, spraying, filling or impounding of natural waters may prevent mosquitoes from laying eggs, or their larvae from developing. Similarly, careful construction of buildings and proper garbage disposal may prevent rats and other disease-bearing vermin from breeding.
3. Sanitary surveillance. As indicated earlier, a number of inanimate materials in the environment may serve as vectors of disease. Meticulous attention to these has been a major factor in making possible the development and continued existence of the modern community. Worthy of particular mention are the adequate and proper disposal of sewage and refuse, the provision of sufficient water purified by filtration and chlorination, the assurance of safe milk by means of dairy and milk processing plant inspection and pasteurization, and the surveillance of all aspects of the food supply, including certain aspects of production, shipment, processing, storage, preparation and service.

II. Increasing the Resistance of Potential Hosts

A. *Maintenance of General Health and Nutrition*

While it is true that specific communicable diseases are caused by specific microorganisms under specified conditions, it nevertheless has been recognized for a long time that an individual's general state of physique, health and nutrition may be a significant determining factor in the chances of infection when exposed, of illness when infected, and of recovery when ill. This relationship is most obvious with regard to the amount and quality of food consumed. More subtle but none the less real are such influences as muscle tone, and posture. Schools are in a peculiarly strategic position to make a most significant contribution in this area of health. Supervised graded exercise and sport, scheduled rest periods, provision of nutritionally sound school lunches, and supplemental feeding are among the more important activities which schools may provide.

B. *Immunization*

The basic concepts of immunization have already been presented briefly in discussing the role of the host in disease. Where individual and group resistance to communicable disease can be increased significantly and safely, it presents probably the most desirable type of control. As pointed out, specific immunizing agents now exist against a substantial number of pathogenic microorganisms. Their use depends, of course, upon circumstances. Generally speaking, everyone should be vaccinated against smallpox. The same is true of poliomyelitis, pertussis and diphtheria. Other antigens should be obtained when specific exposure is anticipated or possible. Thus, if one plans to travel to areas where yellow fever, plague, cholera, typhus fever, and various other diseases are apt to be present, it is wise, if not mandatory to be immunized against them. If one is bitten by a rabid dog, certainly anti-rabies vaccine should be administered. If epidemic influenza threatens, protection by means of immunization is to be recommended.

As far as immunizations against the acute communicable diseases of childhood are concerned, it is best that they be obtained as early as practical. One often hears parents state that they intend to wait until a child is admitted to school before protecting him. For many diseases this is much too late. Most cases of measles, rubella (German measles), pertussis (whooping cough), diphtheria and poliomyelitis occur during the preschool years. It is pointless to purchase insurance after the trip is over. Furthermore, infants and young children tend to have fewer reactions or side effects from immunizing agents.

While there is no universally followed schedule of immunzations, the following is considered practical and desirable.

PRIMARY IMMUNIZATIONS

age	*product*
2 months	0.5 cc. DPT } pertussis vaccine combined with diphtheria and tetanus toxoids
3 months	0.5 cc. DPT
4 months	0.5 cc. DPT
5 months	smallpox vaccine
6 months	1.0 cc. Salk or Sabin Polio vaccine
7 months	1.0 cc. Salk or Sabin Polio vaccine
14 months	1.0 cc. Salk or Sabin Polio vaccine
21 months	1.0 cc. Salk or Sabin Polio vaccine

BOOSTER DOSES

age	*product*
18 months	0.5 cc. DPT
5 years	0.5 cc. DPT, Salk or Sabin vaccine, smallpox vaccine
7 years	0.25 cc. DT (diphtheria and tetanus toxoids)
10 years and each 5 years thereafter	smallpox vaccine, Salk or Sabin vaccine

Reference should also be made to the recent appearance of several new important immunizing materials; live-virus oral poliomyelitis vaccine (Sabin), mumps vaccine, measles vaccine and rubella or German measles vaccine. The first of these is already widely used in place of or in conjunction with the Salk killed-virus injectable vaccine. If Sabin-type live-virus poliomyelitis vaccine is used in place of Salk killed-virus vaccine, each of the three strains should be administered about a week apart. The advantage of live-virus vaccine is a stronger, longer-lasting immunity. Live-virus measles vaccine should be administered at about the first birthday. Gamma globulin should be administered at the same time in order to prevent reactions or symptoms from the vaccine. Mumps and rubella vaccines, if used, should also be given in late infancy since, like measles, these diseases occur essentially in young children.

III. Community Health Education

Last but not least among the measures to be mentioned for the control of communicable disease is as thorough education as possible of the public in matters concerning their health and well being. This should include consideration of nutrition, hygiene, the principles of infection and disease, general symptomatology, first aid, and general patient care. The methods used should include the entire gamut of propaganda, sensitization and educational approaches, and should involve every channel of communication possible. By far the most important, and in the long run the most effective of these methods and approaches is sound, objective and interesting teaching carried out over a planned, period of time in the school classroom. In order that this might be possible, teachers should be encouraged and feel free to call upon the resources of the official and voluntary health agencies, the professional societies and many other sources of assistance that may exist in the community.

While each communicable disease is a biological entity with its own peculiarities, certain similarities among them make it possible to group them into several broad categories. Since control measures depend necessarily upon preferred methods of

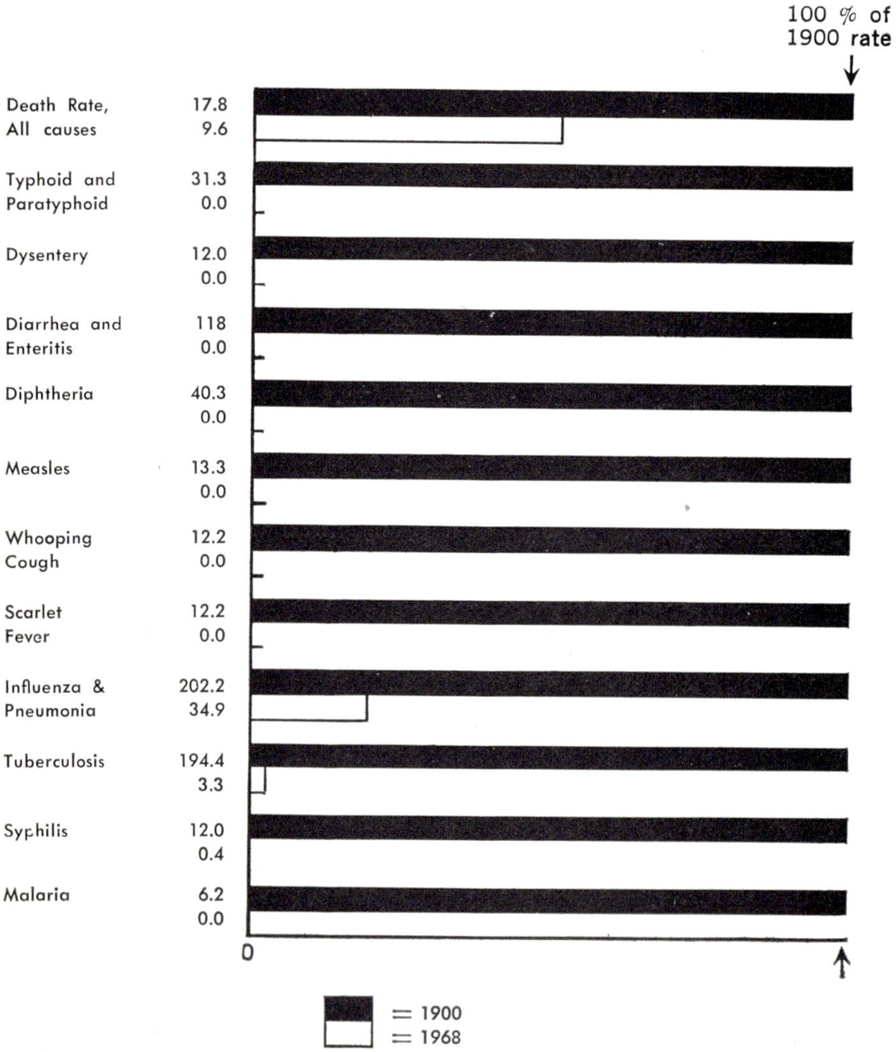

FIG. 25. Changes in mortality, United States (1900-1968).

spread, this factor is also the most convenient basis for grouping. Of practical significance is that by grouping diseases, many control measures may be considered applicable to a group rather than to only a single disease. This makes not only for easier understanding, but also for more efficient and coordinated control activities. This is illustrated in Tables 1 and 2 which present in a summary form the essential epidemiological facts concerning the group of acute upper respiratory diseases and the group of gastrointestinal diseases. Similar group presentations are possible for the insect-borne diseases, the chronic respiratory diseases, and the genito-infectious or venereal diseases. This concept incidentally, is commonly reflected in the method of organization of community health programs. Thus one ordinarily finds, in the health departments of states and of large cities, divisions or bureaus of acute communicable disease control, of tuberculosis or chronic chest disease control, and of venereal disease control.

The Results of Effective Control Measures

As a result of the successful application of various combinations of the foregoing measures, remarkable results have been achieved in the control and even elimination of many of the communicable diseases which affected American communities until quite recently. Figure 25 illustrates what has been accomplished in this respect merely since the beginning of this century in the United States. As a result, during this short period, the average life expectancy at birth has undergone a remarkable increase from 47 to about 70 years. We cannot rest upon our laurels, however, especially in an age of jet travel by large numbers of people. A letup of vigilance would certainly be quickly followed by a resurgence of any or all of these dangerous diseases.

Role of the School in Communicable Disease Control

From the preceding discussion of communicable diseases it becomes obvious that the school is intimately involved in the problem of their control and prevention. School personnel must realize that with large numbers of children in confined space along with the natural susceptibility of children, particularly of elementary school age, to common childhood diseases, the school presents a peculiarly efficient setting for the rapid spread of disease.

Upon the Division of School Health Services falls much of the responsibility for working out cooperatively with the Department of Public Health the most effective arrangements for constant vigilence and effective handling of cases of illness when they occur. This should include the prompt reporting of cases, the observance of quarantine regulations,

Table 1. Summary of Acute Respiratory Diseases

<table>
<tr><th colspan="2">Disease</th><th>Diphtheria</th><th>Scarlet Fever</th><th>Whooping Cough</th><th>Measles</th><th>Smallpox</th><th>Chickenpox</th><th>Mumps</th><th>Meningitis</th><th>Poliomyelitis</th></tr>
<tr><td colspan="2">Cause</td><td>Corynebacterium diphtheriae</td><td>Hemolytic streptococci</td><td>Hemophilus pertussis</td><td>Filtrable virus</td><td>Filtrable virus</td><td>Filtrable virus</td><td>Filtrable virus</td><td>Neisseria intracellularis</td><td>Filtrable virus</td></tr>
<tr><td colspan="2">Incubation Period (Days)</td><td>2–7</td><td>2–7</td><td>7–16</td><td>8–12</td><td>8–16</td><td>14–21</td><td>14–21</td><td>2–10</td><td>7–14</td></tr>
<tr><td colspan="2">Period of Communicability</td><td>Variable, usually under 2 weeks, seldom over 4</td><td>Variable, usually 3 weeks from onset until no discharges</td><td>Catarrhal stage (7–14 days) and 3 weeks of whoop</td><td>Catarrhal stage (4 days) and 5 days of rash</td><td>Catarrhal stage (2–4 days) to disappearance of lesions</td><td>Catarrhal stage (0–2 days) and during 6–10 days of lesions</td><td>Unknown, assumed while glands enlarged</td><td>From onset until 2 weeks after recovery</td><td>Unknown, assumed incubation period and first week of disease</td></tr>
<tr><td colspan="2">Prevalence</td><td colspan="9">World-wide but especially temp. zone—winter and spring except WC (spring), polio (late summer) and diph. (fall and winter). Affects children most. Incidence usually less and older age group affected more in rural than urban.</td></tr>
<tr><td colspan="2">Source</td><td colspan="9">Discharges from nose and throat of cases—Occ. other lesions in Diph. SF, and SP. Carriers in Diph., SF, meningitis, and poliomyelitis.</td></tr>
<tr><td colspan="2">Spread</td><td colspan="9">I° cases, II° fomites. Occ. milk in Diph. and SF (explosive epidemics). Carriers in Diph., SF, meningitis and poliomyelitis.</td></tr>
<tr><td colspan="2">Susceptibility</td><td colspan="9">Everyone after 6 mos. of age not having active or acquired immunity. Exceptions: SF varies geographically. SP and WC susceptible from birth. Some immunity probably acquired without disease by age and contact in all but SP and measles.</td></tr>
<tr><td rowspan="2">Immunity</td><td>Passive</td><td colspan="9">Convalescent serum and gamma globulin give some protection for several weeks in all but smallpox. Whole adult blood in whooping cough, measles, mumps. Placental extract in measles. Antitoxin in diphtheria.</td></tr>
<tr><td>Active</td><td colspan="9">An attack gives long-lasting immunity. Artificial immunity long lasting in smallpox and diphtheria, much shorter in scarlet fever whooping cough, poliomyelitis, measles and mumps.</td></tr>
<tr><td colspan="2">Control Measures</td><td colspan="9">1. Early diagnosis and reporting (laboratory in Diph., WC. Mening., Polio)
2. Isolation: Diph., SF, WC, SP Of little value in the rest
3. Disinfection
Concurrent
Terminal
4. Quarantine like isolation
5. Immunization, q.v.
6. Source finding—D and SF (cases, carriers, milk); SP (cases). Of little value in the rest
7. Pasteurization of milk, especially in diphtheria and whooping cough
8. Prevention of overcrowding, especially in meningitis
9. Education</td></tr>
</table>

Table 2. Summary of Gastrointestinal Diseases

Disease	*Typhoid Fever*	*Paratyphoid*	*Dysentery, Bacillary*	*Dysentery, Amebic*	*Cholera*	*Brucellosis*	*Hookworm*
Cause	Eberthella typhi	Salmonella (several species)	Shigella (several species)	Endamoeba histolytica	Vibrio comma	Brucella (several species)	Necator americanus
Incubation Period	3–38 days, usually 7–14 days	3–15 days, usually 4–10 days	2–7 days	2 days to several months usually 3–4 weeks	1–5 days	6–30 days	None in true sense
Prevalence	World-wide, warm seasons esp; males and young adults esp.		Tropics and subtropics esp. warm season; all ages and sexes		India, China	Mediterranean, U.S., Canada, Scandinavia; warm season	Limited to warm, moist sandy soil; children, esp. white
Period of Communicability	Prodromes, illness, and convalescence until stools negative					20–300 days	While infested
Source	Feces and urine of cases and carriers		Exception: Brucellosis; milk, tissues, blood, and discharges of infected cows, swine, goats				
Spread	Infected water, food, fomites, flies, direct contact		Exception: Brucellosis; milk and contact with tissues and discharges Hookworm; contaminated soil. Neither man to man				
Susceptibility	General susceptibility, decreasing with age		Exception: Brucellosis; most persons have some natural immunity				
Immunity — *Passive*	None						
Immunity — *Active*	One attack gives long-lasting immunity in typhoid. Relative immunity in paratyphoid and bacillary dysentery. Short immunity with vaccines in typhoid and paratyphoid (about 2 years) and cholera (about 1 year)						
Control Measures	1. Early diagnosis and reporting of cases and carriers Laboratory tests 2. Isolation in all but hookworm, am. dysentery, and brucellosis 3. Disinfection—concurrent—terminal in all but hookworm and brucellosis 4. Quarantine—cholera only (5 days) 5. Immunization (q.v.) 6. Source finding—cases and carriers, important in all 7. Water sanitation 8. Excreta sanitation 9. Food sanitation 10. Milk sanitation 11. Shellfish sanitation 12. Prevention of fly breeding 13. Carrier control 14. Education General, cases, carriers						

assistance in special immunization procedures, implementation of procedures for readmission to school after illness, cooperation on epidemic precautions and similar activities. In instances where the administration of school health is vested in the local health department, channels for handling disease control problems are more direct and much time and effort is conserved. Cooperation with the local medical society often leads to better understanding by private family physicians of the total picture and of the complexity of necessary community inter-relations. The school can provide an excellent means of getting a health message across to the general public through both pupils and their parents. Carefully planned cooperation should include education of parents and the general public in regard to specific local problems, their care and prevention, and to possible epidemic precautions. This is an area in which the school health coordinator and the school health council might give valuable help and leadership. Communications media, conferences, speakers, and other educational means should be employed to their fullest extent.

While understandably the classroom teacher wants as complete attendance as possible, undue emphasis upon perfect attendance records has sometimes resulted in having pupils struggle to school despite acute respiratory or other diseases. Fortunately, most states have abandoned a former common but ill-advised practice of basing educational appropriations and the payment of teachers on pupil-attendance figures.

The school environment provides many opportunities for cooperation with the official health agency. The school needs to work closely with the Department of Health in the implementation of sanitary measures relating to water, milk, food supplies, sewage and waste disposal, swimming pools and laboratory tests, and the in-service education of food handlers and other staff workers. Details concerning this will be presented in a subsequent chapter.

The Division of Health Services should also work closely with the guidance counselor, the health coordinator, and the community agencies in the adequate follow-up of cases of communicable diseases and behavioral and mental problems in connection with which those affected may require help other than medical in order to cope with the conditions from which the disease stemmed.

The Role of the Teacher in Communicable Disease Control

Although the control of communicable disease is the concern of all school personnel, the classroom teacher, because of her daily contact with the children, is in a key position to make many significant contributions. It is most important that she possess accurate, scientific understanding of the factors involved in communicable disease, not only that she may prove effective in her teaching but that she herself may live up to her responsibilities and opportunities in the matter of prevention and control.

Nobody else on the school health team duplicates the teacher's precise functions in cooperating with school health services, healthful school living, and health education in the control and prevention of communicable disease. At the same time, she needs to keep constantly in mind the differences in attitudes, practices, and understandings in regard to communicable diseases that exist among the parents of the children she teaches. Differing cultural attitudes toward disease and medical care in general also play a part. If the teacher is sensitive to all of this, she can often contribute through a tactful approach to parents toward the successful solution of problems in this area.

The teacher should be familiar with the written school and health department policies and procedures concerning the discovery and handling of suspected cases, the procedures for reporting, exclusions, quarantine, and readmission as set forth in the handbook usually provided by the Department of Public Health or by the Board of Education as a guide to school personnel. A list of symptoms and conditions which merit suspicion or attention is sometimes included as a guide to the teacher.

Through her own alertness and familiarity with early symptoms, the teacher is often able to detect deviations from normal health in the pupils she sees from day to day. Her promptness in reporting such deviations to the school nurse or physician, and the temporary isolation of the child until the arrival of the parent can be critical factors in preventing the further spread of disease. When a case of communicable disease is discovered in a child who is attending school, or is reported a day or so after the child has been in school, it is often customary to notify parents of the other children in the class of this fact, and to ask that they be especially watchful for symptoms which their children might develop as a result of their exposure. In the case of some diseases, parents of known contacts may be requested to keep their children at home until the period of incubation has passed without the development of signs or symptoms of the disease. A daily morning informal health review by the teacher of kindergarten or lower elementary grades has proved effective in screening deviations from normal health and the development of possible symptoms. Some teachers find it possible to do this merely by standing at the door of the classroom and carefully observing each child in turn as she greets him upon arrival at school.

Other preventive measures whereby the teacher might contribute positively toward communicable disease prevention and control are listed briefly as follows:

1. The teacher herself should present to the children an example of the best possible personal habits. Children usually

imitate, and the teacher's example is a far more potent factor than most teachers realize.

2. The teacher should strive to inculcate her pupils with desirable health habits such as the use of tissues, handwashing before eating and after the toilet; the individual use of toilet articles and drinking cups; the care of wraps and clothing; the careful use of materials shared in common such as library books, equipment, games; the risks involved in smoking, the over use of candy and chewing gum; proper food selection; and the importance of observing safety regulations.
3. The teacher needs to be temperature conscious and to try to maintain room temperature at the desirable 68 to 70 degrees of temperature. Children enjoy carrying responsibility and are very useful as monitors in keeping room temperature charts.
4. During the first few days of the school term it is important that teachers in the preschool and lower elementary grades instruct their small students in the sanitary use of drinking fountains and toilets, proper ways of sneezing, coughing and blowing one's nose.
5. The observance of sanitary handling and serving of foods during the mid-morning feedings and at lunch time is imperative. This includes prevention of fly breeding, the use of straws in milk containers, the provision of paper napkins, the discouragement of the sampling of each other's food, and the insistence on the washing of hands with soap by those who handle the food of pupils and teachers.
6. The teacher needs to stress the use of individual lockers for wraps and clothing, or lacking lockers, individual hooks, the use of individual blankets at nap time, of one's own sneakers during gym periods, and of one's own towel after a shower.
7. Due precautions should be taken in having the pupils wear adequate wraps during outdoor play periods and when cooling off after vigorous play. The teacher should locate outdoor activities with proper regard to the wind, sun, and dust.
8. The proper arrangement of groups of children to prevent undue exposure to droplets and other contacts during class periods, rest periods, and when pupils are working at tables is important. When children use cots or floor mats for rest periods, the teacher should have the children lie in alternate directions to prevent breathing and talking in each other's face.
9. The teacher should cooperate willingly with others in solving the individual child's special health problems as may be re-

quested by a parent or family physician. This includes, if indicated, seeing that prescribed medications are taken and assuring special feedings, rest periods, and limited exercise upon return after illness.

10. As has been pointed out, in teaching her pupils, the teacher in a sense, actually teaches the child's family too. Therefore, she is in a strategic position to pave the way for new immunization procedures or other special health measures which may need the assistance of the school for their implementation.

In secondary schools, booster shots for certain immunizations may be important. Respiratory diseases, skin conditions and other diseases also may present many problems. To cope with these effectively involves investigation of health habits, concepts and attitudes that may be related to their acquisition, prevention, or treatment. At the secondary school level, students are especially prone to come to school with respiratory illnesses in order to maintain grades, to play on athletic teams, or to participate in social activities. Unusually rapid physical growth occurs during this period. However, nutritional status is often lowered through an inadequate or missed breakfast, a poorly chosen or omitted lunch, and a dependence upon snacks. Late hours, inadequate sleep and too many activities also often compound the problem. Guidance by the teacher in appropriate total living, and the budgeting of time, energy and rest are of great value to the secondary school pupil.

Effective assistance to pupils in order that they meet this many-faceted problem lies in the wise utilization by the teacher of the many types of informational and educational aids available from official and voluntary health agencies. These are materials which add to the teacher's own equipment and understanding, for use with pupils, and for distribution to parents. Here too, adequate familiarity by the teacher with community health facilities and resources will prove invaluable.

Questions for Discussion

1. Has your community suffered from any important epidemics during its history? When? What kind?
2. Choose some communicable disease (ex., tuberculosis, diphtheria, pneumonia, typhoid, *etc.*), and trace its history in your community over the years. What factors were involved in any changes in its incidence?
3. What are the predominant communicable diseases in your community at present? How are they spread? Can they be reduced?
4. Study the story of the 1957-58 world wide epidemic (pandemic) of Asian influenza or the 1963 typhoid epidemic in Zermatt, Switzerland, tracing its progress, means of travel and the measures that were taken in the United States to combat it.

5. What are some of the common folk-beliefs and superstitions concerning various communicable diseases; their cause, prevention, and treatment? Do any exist in your community? In your class?

Suggested Reading

1. *Control of Communicable Diseases in Man,* 11th Ed., Am. Pub. Health Assn., New York, 1970
2. ANDERSON, G. W. AND ARNSTEIN, M. G.: *Communicable Disease Control,* New York, The Macmillan Co., 1963.
3. JAMES, G. AND GREENBERG, M.: Bookshelf on Epidemiology and Evaluation, Am. J. Pub. Health, *47*:401, 1957.
4. MAY, JACQUES, M.: *The Ecology of Human Disease,* New York, M.D. Publications, 1955.
5. BETT, WALTER R. (Ed.): *The History and Conquest of Communicable Disease,* Norman, University of Oklahoma Press, 1954.
6. WINSLOW, C.-E. A.: *Man and Epidemics,* Princeton, Princeton University Press, 1952.
7. CAMUS, ALBERT: *The Plague,* New York, Alfred Knopf, 1948.
8. ROUECHÉ, BERTON: *Eleven Blue Men,* New York, Berkely Publications, 1955.
9. ————: *The Incurable Wound,* New York, Berkely Publications, 1955.
10. ROGERS, F. B.: *Epidemiology and Communicable Disease Control,* New York, Grune & Stratton, 1963.

Chapter 5

The World Around Us—Environmental Health

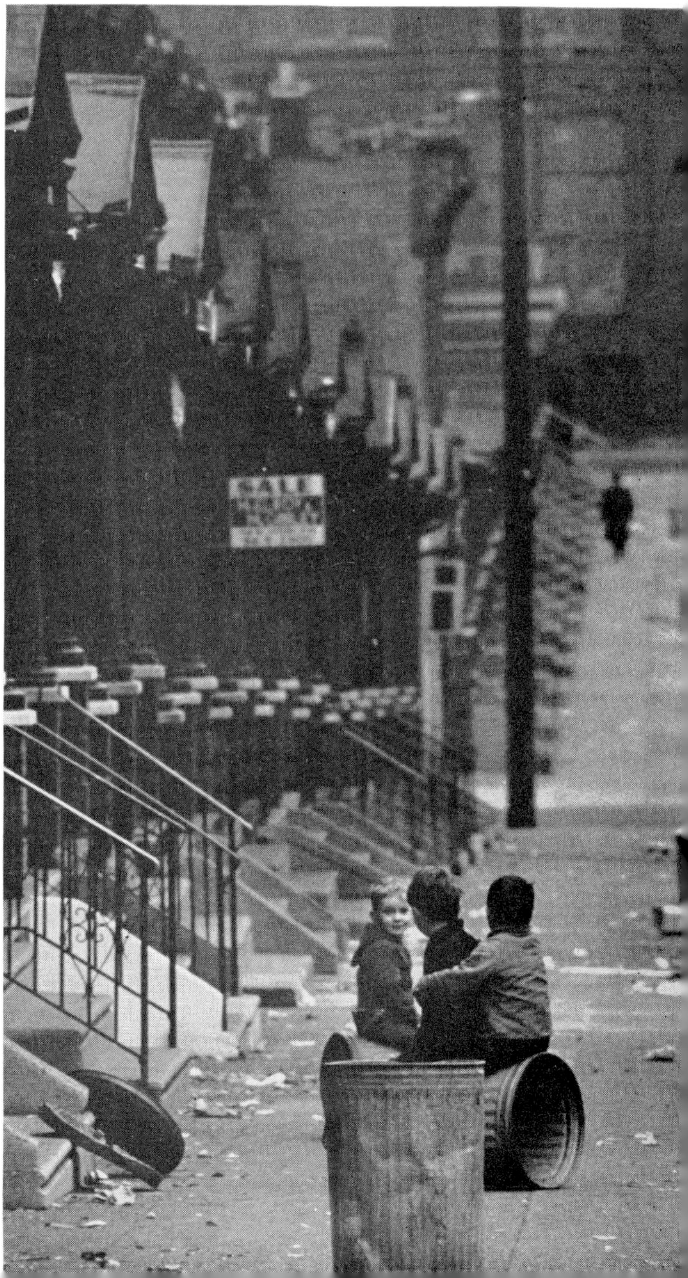

Fig. 26. Our World

The Importance of the Environment

The history of man clearly reveals that his health and survival have always been intrinsically dependent upon his relationship with his environment. Of all the controllable diseases which afflict mankind, those that have their roots in the environment are easily the most widespread and devastating. The chief health problems of the past,—yellow fever, plague, malaria, cholera, typhoid, the dysenteries and certain others,—have all been subdued primarily through the modification of the environment;—eliminating the causal agents of disease or limiting their proliferation in the environment. There is no doubt that if the major health problems of the present,—heart disease, cancer, hypertension, emphysema and chronic bronchitis, accidents, mental illness and many others,—are to be brought under control, modifications of the environment will play a major role.

It is important to realize that the relationship between man and his environment is dynamic and that man is only one of innumerable components of his environment. Unless these truisms are fully taken into account, any efforts to improve public health and welfare are doomed to failure. Until surprisingly recently, man's attitude toward his environment was casual and selfishly utilitarian. The sky above and the earth and the seas below seemed vast, especially when populations were smaller and most people lived rural lives. The deposit of human waste on the ground, the disposal of refuse into a stream, or the setting of a brush fire seemed of little consequence. Furthermore, ownership of land seemed to imply absolute rights of use, even if the health and enjoyment of life of others were affected. A man's house was regarded as his castle, a concept widely misinterpreted to mean that anything within was immune to outside concern or social intervention. As indicated in the discussion of the evolving community, this state of affairs could persist only so long. A social and hygienic break-point was certain to be reached. Population increase, urbanization, technological and industrial progress, and greater interdependence of people have led us close to the break-point. A social and legal re-evaluation of human and property rights became necessary, even under the most democratic circumstances. The safeguarding and conservation of the total environment became recognized as a responsibility of government to all the people, present and future.

One indication of this has been the expansion of interests and types of workers involved in the provision of a safe and healthy environment. As mentioned in the brief historical summary, public health had its origin in a concern about environmental problems, essentially incidents of gross insanitation. Through time, the significance of such problems has tended to be downgraded, and concern about them has been pushed into the background. Meanwhile, there has been added to the older more prosaic environmental concerns, a far more extensive, complex and potentially much more dangerous group of problems. One might generalize the changes in the types of environments that affect man to have been essentially as follows. Before the 1700's, the chief environmental concerns were biological or natural physical factors such as wild animals and floods. During the 1800's, due to industrial and urban growth, matters of gross insanitation commanded most attention. During the 1900's and especially since the end of World War II, chemical and physical factors developed and used by man have become the prime environmental concerns. These changes in the nature of the problems are reflected in the types of personnel required to solve them. Where once only sanitary inspectors with little training seemed adequate to meet the hygienic needs of the environment, the modern environmental health program now requires engineers and sanitary scientists with various specialized backgrounds, veterinarians, experts in food and milk production and control, entomologists, radiological and meteorological scientists, and individuals from many other disciplines.

What is the Environment?

The environment should be regarded in an all inclusive sense. Physically, attention must be given to the earth's substrata and surface, its waters, its plants and animals, the foodstuffs produced, transported, processed and served, and the atmosphere around us. With regard to contaminants, until recently, prime if not exclusive consideration was given to bacteria. The goal of environmental health was limited to the control of certain excreta-transmitted communicable diseases such as cholera, typhoid and dysentery. In this and in many other countries, these diseases have been largely conquered, essentially by the application of sanitary science and engineering. In addition to these filth-borne bacterial diseases, workers in environmental health in company with medical researchers and public health administrators have achieved notable success against certain other diseases such as yellow fever and malaria spread by insects which breed in the environment. While the diseases mentioned may seem exotic to us now, it is important to appreciate that they were devastatingly common only a short time ago and require a never-ceasing vigilance against them. In this shrunken world of rapid travel and extensive population increase and movement, their reintroduction and recrudescence with explosive violence is an increasing possibility.

While the bacterial infection of the environment in itself is of great importance, there has come about during recent years an awareness of a number of other adverse factors that may affect the environment of man. There have now been identified more than 200 viruses, most of them since 1948, many of which may infect man by way of water, food, milk, air, insects or rodents, and cause illness. Beyond this, we must be increasingly concerned with non-viable as well as viable elements in our environment. Newly discovered synthetic chemicals are being added as preservatives, flavoring and coloring agents, and detergents to our foods, drugs, cosmetics, and soaps. Still other materials are widely used in spray or powdered form as insecticides, herbicides, pesticides, fungicides, frost preventatives and for many other purposes. Chemists can synthesize and produce, and salesmen can merchandise a dozen or more products, while those concerned with protecting the public's health are trying to determine the safety of one.

In addition, technological developments and industrial expansion have resulted in extensive pollution not only of the soil, but of the air and water. Atmospheric and water resources serve many purposes, but in the final analysis the most important is to sustain life. The vast array of new chemicals and waste products which increasingly are discharged into these natural resources presents workers in environmental health with one of their greatest and most complex problems. A major cause for concern at present is the threat of excessive ionizing radiation in the environment. How much do we normally receive, and how much more can we tolerate? At what point must we forfeit further technological, industrial, economic and military progress or personal pleasures and conveniences for the survival of our species as we know it? What protective measures are necessary in relation to the increased use of fissionable material in industry? How can the waste products of nuclear fission be disposed of safely? How can the public's demand for ever more power be met without irreparable contamination of the environment and destruction of the earth's ecosystems? These are some of the questions which command the attention of the present day worker in environmental health. They are a far cry from the garbage and refuse heaps which so many of the public still identify erroneously with public health.

The Consequences of a Poor Environmental Relationship

For public health and other purposes, the environment should also be regarded from the social and psychological as well as from the physical point of view. Man, especially modern urbanized man, actually lives in several types of circumstances or environments. Variations depend essentially upon such fundamental characteristics as age, sex, education and training, occupation and economics. The child, for example, divides his hours, interests and activities among his family in the home environment, his teachers and peers in the school environment, his intimate friends of similar age in the community and especially the recreational environment, and the broader outside world and the world of imagination through the environment presented by books, motion pictures, radio and television. Each of these groups and their respective environments is necessary to the total development of the child and, depending upon their nature and quality, may influence his present and future life to his benefit or to his detriment. It is neither practical nor possible to separate out any one of these influences or to ignore it.

In like manner the adult divides his existence among a number of different environments in the company of a number of different groups of people. One of the most important of these, of course, is the work environment. Depending upon its nature, it may enhance his total personal, family, and community life or act quite to the contrary. By like token, of course, the circumstances of the wage earner's home environment and the total neighborhood and community environment can contribute to his work efficiency and productivity or seriously limit it. The most cursory observation indicates a direct or indirect relationship between undesirable living circumstances; personal, behavioral, and medical problems; and social and work performance. This is especially true and evident in lower income, urban situations which by dint of sheer numbers of persons and because of excessive crowding accentuates all such problems. The numerous social and economic difficulties of cities are of course most commonly seen concentrated in the slum or substandard neighborhoods. In view of this, it is interesting to note the original Latin word for town-dweller—pagani.

Recently environmental insalubrity has been recognized to have undesirable psychological and mental effects as well as contributing to the persistence of numerous other social ills. Among those are the development and continuance of slums, juvenile and adult delinquency, and apathy toward personal or community improvement and progress. There has evolved, therefore, a new attitude concerning the significance of environmental cleanliness. This philosophy has been well stated in the credo of the National Sanitation Foundation:

> Sanitation is a way of life. It is the quality of living that is expressed in the clean home, the clean farm, the clean business and industry, the clean neighborhood, the clean community. Being a way of life it must come from within the people; it is nourished by knowledge and grows as an obligation and ideal in human relations.

The role of population increase and population density in the genesis and intensification of public health, environmental health and social problems is no longer subject to question. Perhaps the clearest and most dramatic way to emphasize this relationship is to call attention to some of the work of Dr. John B. Calhoun, of the National Institute of Mental Health[1,2,3] with colonies of mice and rats. In a provocative series of long-

[1] Calhoun, John B.: Population Density and Social Pathology, Sc. Amer., *206*: 139, Feb. 1962.

[2] ————: The Role of Space in Animal Sociology, J. Soc. Issues, *22*:46, Oct. 1966.

[3] ————: A Behavioral Sink, in, *Roots of Behavior,* (Ed. Bliss, E. L.) New York, Paul Hoeber, 1962 (p. 295-315).

term studies, Calhoun has been able to illustrate the ultimate effects of uninhibited breeding and the resulting excessive crowding. Given a healthy breed of laboratory animals, provided with constantly ample supplies of food, water, and nesting material, and unhampered opportunity to propagate in quarters carefully designed to be spatially adequate for 144 animals, well before reaching an eventual naturally imposed ceiling of about 2,500 animals, there develops a breakdown of practically all aspects of normal behavior.

Ordinarily, laboratory rats are naturally clean about themselves and their environment. When limited in numbers they typically avoid soiling each other or their nesting places. Under the conditions allowed in these experiments, however, gross insanitation from bodily discharges becomes ubiquitous, and the tendency for personal grooming is lost. Territorial prerogatives are ignored. The strong attack the weak, and groups of the strong drive off groups of the weak. As a result, in each large experimental pen, masses of essentially outcasts which Calhoun refers to as "behavioral sinks" appear. The members of the outcast behavioral sinks become excessively violent, but only among themselves,—not with the strong overlords. Marked aggressive behavior appears among many of the females. Scattered throughout may be seen individuals who clearly demonstrate various signs and symptoms of regression, confusion, withdrawal, and mental disturbance. Throughout, and even among the dominant animals, sexual desire and the ability to mate decline markedly. Homosexuality appears, with males trying to copulate with males, and females with females. Increasingly the group becomes non-productive. Such normal mating as does occur becomes increasingly infertile, such conceptions as do occur terminate increasingly in spontaneous abortions, such cubs as are born are typically premature and weak, and are typically ignored and cannibalized. Incidentally, it has been disturbing to note that once arriving at this state, removal of animals to more "normal" circumstances does not typically result in "recovery." Permanent damage, probably through permanent endocrine glandular change has resulted.

One has only to read one's daily newspaper to recognize that a reasonable amount of interpolation from such studies to man, his numbers, concentration, living circumstances, and total environment seems valid. As mankind becomes overwhelmingly numerous and more densely crowded, as he continues to use up and abuse his environment at an ever more rapid rate, as in the process he produces ever more physical, chemical, biological, and psychological hazards and stresses on the land he lives on, in the food he ingests, in the air he breathes, and in the water he drinks, one has ample cause for concern about the immediate and long-range consequences. Already on all sides we see a dangerous interplay of forces between man and the biocommunity of which he is a part. We seem in danger of being overwhelmed by a torrent of technological change which we have set in motion but increasingly seem incapable of controlling. As a nation and as a world, we must face a harsh and frightening reality. Despite dramatic advances in medicine, science, engineering, and technology, despite improved economic standards of living and perhaps even because of them, we have not succeeded in creating a physical, psychological, and social environment in which can be found a true total quality of life for the "whole man." Surely, this must be the purpose and the goal of all our strivings.

As a result, increasingly, and especially among the young, we hear the cries, "Where does this all lead? What does it all mean?" We have landed men on the moon and have even fathomed the mysteries of cellular physical-chemistry, while we are unable to determine what to do about the mountains of trash that litter our cities and countryside breeding disease and disaffection. We are excited by the miracles of extremely expensive organ transplant operations, while we continue to lose our standing among the nations in infant mortality and life expectancy. With specific reference to the latter, it is notable that there has been no significant improvement in life expectancy after the age of forty since the beginning of the century. There is much left to be done on this planet. Currently there is much concern about expenditures for "health care." The fact is that all but a small fraction of the concern and resulting effort is devoted to "sickness repair"—vast expenditures largely for things allowed to go wrong. Certainly no reasonable person would deny the necessity of providing the best possible therapy or custodial care to those who need it, but it should be recognized more fully that the prevention of illness and injury and the promotion of positive health are more fundamental concerns and provide the only sound ultimate solution to the medical care and many other social problems.

The Cost of Environmentally Related Illness

The cost to the Nation for the treatment of illness is already substantial and mushrooms every year. It now stands at about $53 billion per year and has been rising by more than 8 per cent annually since 1950. The average worker currently loses seven work days yearly because of illness. Thousands of productive people die prematurely or become disabled every year because of accidents, heart disease, cancer, emphysema and other major causes of death. As will be indicated in the chapter on medical care, the need for treatment facilities, hospitals, clinics, nursing homes, far exceeds what is available or what can be supplied within the foreseeable future. The need for physicians, nurses, and other health workers is acute and will continue to grow greater.

Much of this expenditure and much of this sickness and loss of life is preventable. The contributory relationships to specific diseases by such environmental hazards as air and water pollution, occupational hazards, overcrowded housing, and poor sanitation are difficult to identify with exactness. They are known, however, to be substantial. For example, the current health costs of air pollution alone are estimated conservatively at $2 billion per year. The direct cost of absenteeism or restricted activity caused by occupationally related illness and injury amounts to billions of dollars annually. Non-occupationally related accidents cause about 100,000 deaths and 9 million injuries each year. While more than half these deaths are caused by highway accidents, a substantial proportion are attributable to the home and school environments. The major diseases closely related to environmental hazards include the chronic respiratory diseases, especially emphysema, heart disease, mental illness, and cancer. Chronic respiratory diseases, associated with occupational conditions, air pollution, and smoking (a self-imposed environmental hazard) constitute the Nation's second leading cause of disability. Social Security payments to victims of these diseases or to their families total $90 million annually. Emphysema, the major chronic respiratory disease, and the most rapidly increasing cause of death, results in nearly 50,000 deaths per year. Heart disease, the leading cause of death, which results in the loss of about 700,000 lives annually, is due at least in part to the stresses of the modern environment. It is the leading cause of Social Security compensated disability, and costs the Nation more than $25 billion each year. The mentally ill, many of them victims of an assortment of environmental stresses, occupy more than half of the Nation's hospital beds. Occupational exposures are believed to be related to a significant, though not yet precisely determined, number of the 320,000 cancer deaths which occur each year in this country.

Are all of these casualties really necessary? A brief look at the past may provide some guidance. It is instructive to see where our successes have been up to now. In 1900, our death rate was 17.2 as compared with 9.5 per 1,000 population at present. If the earlier rate applied now we would experience an annual loss of life of almost 3,500,000 instead of the current 1,850,000. This represents about a 50 per cent improvement in two-thirds of a century. But analysis will show at least three-quarters of the improvement in the death rate since 1900 is because of the lowering or eradication—essentially through public health measures—of infant mortality, maternal mortality, typhoid and paratyphoid, dysentery, diarrhea and enteritis, smallpox, measles, diphtheria, pertussis, hemolytic streptococcal infections, tuberculosis, malaria, and syphilis and its sequelae. In many of these, environmental health measures played dominant roles. Thus, with proper deference to the pediatric and obstetrical professions, more infants have been saved through pure milk, food, and water than anything else. Housing has long been known to be one of a number of factors in tuberculosis and some hemolytic streptococcal infections. These relationships are difficult to measure but are nonetheless existent. Much clearer is the role of environmental health in the control and elimination of enteric infections. To express it another way, 1,300,000 of the 1,650,000 lives saved each year is attributable to the successes of previous decades over the conditions listed. That leaves only about 25 per cent for all of the remaining causes of death, many of which have been increasing. This, incidentally, is why the spectacular decline in the death rate has plateaued in recent years.

The question arises, therefore, can anything significant be done about the latter group of diseases? It is often stated that the first group of diseases by their nature were subject to prevention and, therefore, have declined probably as far down as they are going to go but that the remainder is not subject to control and prevention. Some years back, an analysis was made of further achievable gains in both groups of diseases.[4] Listed under each cause of death were suggested activities that might produce the improvements. Using the 1,715,900 deaths which occurred in the United States in 1960 as an example, it was indicated that the residue of the first group of diseases could now reasonably be expected to be reducible by close to 100 per cent and the remainder, including among others most of the so-called chronic, non-communicable diseases, were considered subject to a reduction of about 25 per cent in the then existing state of knowledge. Accomplishments, of course, would depend upon appropriate determination and action. Overall, it was calculated that conceivably about one-third of the current illnesses could be subject to control and the ultimate deaths of those involved postponed. It is immediately apparent that any present and future achievements of this nature must depend upon high priority emphasis on primary and secondary prevention and a forthright approach to the hazards of the environment. With reference to the latter, members of the medical profession must become much more cognizant of the fact that a significant proportion of the so-called chronic, non-communicable diseases as well as mental illness has its genesis in the environment and that not only can more attention to the environment prevent many of these illnesses, but also that the expenditure of money and professional effort merely to treat these clinical conditions after they occur, without concern for their environmental sources, is fruitless.

The Magnitude of the Problem

With specific reference to the physical environment, we are rapidly approaching a most critical point. Threats from unsafe food, water, drugs,

[4]Hanlon, J. J.: *Principles of Public Health Administration,* 5th ed., St. Louis, C. V. Mosby Co., 1969, pp. 124-127.

chemicals, and a variety of consumer products are rapidly increasing. The quality of American life, particularly urban life, is deteriorating into a morass of environmental problems so complex as to appear almost beyond solution. A brief review of a few that demand attention is appropriate. Toxic matter is being released into the air over the United States at a rate of more than 200 million tons a year, or almost a ton for every American. It comes from 90 million motor vehicles, from factories, power plants, municipal dumps, and private incinerators. About 60 per cent derives from the internal combustion engine. The use of artificial additives to impart flavor, color, or other aesthetic qualities to food has increased fifty percent in the past ten years, and with an average annual consumption of three pounds. As yet we know little if anything about their possible long-range effects but there are indications already that some involve risk to our own and future generations. Pesticides leave residues on food crops, and have already been broadcast throughout the ecological systems of the earth. Measurable amounts of DDT are found in arctic seals and antarctic penguins. By now, the body fat of the average American contains about 12 parts per million of DDT, and is now a component of mother's milk. The vast amount of pesticide that ultimately ends up in the seas is known to have potential effect on the ability of the microscopic plankton of the oceans to produce oxygen. Add to this the layer of oil, thin though it may be, on the surface of the oceans of the earth tending to limit the energizing rays of the sun that reach the plankton. And bear in mind that we depend on that plankton for about 60 per cent of the oxygen in our atmosphere.

Not counting industrial and agricultural wastes, we discard more than 165 million tons of solid wastes every year. Auto graveyards mar our landscapes; smoking, foul-smelling dumps pollute the air; no-return bottles, non-degradable aluminum cans, plastic and other packaging that cannot be recycled create ever-growing mountains of trash, the complex contents of which increasingly pollute our surface and ground waters. In low-income urban areas, accumulated garbage and refuse breed rats, vermin, and disease.

Each year more than 500 new chemicals and chemical compounds are introduced into industry, along with countless operational innovations, many of them without adequate knowledge or concern for potential hazard. Thousands of workers suffer from preventable industrial diseases, cancers, hearing loss, skin diseases, and lung diseases such as coal miner's "black lung" (Pneumoconiosis), cotton worker's "brown lung" (byssinosis), asbestos miner's disease (asbestosis) as well as lung cancer of uranium miners. These are only a few of a long list of occupationally related illnesses.

Much of the drinking water available to our Nation's communities is of unknown quality. Over 19 thousand communities serve about 60 million people with public water supplies which are not yet covered by

U.S. Public Health Service safe water standards. A recent (1969) survey indicated that over 90 per cent of domestic supplies for which States and localities are responsible do not receive adequate surveillance to provide accurate information on chemical quality. In fact, 27 per cent of the samples taken exceeded one or more of the Public Health Service's recommended limits for chemicals. Meanwhile many streams and lakes, such as Lake Erie, have been practically killed and are relatively lifeless except for algae and trash fish.

Accidents take the lives of 100,000 Americans every year and injure 52 million more; 18,000 of the deaths and 20 million of the injuries are associated with consumer products. Some 3,000 deaths occur every year from accidental ingestion of poisons. Pathetically most of these victims are very young children. Radiation sources now exist throughout the environment. They range from the large-scale applications of nuclear energy, particularly for electric power generation, through laser and microwave technology in industry, to the use of radionuclides and x rays in the healing arts, and the use of microwave ovens and other electronic equipment in the home. Our scientific knowledge and protection against these growing hazards to ourselves and to future generations is still in an early stage.

The world clamors for the thousands of new miracle drugs which pharmaceutical research produces to treat specific disease problems. Yet, despite the best efforts at testing, labeling, and other controls, they often produce unforeseen side effects and some may even offer potential genetic threats. What these new chemical formulations may contribute in terms of the total body burden and synergistic chemical barrage to which modern man is being exposed has hardly begun to be explored. As Barry Commoner of Washington University in St. Louis has put it, "the new Technological Man carries Strontium 90 in his bones, Iodine 131 in his thyroid, DDT in his fat, and asbestos in his lungs."

It is now quite clear that unless man obtains and promptly applies the necessary knowledge to the burgeoning problems of the environment, we are courting inevitable disaster. The importance of this was emphasized by James A. Shannon while Director of the National Institute of Health when he said:

> "At the moment of our great victories over many . . . diseases . . . we are now confronted with the realization that the most formidable and pervasive challenges to the well being of man lie in . . . the hazards man has created for himself in the products, processes, and living patterns of his increasingly technological world."

In summary, man's current problems derive from three sources. His ability to acquire and apply technical knowledge has far outstripped (1) his biological and physiological ability to adapt to the changes that result; (2) his ability to relate properly and in a planned sense to his environment as part of a delicately balanced ecologic system; and (3) his ability to relate properly to himself and his fellowman.

The Field of Environmental Health

The school child spends his time more or less equally among the three environments of the home, the neighborhood and the school. Generally he is affected by work environments only to the extent that they directly affect his parents and teachers and through them may indirectly affect him. Specific attention will be focussed later on the importance of the school environment. At this point it is well to consider the broader community aspects of environmental health.

Public health concern and action with regard to the environment is commonly misconceived to be restricted essentially to the disposal of garbage and refuse. Ironically, it is rare that this is a function of a health agency. Typically, it is a Department of Public Works, or some similar unit of government that is given the responsibility for such matters of community housekeeping. The only valid concern of Departments of Health in this respect is in relation to the extent to which the handling and disposal of such materials may allow breeding and harborage for rodents and other disease transmitting vermin. In contrast, most people tend to be surprised to learn of the broad spectrum of environmental interests and activities of the modern official community health agency. Today they present an imposing array which includes the sanitary control and surveillance of the production, processing, packaging, distribution and serving of milk, milk products, meats, fish, shellfish and other foods; the control and surveillance of certain drugs, cosmetics and chemicals; the elimination of insect and rodent vectors of disease; the surveillance of atmospheric quality, with consideration given under various circumstances to temperature, humidity, dust, smoke and bacterial contamination, and to control measures in particular instances by means of smoke exhaust or effluent abatement, air conditioning and air sterilization; the sanitary surveillance of domestic water supplies and the prevention of their pollution by man, animals and industry; the production in company with a Department of Public Works or Water Department of a safe drinking water, filtered, chlorinated and preferably fluoridated for the reduction of dental caries; the assurance, again in cooperation with a Department of Public Works, of the safe and satisfactory disposal of human and solid wastes; the sanitary supervision of recreational areas such as playgrounds, parks, camps, picnic grounds, swimming pools and beaches; the promotion of occupational health and safety measures; the study of accidents and the development of accident prevention programs in cooperation with police, fire, housing and community planning agencies; the surveillance of the amount of ionizing radiation and the protection of indi-

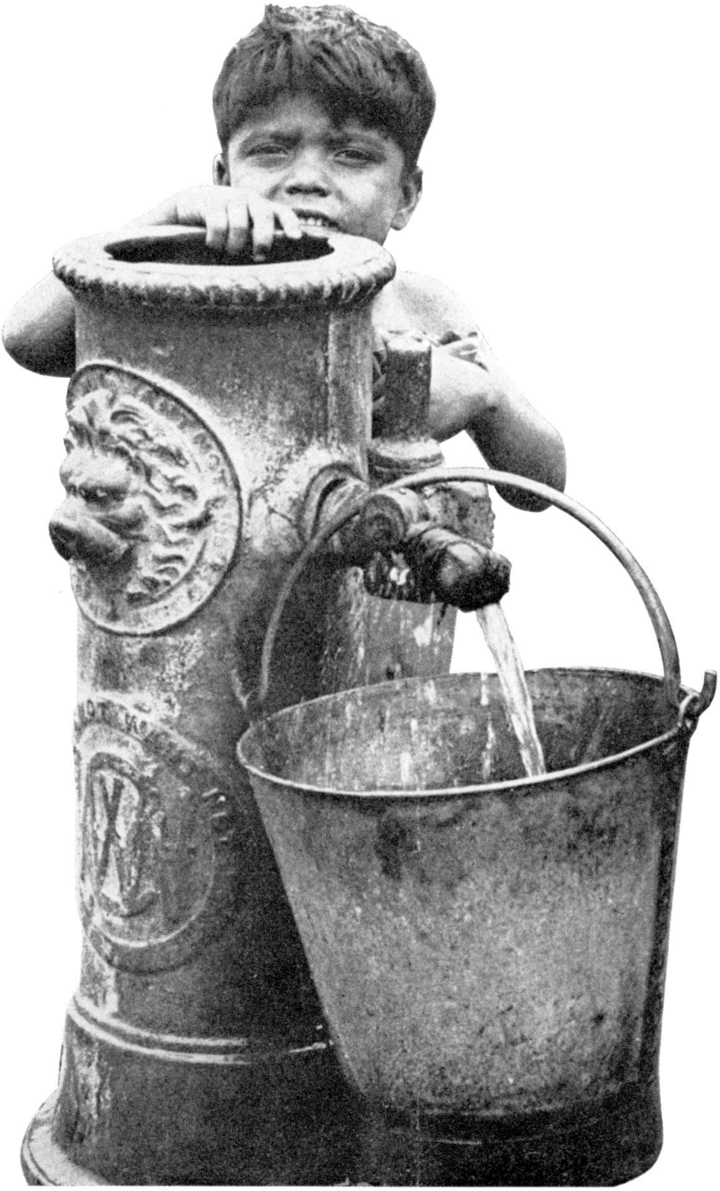

FIG. 27. Water, a universal necessity.

viduals from accidental or undue exposure from professional x-ray equipment, industrial installations and unwarranted sources such as shoe-fitting fluoroscopes. As extensive as this summary appears, it is actually only a partial list which is constantly growing in company with our expanding technological culture. It is obviously not practical to consider each of these activities here in the extent of detail they really merit. In lieu of that, certain aspects of them are presented under the general headings of Water, Waste Disposal, Food and Milk, Air, Radiation, Housing, Vector Control, Accident Prevention, and Occupational Health.

Water

Safe water in sufficient amount is one of the prime necessities of existence, as well as a necessity for the social, economic and industrial life of a people. Its uses are many, for consumption by man and animals; for cooking; for cleaning and cooling of the body, of objects and materials used by man, and of the environment; for agricultural purposes; for many industrial processes; for recreation; for fire protection and for the disposal of human and industrial wastes. It is estimated that each day, the United States consumes about 310 billion gallons of water; municipal consumers, 24 billion; rural consumers, 4 billion; industry and all other, about 152 billion; and agricultural irrigation, 130 billion. The per capita domestic use alone, with which we are chiefly concerned is about 150 gallons per day.

About two-thirds of the population of the United States are served by public water systems. Despite this, 35,000 communities of 25 or more people, totalling 40 million people lacked service from public (whether privately or publicly owned) water systems. In addition there are about 27 million rural dwellers who need improved safe private water supplies.

Public water supplies come from either of two primary sources, surface waters including streams and lakes, and ground waters including wells and springs. Generally speaking, surface waters are more apt to contain bacterial contaminants, while ground waters are more apt to contain dissolved chemicals. However, it must always be borne in mind that streams and lakes are increasingly polluted with industrial, agricultural and domestic chemicals, and that springs and wells may easily receive dangerous bacteria either from their immediate surroundings or through underground seepage or fissures. Appearances can easily deceive, and crystal clear water from any source can contain considerable numbers of dangerous microorganisms. Accordingly, especially when a water is used by many people, treatment is always indicated.

The assurance of a safe and satisfactory public water requires consideration of the following:

1. The watershed of surface waters, *i.e.*, the land adjacent to all contributing streams and lakes, should be protected and its use controlled to the extent practical.
2. The community water intake should be located so as to minimize contamination and pollution.
3. Provision should be made for primary sedimentation and clarification by means of storage reservoirs and exposure to light and air.
4. Bacteria, algae, and any residual turbidity should be removed by means of a coagulant (alum) followed by passage of the water through a sand filter.
5. A disinfectant, usually chlorine (0.2 to 0.5 parts per million) should be added to eliminate any residual or subsequent bacterial contamination.
6. A fluoride salt up to a concentration of from 0.7 to 1.5 parts per million should be added to prevent dental caries. The amount to be added depends upon the amount of fluoride naturally present in the water, and the average consumption of water per individual.
7. The use of the supervised public water by all of the people in a community should be encouraged and assured by an adequate distribution system, housing requirements and reasonable water rates.
8. Contamination of the community water after its treatment should be prevented by elimination of all cross connections between the system carrying the purified water and any other systems, and by prevention of back-siphonage of contamination into the pure water distribution system.

Rural water supplies for human consumption present quite a different situation. The use from each source is usually restricted to only one or two families. Therefore, the direct consequences of contamination of rural water supplies tend to be limited. Occasionally, however, indirect consequences of greater importance may result as in the case of infection of a dairy farmer who supplies milk to a large number of rural families or to an urban market. In the rural setting, domestic water is usually obtained from relatively simple wells which often are shallow and unprotected. They may be polluted by surface washings, or by underground seepage from improperly located privies, poorly constructed septic tanks, or adjacent barnyards. Sometimes contamination occurs over a considerable distance through underground fissures and streams. These problems can be prevented or solved only slowly by means of persistent school and community health education in conjunction with sanitary consultation from county or state health departments and agricultural

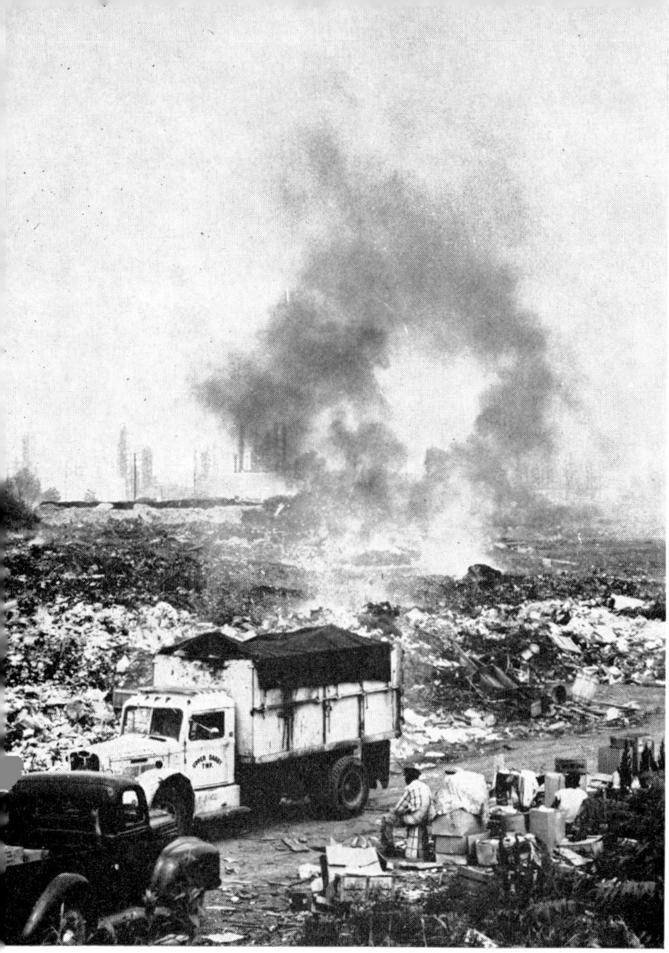

FIG. 28. Improper refuse disposal.

or farm agents. Farm families should be encouraged and guided in the proper location of wells and sanitary facilities, proper construction of wells, and the installation of a pump in a tightly sealed, curbed and drained well top.

Waste Disposal

The problem of waste disposal is intimately related to those of water sanitation and stream pollution. The waste of a modern community is complex in nature, including human excretions, garbage, refuse, surface runoffs from rains and street washings, and unwanted materials from industrial processes. The basic purpose for sewerage systems is to get rid of human excretions and surface runoffs. Increasingly, however, kitchen-ground garbage and detergents from home dish and clothes washers are added. If industrial wastes are discharged into the sewerage system, the situation is further complicated.

In general, community wastes may be disposed of in any of four ways: (1) discharge into bodies of water, with or without treatment (2) deposit on the surface of the ground, (3) burial in the ground, and, (4) incineration. Each of these has its advantages and disadvantages as well as potential hazards to health.

Satisfactory waste disposal should take the following factors into consideration:

1. There should be no pollution of ground water that may enter wells or springs.
2. There should be no pollution of surface waters.
3. There should be no pollution of the surface soil.
4. Excreta should not be accessible to flies or animals.
5. Odors and unsightly conditions should be prevented.

6. Construction and operation of any waste disposal facility should be simple and inexpensive.

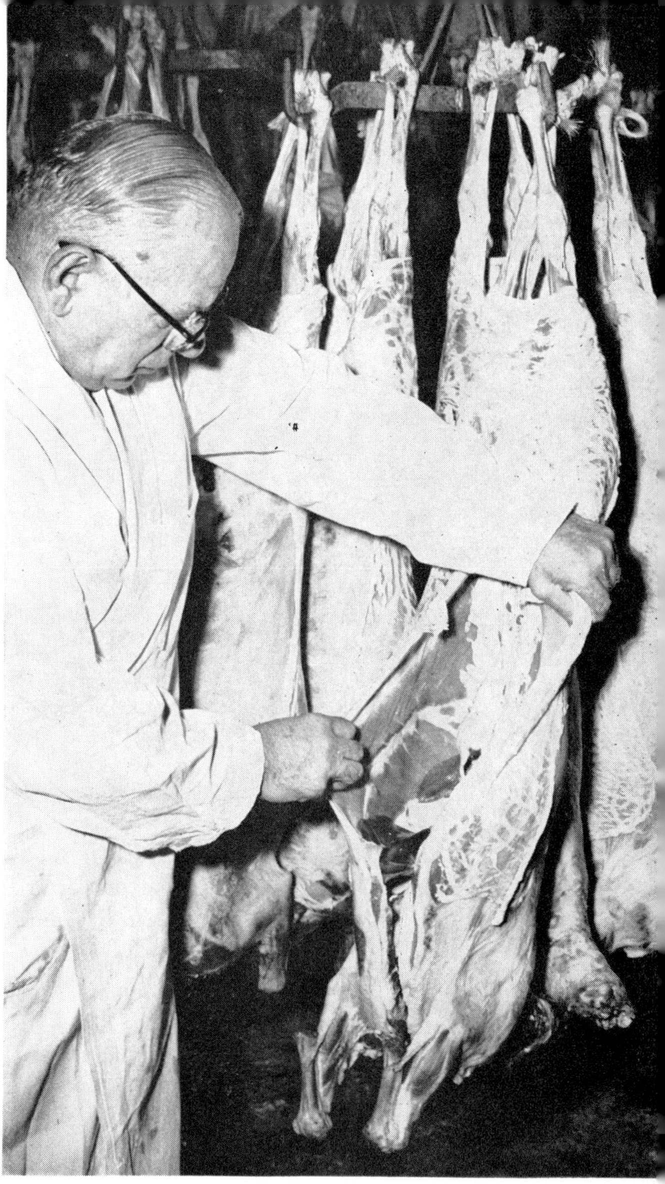

Fig. 29. Protecting the food we eat.

Of the various types of waste products, human excreta is by far the most important and potentially dangerous. The method of its disposal depends in large part on socio-economic circumstances that may be considered in three categories. In the simplest, that usually found in rural situations, there is no water carriage possible. Use is made of the pit privy, the bored hole latrine, the vault privy, the chemical toilet, the septic privy or the box and can toilet. Then there are situations, most commonly observed in small towns and suburban areas, where a public water system exists, making water carriage of waste eventually possible, but where no public sewerage system has yet been constructed. Here, individual cesspools or septic tanks are commonly used. The method of their design and construction, the nature of the soil, and the number and proximity of installations are key factors in determining their suitability. Finally, there are situations where both a public water system and a sewerage system exist, making possible the water carriage and disposal of human wastes. The problem that arises here is the production and concentration of tremendous quantities of waste, complicated by the possibility of cross-connections and back-siphonage between the two systems.

Under such circumstances it is most desirable that sewage be treated before its ultimate disposal. This is accomplished in different situations by combinations of the following procedures: (1) screening and/or sedimentation to remove large and settleable materials, (2) anaerobic digestion of settleable solids in a septic tank, Imhoff tank or sludge digestion tank, (3) oxidation of nonsettleable organic matter by filtration, activated sludge, or irrigation methods, and (4) disinfection with chlorine or other disinfectants.

Food and Milk

Like water, food is essential to life. Also like water, food can be a two-edged sword, a blessing or a disastrous hazard. Milk may properly be regarded as a specialized food with special benefits and special problems. An interesting shift has occurred in the United States in the relative sanitary importance of these three necessary elements—water, milk and food. Through the first quarter of this century polluted drinking water accounted for a major proportion of the known epidemic gastrointestinal infections. Since then, due to remarkable strides in the provision of pure water and safely produced and pasteurized milk, the number of epidemics and cases of illness attributable to them have declined dramatically. This has not been true, however, of foods (Table 3).

It is interesting that while milk and dairy products are the most perishable and potentially dangerous foods, and while they are consumed in increasing quantities, they have become a relatively unimportant source of disease. The reason is that their very perishability and danger forced great attention on assuring their safety. In 1924, the Public Health Service developed a Recommended Milk Ordinance and Code in an attempt to promote scientifically sound standards and uniform legislation. It has now gone through nine revisions, each based upon the opinions and experience of public health officials, the milk and dairy industry, veterinarians, scientists, consumer interests and others. By now it forms the basis of regulation and action in the majority of states and a large number of local communities. A similar document has been developed for frozen desserts. The widespread adoption of the simple process of pasteurization has played a very significant role in the safety of milk and dairy products. By now, almost all of the fluid milk sold in the United States is protected by pasteurization.

The supervision and control of the production, processing and distribution of milk and milk products requires the ever vigilant cooperative activities of individuals from local and state public health agencies, departments of agriculture and responsible representatives of the milk and dairy industry.

As may be inferred from Table 3, the problem of safeguarding food is a matter of considerable concern to public health authorities. An analysis of 371 food-borne epidemics during 1969 presents an interesting picture. In terms of their nature, they were distributed as follows: Clostridium botulinum, 10; Clostridium perfringens, 65; E. coli, 5; Staphylococcic

Table 3. Annual Average Reported Water, Milk and Food-Borne Epidemics and Cases, U.S. 1938–1960

	Water		Milk and Milk Products		Other Foods	
Period	Epidemics	Cases	Epidemics	Cases	Epidemics	Cases
1938–42	49	20,688	42	1,823	181	5,819
1943–51	23	3,594	23	806	308	11,274
1953–57	7	609	11	308	216	10,694
1958–60	7	845	10	179	247	9,318

infection, 94; salmonellosis, 49; shigellosis, 10; streptococcal infection, 4; viral, 9; trichinosis, 11; chemicals, 27; other 7; and unknown, 80. The sources of the epidemics help to pinpoint the problem: public restaurants, 110; food shops, 1; private homes, 157; picnics, 3; schools, 38; churches, 3; camps, 11; and others, 43. It is notable that more than half of these outbreaks occurred in public or semi-public places which should be subject to control by public health, school or institutional authorities. It is also of note and concern that of the total of 28,563 persons affected by these outbreaks, two-thirds or 19,842 were in schools.

Nevertheless, the problem as it exists is not due to lack of effort. As early as 1879, federal legislation was proposed to prohibit adulteration of food and drink. It was not until 1906 that such a bill was finally enacted. In the ensuing 20 years, other acts were passed which related to proper weights, packaging, labeling, food purity, meats, and standards for butter. In 1927, a federal Food and Drug Administration was established in the Department of Agriculture to administer all of the accumulating provisions. As time passed, more legislation appeared, and in 1938 they were all brought together in a federal Food, Drug and Cosmetic Act. Two years later the Food and Drug Administration was relocated in the Federal Security Agency which in 1953 became the Department of Health, Education and Welfare. At present, the Food and Drug Administration is one of the four basic components of the Public Health Service of H.E.W. Even now, however, federal food control activities are complicated by the fact that responsibility for meat inspection and some dairy responsibilities remain with the Department of Agriculture. Fortunately, the two agencies work in close collaboration, each fulfilling its respective duties.

Responsibility for the surveillance and protection of food is quite confused on the state level. All but four states have some food control agency, but there is no uniformity. In about half of the states it is the department of agriculture. In most of the remainder it is the state department of health. In two states, a food and drug commission, in one the state chemist, and in another a public service department have responsibility. If organizational responsibility is confused, the legislative provisions and requirements of the States are even more so. Effort has been made in recent years to bring about revision and modernization of state laws to bring them into conformity with the federal Food, Drug and Cosmetic Act. Progress has been made in about one-third of the states.

Almost all municipalities and many counties engage to some extent in the supervision of food. Customarily it is done by personnel of the local health department. Their activities include inspection, rating and certification of food processing and serving establishments, the sampling and analysis of foods, physical and laboratory examination of food handlers, the provision of indoctrination courses in personal hygiene and acceptable food handling to employees of restaurants and similar establishments, and the prosecution of infringements of local food ordinances and laws. The Public Health Service has developed a Recommended Ordinance and Code Regulating Eating and Drinking Establishments in an attempt to bring about a more consistent and scientific local approach. By now it has been adopted by the majority of local communities in the nation.

Mention should be made of the efforts of certain segments of the food industry itself to improve conditions. Notable among the organizations through which they variously support employee training, public education, research and "self regulation" are the National Consumers Association, the Food Industries Sanitation Association, the National Dairy Council, the Ice Cream Merchandising Institute, and the American Institute of Baking. Attention is called especially to the National Sanitation Foundation, a multi-industry sponsored and supported organization which conducts research, training, and educational activities, planned and developed jointly by representatives of industry and public health.

Air Pollution

Man's first concern about the purity of the food and water he consumed is lost in prehistory. By comparison, it is only relatively recently that the importance of clean air has been recognized. It is true that a few early legislative curiosities exist. Thus, Edward I of England banned the use of sea coal (soft coal) in towns and cities. In 1306, a royal proclamation prohibited the use of coal as fuel by artisans, and there is recorded the execution of a violator the following year. The smogs of London, one of the oldest and largest industrial centers, are by no means of recent occurrence. In fact, in 1661 a report claimed that almost one-half of the deaths in that city were "phthisical and pulmonic distempers" which resulted from the pollution of the atmosphere by the chimneys of homes and industries.

It was not until large numbers of people began to be concentrated in large industrial centers that the pollution of the atmosphere became a matter of real concern. Until recently, however, attention was focused

Table 4. Tons of Air Contaminants Emitted Per Day Los Angeles, 1961

	Type of Air Contaminants				
Source	*Hydro-Carbons*	*Nitrogen Oxide*	*Sulfur Dioxide*	*Carbon Monoxide*	*Aerosols*
Automobiles	965	250	19	6850	27
Other modes of transportation	223	88	8	2102	10
Petroleum industry	250	10	40	700	5
Industrial organic solvents	300	0	0	0	7
Combustion of fuels	11	395	410	2	52
Metals	0	0	*	180	6
Chemicals	16	*	51	0	8
Incineration of Refuse	*	3	1	4	4
Minerals	2	0	*	0	4

* less than ½ ton per day.

Dickinson, J. E.: Air Quality of Los Angeles County, Tech. Prog. Rep., vol. 2, Los Angeles County Air Pollution Control District, Feb. 1961.

essentially upon smoke and soot which reduce the amount of sunlight, and which soil clothing and buildings, damage crops, and irritate the eyes and upper respiratory system. Additional knowledge and technological change have combined to broaden the area of concern. As populations have multiplied, urbanization and metropolitanization progressed, industry and technology expanded, and the motor vehicle was developed and became commonly used, the types and amounts of emissions into the air have increased enormously.

For example, about 13,000 tons of material contaminate the air of Los Angeles each day (Table 4). As a result, earlier programs that were conducted under the name of "smoke control" have now expanded to become "air pollution abatement programs" which must give attention to a wide variety of materials. In general they fall into two classes: (1) particulate matter and aerosols, the most common of which are metallic oxides, sulfur trioxide, fumes, mists, fogs, carbon, tar, and fly ash, and (2) gases and vapors, especially sulfur dioxide, carbon monoxide, and ozone. Air pollution may result from many sources. In cities, household and business heating facilities, industrial processes, railroad yards, incinerators and burning dumps, and especially the exhaust from motor vehicles are most

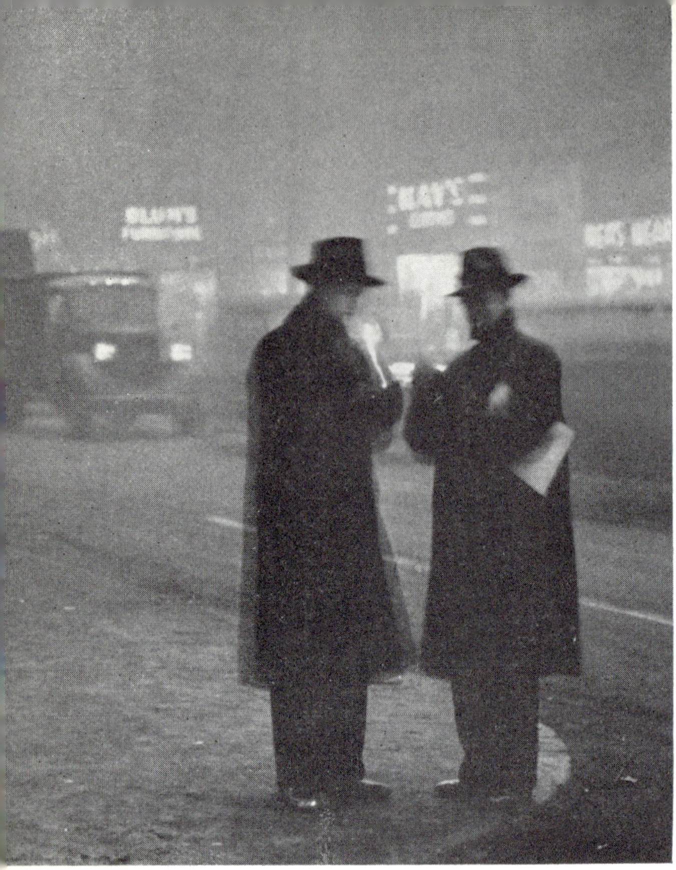

Fig. 30. Darkness at noon.

important. The internal combustion engine of vehicles accounts for 60 to 70 per cent. In suburban and rural areas, brush fires, agricultural and insecticidal sprays, and pollens may be significant. So great has the problem become that increasingly one hears reference to our "aerial sewerage system."

Important also to our increased awareness of air pollution has been a more realistic recognition of the degree of our dependence upon pure air, the fact, for example, that pound for pound we consume about ten times as much air as water, and the recognition of the increased amount of illness attributable to polluted air.

Attention was focused upon the latter by several unusually dramatic incidents of an epidemic nature in recent years. During four days in 1930, the inhabitants of the heavily industrialized Liège area of the Meuse Valley of Belgium were exposed to particularly heavy pollution of the air with sulfur dioxide, sulfuric acid and other chemicals. Thousands became acutely ill and 63 died. In 1948, there occurred the famous Donora, Pennsylvania incident. This industrial town of 14,000 people was subjected to fog laden with smoke, fumes and gases for four and one-half days. About 43 per cent of the population became ill and 20 people died. As in Liège, the aged, infirm, chronically ill, and infants were especially affected. Recent retrospective epidemiological studies indicate that such "epidemics" occurred much more frequently and of greater severity than suspected. A measure of this is a comparison of the effect of London's smog episode of 1880, with its great cholera epidemic in which deaths reached a rate of 876 per million inhabitants as compared with a rate of 896 during the smog. Two unusually serious episodes of smog occurred in London in the recent past. During the winter of 1952 there occurred a prolonged period during which the amount of smoke in the air was ten times normal and the sulfur dioxide concentration fourteen times normal. The condition was blamed for 4000 deaths. Planes were

Table 5. Relationship of Atmospheric Sulfates to Respiratory Disease

City	*Atmospheric Sulfates, (micrograms per cubic meter)*	*Av. Ann. Insurance Claims for Resp. Dis. per 1000 Females*
A	19.8	85.7
B	17.1	58.3
C	13.6	50.3
D	13.2	44.2
E	7.4	18.5

Dohan, F. C. and Taylor, E. W.: Am. J. Med. Sc., *240*, 337, 1960.

grounded for several days, 100 ships were fogbound in the harbor and all of the busses of that great city were out of operation because of poor visibility. More recent was an episode during four days of December 1962, which hospitalized about 1000 and accounted for the deaths of about 100 persons. During the Thanksgiving holiday in 1966, a large area with an epicenter in New York City was severely affected. The consquences were not determined with exactness but are known to have been extensive.

These are only a few of many similar incidents that might be mentioned. Of increasing concern, however, are the less dramatic and more difficult to determine long-term effects and potentials of air contaminants on the incidence of certain respiratory diseases ranging from allergies and emphysema to chronic bronchitis and pulmonary carcinoma. Table 5, however, presents some evidence of the relationship which exists. It is known that emphysema and chronic bronchitis are the most rapidly increasing causes of respiratory deaths. For example, during the past decade in New York City, emphysema deaths increased about 500 per cent and chronic bronchitis deaths about 200 per cent. In fact it has been said that to live in Manhattan and to breathe its air is the equivalent of smoking a pack of cigarettes per day. To the foregoing may be added the effects of air pollutants on the skin, the eyes, and even the psyche. One indication is the relationship between the amount of air pollution and the amount of these illnesses in different communities.

In the past decade, increased awareness of the human hazards as well as economic losses from air pollution has caused the majority of states to adopt new or to strengthen existing legislation relating to the problem. In general, state action has (*a*) permitted the establishment of air pollution control districts under local option, (*b*) provided research and technical assistance, and (*c*) established state-wide programs. More recently, in recognition of the fact that air pollution respected no boundaries and that the problem must be attacked on a broader front, the Congress during recent years passed a National Air Quality Act (with several subsequent amendments). This has established a National Air Pollution Control Administration, provided for extensive research which has led to the development of practical criteria and suggested standards for a number of the critical air pollutants. In addition, Air

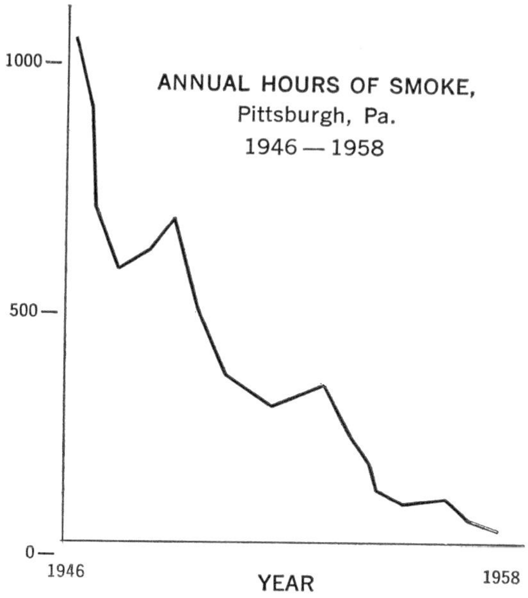

FIG. 31.

Quality Regions which may encompass parts of several states contributing to an air problem shed have been designated as the geographic and political action units.

An excellent example of what a community can accomplish is presented by Pittsburgh, Pennsylvania, which for generations was notorious for its air pollution problem. Beginning in 1946, incineration of waste in the open was prohibited, fuel for heating homes was changed from coal to gas, rail and river transportation in the area was shifted from coal to oil burning diesel engines, and industrial emission standards were developed and enforced. The effect of these measures may be seen in the accompanying chart (Fig. 31) which shows the reduction in the annual hours of smoke since the program began. During the same period, dust-fall dropped from an average of 58.6 to 30.5 tons per square mile per month.

Radiation

The accomplishment of nuclear fission by man has produced within only a few years profound changes in history, technology, and many other aspects of our lives. Many of the achieved or potential effects are beneficial and far reaching in many fields, in medicine, industry, power production and food preservation, to mention a few. On the other hand, certain potentials are not so desirable. Among these are not only the large scale sudden destruction and death, were this tremendous source of energy released for military purposes, but also, and of more

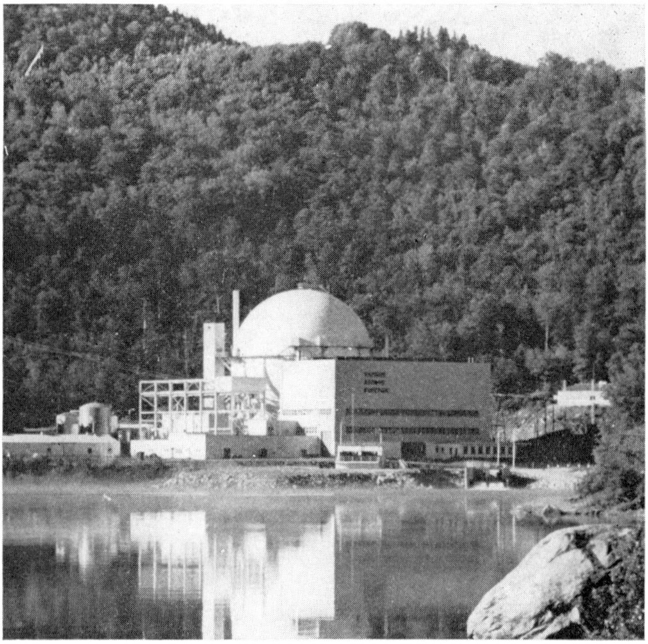

FIG. 32. A nuclear electric power plant.

immediate concern, the possible consequences of radioactive fallout from military testing activities, industrial leakages or accidents which might cause a significant increase in the amount of fissionable material in our environment, and the problems inherent in the disposal of radioactive wastes. As a result, world-wide attention has been focussed upon these problems. Yet exposure of humans to radioactivity is by no means new. It should be recalled that Roentgen discovered x rays in 1895, and the Curies isolated radium three years later. Even these events were recent, since man has been exposed to radioactivity throughout his entire existence on this planet. Because of this, it is strangely impossible to know for sure whether a certain constant low level of radiation is harmful, or even desirable and necessary.

Natural radiation is from two sources; cosmic radiation and naturally occurring elements in the earth's crust. Cosmic radiation, which originates in outer space, is more intense the higher one is above sea level. Radiation from elements in the earth's crust varies considerably from place to place. For example, it is practically absent on the surface of the ocean, whereas some types of mineral deposits and geological formations contain much more than others. As time passes, man accumulates a certain amount of these elements in his body by way of exposure to his environment and the consumption of various foods and waters, augmented sometimes by medical therapy. Often these elements tend to concentrate in particular parts of the body. Thus, some radium and radiothorium are normally found in the skeleton, radioactive potassium and carbon are present in soft tissue, radioactive iodine is deposited in the thyroid gland, and radon and thoron from the atmosphere concentrate in the lungs.

A great deal of attention has been focussed upon the question of radioactive fallout which results from the testing of atomic and hydrogen bombs in the atmosphere. The determination of the amount of radioactive strontium 90 in milk provides a convenient method of measuring the amount of fallout since, under testing circumstances, particles of radioactive material are broadcast over a wide geographic area. Cattle in the area feed widely and the strontium 90 which they pick up from the grass they eat is concentrated in their milk. Actually, fallout has not yet become a significant aspect of the radiation problem. Currently, exposure to radiation in the United States as to source is about as follows:

Medical (x rays, radium, *etc.*)	45%	
Industrial and occupational	7	
Fallout from testing	<1	
Television screens	<1	
Luminous clock and watch dials	<1	
Total man-made sources		55%
Natural sources (minerals & cosmic)		45%
		100%

In terms of control and the future, little or nothing can be done about natural sources. Television and the use of luminous dials, now part of our way of life, are apt to increase in use, but contribute relatively little to the total problem and are subject to technological safeguards. Industrial use of fissionable materials, which is certain to increase greatly, will require and is subject to careful controls. The use of medical sources of radiation, a major factor, will probably increase, but much is subject to control and limitation and the remainder represents a calculated risk in relation to the diseases for the diagnosis and therapy of which it is used. Most risks and injuries from radioactive materials that occur in medicine and industry result from inexperience, inadequate instruction and carelessness. The few accidents that have occurred in industry have been very quickly and well controlled. Over a 15-year period, of about 66,000 workers in programs of the Atomic Energy Commission, only 12 have received radiation doses exceeding 15 rems in a single year. (Present maximum permissible dose per year is 5 rems multiplied by the number years of age beyond 18.) Whether or not the still relatively insignificant amount of radioactive fallout continues, or worse, assumes major importance, will depend upon the good sense and good faith of mankind.

During the past few years, many health agencies have developed programs in the field of radiation. Logically, they have focussed attention on the most significant controllable sources of radiation: *i.e.*, industrial and medical. The Atomic Energy Commission, the Public Health Service, and industry cooperatively have developed standards relating to design, installation, operation and maintenance of reactors and devices using radioactive isotopes, as well as standards of maximum permissible exposure of workers. Similarly, they are working cooperatively on the difficult problem of the disposal of radioactive wastes. A network of stations has been established, involving health agencies, for the constant monitoring of the amount of radiation in the atmosphere, and in milk and food. Health agencies in many places have been successful in outlawing the unwarranted and dangerous use of fluoroscope machines for the fitting of children's shoes. Developing bones are especially sensitive to radiation. Health agencies increasingly have offered consultant testing and advisory service to physicians, dentists, hospitals and others who use x-ray or fluoroscopic equipment in order to minimize radiation leakage and undue exposure of those who operate the equipment. The Public Health Service has also developed a device called a collimeter which attached to x-ray equipment limits the area exposed to that which is really necessary. In partnership, the medical profession, hospitals, clinics and health departments have brought about significant limitation of the use of fluoroscopes and x rays for diagnostic purposes, where other approaches are possible. Thus, the practice, once not too uncommon, of fluoroscoping or x raying the abdomens of pregnant women to determine the position of the foetus is now strictly limited to the most necessary cases. Similarly, the marked reduction in the amount of tuberculosis in many localities has made it practical to apply a simple skin test to large numbers of people, especially school children, thereby restricting chest x raying to only those who have a positive skin reaction.

Housing

While a relationship between housing and health has long been recognized to exist, its definition or quantification is very difficult. It is a common observation that individuals who live in poor housing or in slum neighborhoods have a much greater and more complex amount of illness as well as other social problems. How much is cause and how much effect is difficult to say. Despite the generalities, many studies have indicated some very specific and direct relationships. For example, poorly designed and constructed dwellings or those in a state of ill repair have been shown to be conducive to much higher rates of accidents, diseases spread by vermin and even some respiratory diseases. Older houses with many layers of lead-bearing paint understandably give rise to all of the incidence of lead poisoning in very young children

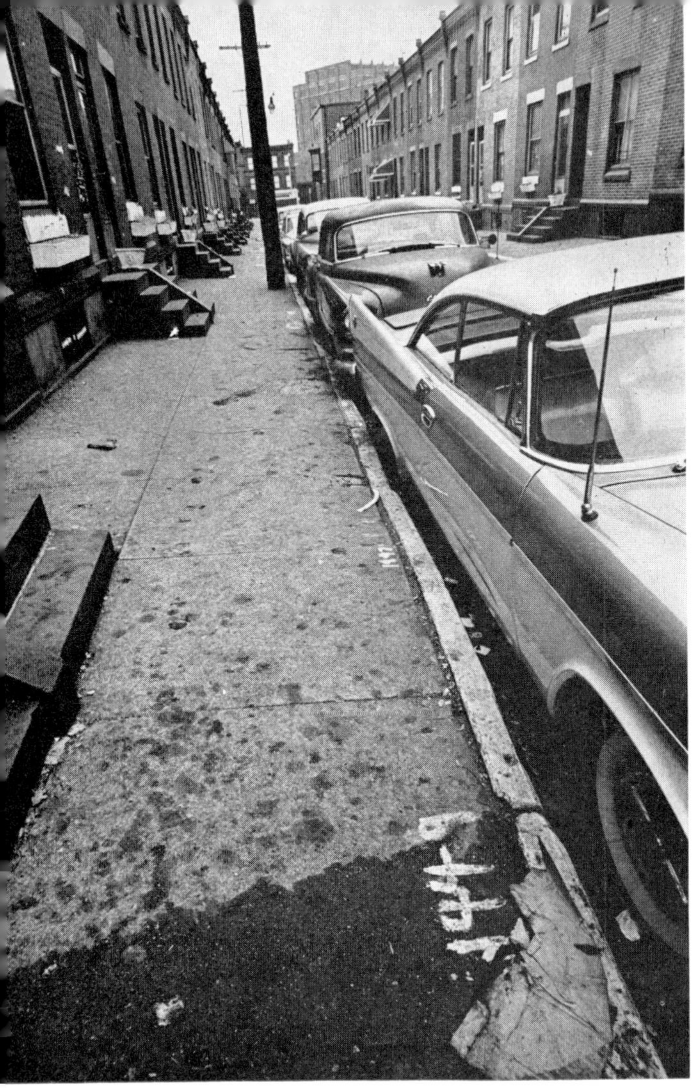

FIG. 33. Home sweet home!

who may gnaw on the woodwork. This "silent endemic," incidentally, is an inadequately recognized phenomenon both with regard to extent and consequence. For example, during the first six months of 1970, about 1,000 children in New York City were hospitalized because of it. There is increasing evidence that it takes a high toll in children, not only in terms of deaths but also in mental retardation, cerebral palsy, convulsive seizures, blindness, learning defects, behavior disorders, kidney diseases, and other handicaps. Overcrowding, so common in the poorer sections of large cities, favors the transmission of serious, person-to-person illnesses such as tuberculosis, pneumonia, and acute respiratory communicable diseases of childhood.

It is estimated that about 10 per cent of the more than 52 million dwellings in this country (1966) have basic health or sanitary deficiencies, such as dilapidation, or lack of hot running water, flush toilet, bathtub or shower.

Beginning in the 1930's the Committee on the Hygiene of Housing of the American Public Health Association, later joined by the Public Health Service, conducted a number of studies and published several documents which enunciated basic principles upon which suggested standards, methods of housing evaluation and proposed ordinances were based. These studies and resultant documents have played an important role in guiding efforts toward the improvement of housing and neighborhood planning. The basic principles that were listed are as follows:

Fundamental Physiological Needs

1. Maintenance of a thermal environment which will avoid undue heat loss from the human body
2. Maintenance of a thermal environment which will permit adequate heat loss from the human body
3. Provision of an atmosphere of reasonable chemical purity
4. Provision of adequate daylight illumination and avoidance of undue daylight glare
5. Provision for admission of direct sunlight
6. Provision of adequate artificial illumination and avoidance of glare
7. Protection against excessive noise
8. Provision of adequate space for exercise and for play of children

Fundamental Psychological Needs

1. Provision of adequate privacy for the individual
2. Provision of opportunities for normal family life
3. Provision of opportunities for normal community life
4. Provision of facilities which make possible the performance of tasks of the household without undue physical and mental fatigue
5. Provision of facilities for maintenance of cleanliness of the dwelling and of the person
6. Concordance with prevailing social standards of the local community

Protection Against Contagion

1. Provision of a water supply of safe, sanitary quality, available to the dwelling
2. Protection of the water supply system against pollution within the dwelling
3. Provision of toilet facilities of such a character as to minimize the danger of transmitting disease
4. Protection against sewage contamination of the interior surfaces of the dwelling
5. Avoidance of insanitary conditions in the vicinity of the dwelling
6. Exclusion from the dwelling of vermin which may play a part in the transmission of disease
7. Provision of facilities for keeping milk and food undecomposed
8. Provision of sufficient space in sleeping rooms, to minimize the danger of contact infection

Protection Against Accidents

1. Erection of the dwelling with such materials and methods of construction as to minimize danger of accidents due to collapse of any part of the structure

2. Control of conditions likely to cause fires or to promote their spread
3. Provision of adequate facilities for escape in case of fire
4. Protection against danger of electrical shocks and burns
5. Protection against falls and other mechanical injuries in the home
6. Protection of the neighborhood against the hazards of automobile traffic

One of the leaders in the field has pointed out that solution of the problem involves three areas of activity:

> First, prevention of accelerated rates of deterioration of dwellings and their environment, thereby forestalling the formation of new blighted and slum areas; second, the rehabilitation of existing substandard housing, if salvage is economically feasible, and its demolition—which is part of rehabilitation in its broader sense—of substandard dwellings that are beyond repair; and, third, the production of enough new housing to provide for population increase for families now overcrowded, for replacement of demolished and decayed structures, and for the normal vacancy cushion.[5]

Poor housing is not limited to either the strictly urban or rural situaations. Recent years have witnessed the unfortunate development of what have become known as suburban or fringe slums. These have come about in one of two ways, the development of squatter settlements in undeveloped areas close to cities, or the mushrooming of poorly planned and constructed forests of suburban real estate developments that rapidly deteriorate. Water and sewage problems in these situations tend to become particularly acute. These may be listed among the many other reasons for needed state and national land-use policies.

While much of the nation's effort to improve the quality of housing originated with public health agencies because of their concerns with disease, lighting, ventilation, plumbing and the like, gradually responsibility for on-going programs has tended to be centered in housing or inspection departments. Actually many departments of government and many disciplines must be concerned with the problem; health, building inspection, plumbing, water, public works, law, schools, recreation, fire protection, traffic engineering, public welfare, and redevelopment authorities. The problem is so complex that it is most desirable that there be established some form of coordinating housing board or commission with representation of the many agencies concerned with the problem and with contributions to make toward its solution. The need was recognized on the federal level by the establishment in 1965 of a cabinet Department of Housing and Urban Development.

[5] Johnson, R. J.: Health Departments and the Housing Problems, Am. J. Public Health *42*:1583, 1952.

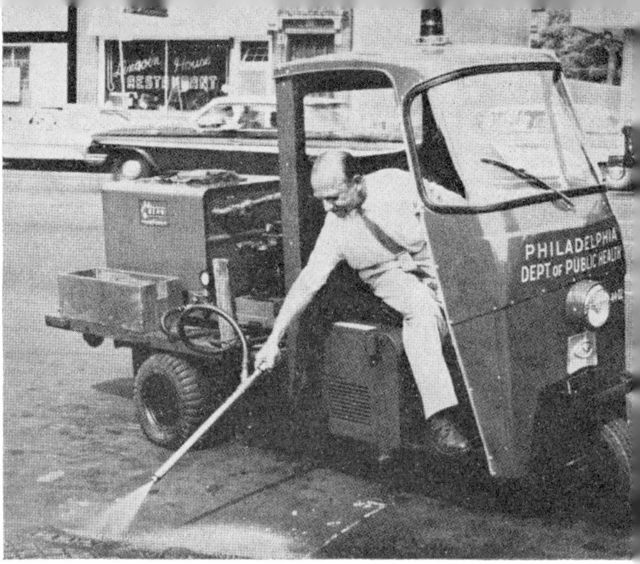

FIG. 34. Kill those mosquitoes!

The most important activities of the public health agency in the field of housing include, (a) the development and promotion of practical and desirable housing standards, (b) participation in the inspection and enforcement activities of the community in relation to building codes and housing ordinances, (c) determination by studies and surveys of the quality of housing in the community, (d) participation in the community's efforts in relation to housing rehabilitation and slum clearance, (e) participation with other agencies in the assurance of the production of suitable new housing including the requirements and administration of permits and licenses as may be indicated, and (f) public education concerning the importance of housing to health.

Vector Control

Of the many diseases that may afflict man, there are some which man shares with certain other animals such as insects and rodents. The majority of these diseases have their primary home in the other species from which they may either occasionally or epidemically surge forth to affect man. The control or eradication of diseases of this type, therefore, depends in large measure upon the elimination of the other species that may be infected, or the elimination of vectors that may transmit the infection from the other species to man. A few examples will serve to illustrate. Rabies is primarily a disease of dogs, wolves, foxes, and bats. Occasionally, a human may be bitten by one of these and thereby acquire this dreadful disease. The obvious way to eliminate rabies is to search out and eliminate all of the members of the other animal species that are affected by the disease so that even if a human is bitten by an animal, that animal will not be infected with rabies and therefore cannot transmit it.

There are a great many diseases that are spread by insects such as mosquitoes, flies, fleas, lice, roaches, ticks and mites. The insects pick up the infection from some other species or occasionally from another human and pass it on by biting the human host. One of the most effective approaches to control is to eliminate the transmitting insect.

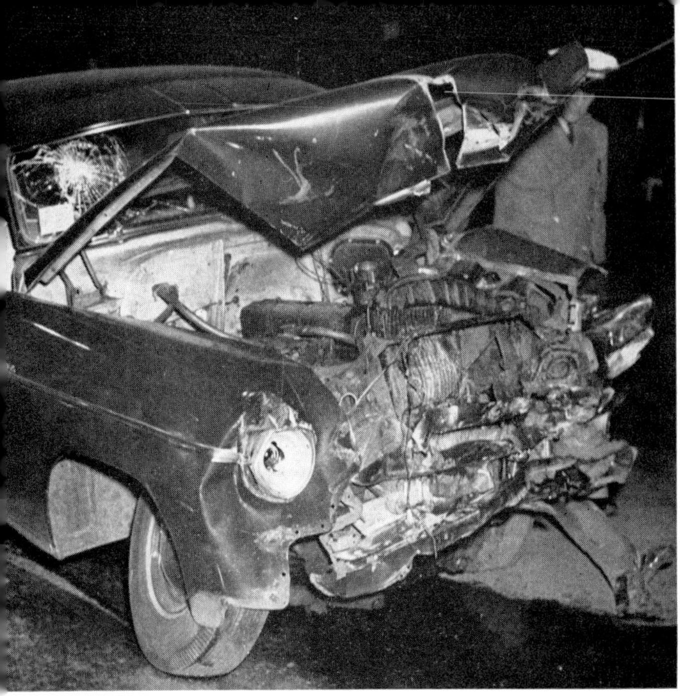

FIG. 35. Requiem for a driver!

This is the basis of the attack on malaria, yellow fever, and typhus fever, as examples. Still another approach, of course, is to eliminate, if possible, the other animal species upon which the insect feeds. A common example of this is represented by concerted attacks upon the rat population.

Depending upon local circumstances – economic, climatic, and the like—health departments variously have established vector control activities as part of their environmental health programs. In addition to general educational and promotional approaches, they may engage in the conduction of vector surveys, application of insecticides or rodenticides to vector breeding places, insistence upon rat-proofing in relation to housing, the supervision of refuse and garbage disposal, and similar activities. In order to carry out such functions, various types of personnel may be employed—sanitary engineers, sanitarians, sanitary inspectors, zoologists, entomologists, biologists, chemists and laboratorians.

Accident Prevention

People in general are quite conscious of the problem of accidents. However, there tend to be two blind spots in their thinking: the over-all importance and the extent to which all ages are affected, and the fact that automobile accidents account for only one part, in fact, less than half of this great problem. In 1968, 115,000 people were killed in the United States by accidents. This was at the rate of about 13 deaths each hour. About 55,000 of these were killed in automobile accidents while 28,500 died from home accidents, about 14,300 from work related accidents and about 20,500 from other types of accidents. With reference to non-fatal accidents, there occurred a total of 11 million, of which 400,000 resulted in permanent impairments. As to location of the non-fatal accidents, 2 million involved motor vehicles, 4.3 million were in the home, 2.2 million occurred at work and 2.6 million occurred under other circumstances. It usually comes as a surprise that accidents constitute the fourth leading cause of death in infants. Between the first birthday and the 35th year of age, accidents are the leading cause of death. From 35 to 54 years of age they are the third leading cause of death. From 55 to 64 they are in fourth place and from 65 years on in sixth place.

Unfortunately, there is a common fatalistic attitude toward accidents. In fact, a great many people equate the word "accident" with "chance." However, to quote an increasingly well-known slogan, "Accidents don't just happen." There is an epidemiology of accidents and by now there is a great deal known about it. It is known, for example, that almost 50 per cent of vehicular deaths of drivers, passengers or pedestrians involves someone who is significantly under the influence of alcohol. Certain types of accidents tend to occur at certain times of the day much more than at other times and to affect certain types of people. It is well known that more males are killed in automobile accidents than are females, and that more of the elderly are killed by falling down stairs or in the bathtub than younger persons. As far as home accidents are concerned, contrary to what might be expected, the bedroom is the most dangerous room in the house being the location of 53 per cent of all fatal home accidents—slipping and falling, suffocation, fire, and poisonings especially. Living and dining rooms account for 15.5 per cent, kitchens for 14.5 per cent, stairs for 5.7 per cent and bathrooms for 5 per cent.

By now it has been well demonstrated that there are certain types of people who are "accident prone." They are involved in one type of accident after another in contrast with certain others who never become involved despite the circumstances. This is true among school children (and teachers), a factor which teachers and school superintendents should bear in mind. As to reasons, there may be mentioned training and education, example in the home and community, safety engineering on the streets and at work as well as a spectrum of mental hygiene factors. There is increasing evidence that many "accident prone" persons subconsciously seek and put themselves in situations where they may be involved in accidents in order to obtain sympathy, attention or indeed even as evidence of a submerged suicidal or death wish. On the basis of these and many other facts, an increasing number of community health organizations have become engaged in programs aimed at the reduction of accidents of all types. Where such specific concerted attention has been given to the problem, improvement invariably follows. As is so often the case in public health, a multidisciplinary approach is required involving engineers, educators, statisticians, and various other professional persons. An important place to start is with an accident survey followed by some mechanism for reporting accidental injuries which may be followed up in order to determine the variables.

There are several specialized types of accidents that recently have commanded the attention of health agencies—accidental poisonings in the home of children, and the suffocation of infants and young children by sheet plastic used for packaging goods and protecting clothing. In cooperation with industry, significant steps have been taken to remove the potential dangers of sheet plastic. This has involved both public and industry sponsored education on a wide scale, the use of perforated sheet plastic, and the encouragement to destroy the material after it has served its primary purpose. Accidental poisonings are particularly difficult by virtue of the fantastic proliferation of all types of chemicals and drugs which now find their way into the household. Every day that passes sees several new products on the market, many of them quite toxic. They are designed for cleansing, bleaching, cosmetic, medicinal, and various other laudable purposes. However, all too frequently they get into the hands of the curious "crawler" or "toddler" who follows a natural instinct to investigate, and tasting is one of the most interesting methods of investigation for young children. In order to combat this problem a great many health agencies have established "Poison Control Programs" or "Poison Control Centers" which develop files, as up-to-date as possible, of the many products available in the community that may have a deleterious effect. Parents, teachers, physicians, hospitals or indeed, anyone may telephone such centers and provide either the names of the ingredients on the label of a package or the signs and symptoms which have appeared in the child. With this information it is usually possible to provide quickly first aid advice concerning the type of antidote and treatment which should be used. A well-designed program follows this up with home visits for the investigation of the circumstances in order to advise the parents concerning the proper use and storage of the responsible and potential offending materials.

The most effective attack upon the accident problem involves everyone in the community including, very much, the teacher. Among the many approaches and techniques that should be considered and included are:

1. Teaching in the schools the facts about accidents and the factors involved in their occurrence and their prevention
2. Driver training in the schools in conjunction with other community agencies and organizations
3. Further research and investigation on the prevalence and incidence of accidents by means of research, reporting, and surveys
4. The promotion of the use of safety devices in the home, public buildings, places of work, on the farm and in vehicles. Of particular pertinence in connection with the last is the promotion of the use of seat belts in automobiles.
5. The inclusion of accident prevention factors in building codes.
6. City planning, traffic studies and highway design
7. Careful consideration of physical and mental factors in the issuance of drivers licenses

8. Improvement of the design of toys, household equipment, furniture, and industrial equipment with particular consideration given to the special needs and habits of the very young, the handicapped and the elderly
9. The development of a poison control program with an up-to-date poison control center

Occupational Health

One of the characteristics of our 20th century society is a concern by our communities and governments for the health of the worker. There are a number of valid reasons for this. In the first place, a large proportion of our population spends a considerable period of their daily life in their work environment. Many of the products produced in such work situations may affect the well being of the community as a whole and therefore, must be supervised by the community through its public health workers. Many types of work, especially in the heavy industries involve actual or potential physical or chemical risks, many of which are preventable. Still another reason is the fact that the working population presents a large group, relatively easily reached and influenced for health purposes and may therefore be benefited by various types of health programs. Furthermore, if the wage earner is properly motivated by such activities, they influence the health patterns of their homes and neighborhoods.

The field of occupational health, sometimes referred to as industrial health or medicine, may be regarded as consisting of two three-legged stools. In terms of disciplines involved, there is a stool with one leg representing medical science, another leg representing engineering and chemical science, and the third representing the social sciences. In terms of interested parties and participants in the activities, there is another three-legged stool with one leg representing government (the health agency), a second leg representing the employing agency, and the third leg representing organized labor. In the best of situations, the fields represented by the three legs of each respective stool would work intimately and cooperatively together.

As to purpose of such activities, the following definition of the Council on Industrial Health of the American Medical Association states:

> Occupational medicine deals with the restoration and conservation of health in relation to work, the working environment and maximum efficiency. It involves prevention, recognition, and treatment of occupational disabilities and requires the application of special techniques in the fields of rehabilitation, environmental hygiene, toxicology, sanitation and human relations.[6]

[6] *Medical Services in Industry and Workmen's Compensation Laws,* Rev. ed., Chicago, Am. Coll. Surgeons, 1946.

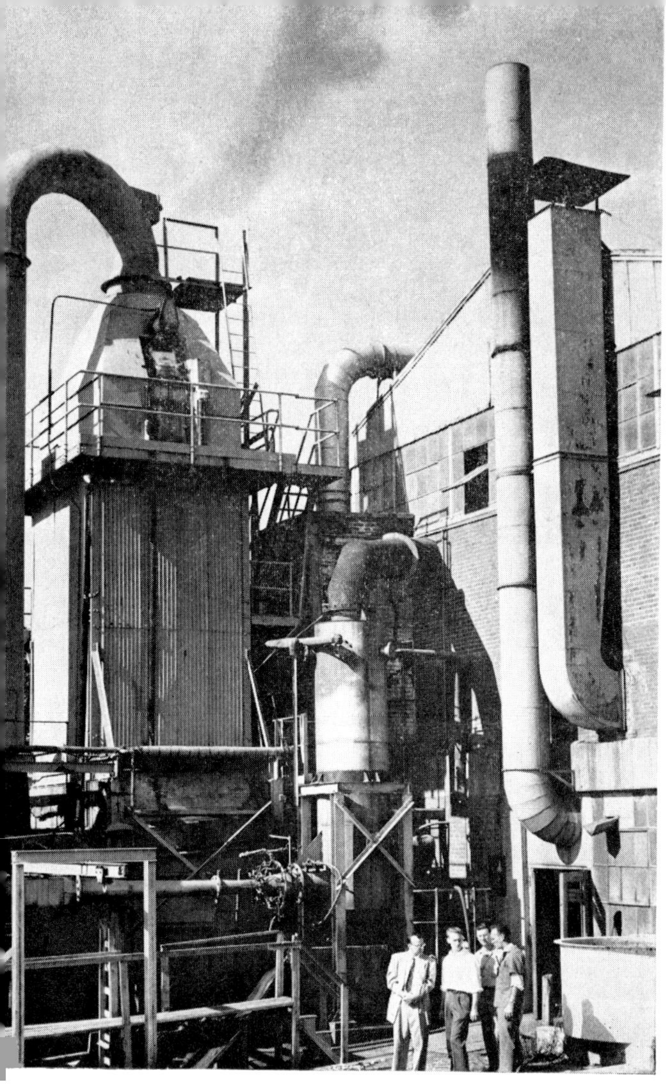

FIG. 36. The worker's health.

The value of attention to occupational health is relatively easy to prove. More than 500,000,000 work days are lost each year by the working population as a result of illness. This represents an annual wage loss of about $4,200,000,000, about 10 per cent of which may be considered to result from the approximate 390,000 annual cases of occupationally related illness. Accidents on the job account annually for over 2.2 million injuries which result in over 14,000 deaths as well as 90,000 permanent impairments. In addition about 2 million are disabled for one day or more. The price is estimated at about 3½ billion dollars per year, of which $1.6 billion is wage loss and $800 million is for medical care. Industry has long since learned the value of occupational health programs. A study by the National Association of Manufacturers of about 1,000 industrial plants that had developed such programs indicated that more than 20 per cent experienced a reduction in absenteeism, 14 per cent of the plants reported reductions of about 30 per cent. Nearly 90 per cent demonstrated a reduced labor turnover with an average reduction of 27 percent, while 92 per cent of the companies reported reduced incidence of occupational injury and illness.

The objectives of an industrial health program may be listed as follows:

1. The assessment of a worker's physical and psychological assets, as well as his liabilities, to facilitate proper selection and placement
2. The prevention of occupational and non-occupational illnesses

3. The provision of treatment, the type and extent of which depends on the policy of the organization
4. The fostering of a personal, physical, mental and social ability to work and enjoy life beyond the mere absence of disease or infirmity[7]

In order to accomplish these objectives, the Council on Industrial Health of the American Medical Association suggests the following scope of services:[8]

1. Regular appraisal of plant sanitation
2. Periodic inspection for occupational disease hazards
3. Adoption and maintenance of adequate control measures
4. Provision of first aid and emergency services
5. Prompt and early treatment for all illnesses resulting from occupational exposure
6. Reference to the family physician of individuals with conditions needing attention, cooperating with the patient and physician in every practical way to remedy the condition
7. Uniform recording of absenteeism due to all types of disability
8. Impartial health appraisals of all workers
9. Provision of rehabilitation services within industry
10. The conduct of a beneficial health education program

Government, one of the three legs of the stool, has certain responsibilities in the protection of the health of the working population, including occupational health and safety surveys and field investigations of environmental conditions in industry, the collection and analysis of data relating to occupational ills and injuries and to absenteeism, the surveillance of atmospheric pollution by industrial plants, the development of techniques for the detection of occupational diseases, their prevention and control, and the development of specific treatment, and the proposal of needed legislation. Health departments concentrate on the supervision of environmental conditions conducive to employment-related illness. They suggest measures for control, promote in-plant sanitation and medical services, provide advisory engineering and nursing services, and conduct health educational activities. Departments of labor and mines are primarily concerned with safety measures and the regulation of working conditions. The industrial or occupational health units of these agencies, in addition to their specific functions, coordinate their activities and services with those of units concerned with sanitation, health education, preventable and chronic disease, thereby attempting to bring to industry a well-rounded health program. In addition, they usually maintain coop-

[7] Cameron, D. C.: Human Relations in Occupational Health, Pub. Health Rep., 67:686, 1952.

[8] Council on Industrial Health of the American Medical Association: Scope, Objectives, and Functions of Occupational Health Programs, J.A.M.A. *164*:1104, 1957.

erative working relations with labor, management, and various pertinent professional societies.[9]

Recent Actions in Environmental Health

As a result of the accelerating abuse of the environment, its impact on man's health and the quality of life, as well as a growing awareness of its dangerous impact upon the total ecosystem of the nation and the entire planet, some important and definitive steps have recently been taken. During the late 1960's large numbers of individuals and organizations became more aware, concerned and vocal especially about the ever worsening problems of pollution of the air, land, and waters. The students of the nation and their teachers and schools played a significant role in what culminated in April 1970 in the remarkable nation-wide phenomenon called "Earth Day." Meanwhile, many members of the Congress proposed and obtained the passage of an impressive list of bills aimed at the improvement and preservation of the environment. Especially important was the passage of the National Environmental Policy Act of 1969. It is of historic significance that this was signed on January 1, 1970 as the first official act of the decade by President Richard M. Nixon who indicated that it could well represent the single most important action taken by his administration. Among other things, the Act established a high level three man Council on Environmental Quality to advise the President in the same manner as does the important Council of Economic Advisors. Included in its many responsibilities is the review of all existing and proposed national actions and legislation that may in any way have an impact upon the environment. This led the way to the Message on the Environment containing 37 action points, sent by the President to the Congress on February 10, 1970. Meanwhile, truly efficient and effective efforts on the Federal level were handicapped by the extensive diffusion of programs and responsibilities. Recognizing this, on July 9, 1970 the President sent to the Congress a proposal for the integration of many of the environmental programs and responsibilities of various Federal Departments and Agencies into a new Environmental Protection Agency, the Administrator of which reports directly to the President.

During this same period, similar steps were beginning to be taken by an increasing number of States and localities, some of which have already established new operational entities in which many environmental protection and pollution abatement activities are coordinated. All of these efforts, however, will be of limited or no ultimate effect unless the community of nations agrees to work together to preserve the environment while enjoying the ever multiplying fruits of scientific and

[9] Hanlon, John J.: *Principles of Public Health Administration,* 5th ed., St. Louis, C. V. Mosby Co., 1969.

technological development. Accordingly, the Director General of the United Nations has called for a World Conference on the Environment. This will be held in Stockholm in 1972. Already, many of the nations are preparing for this important precedent-setting international meeting which, it is anticipated, may bode well for the future of the world and mankind.

Questions for Discussion

1. What provisions have been made in your community to assure an adequate supply of pure water?
2. What are the advantages and disadvantages of fluoridation of drinking water and of the topical application of stannous fluoride to the teeth of children?
3. From what areas does your local milk supply come? What agencies are involved in supervising its purity?
4. In your community is there an air pollution problem?—a radiological health problem?—a sewage and refuse disposal problem? Are there programs dealing with these problems and if so, who is involved? Can you find instances here of local, state, and federal partnership?
5. Review generally the adequacy of housing in your community. If possible make a map which shows the location of slums, encroaching blight, central rot, and similar land use problems. Walk around some of these areas and consider how these problems may be related to the public health.
6. Are there any diseases present in your community which are spread by animal vectors? What are they? How serious are they? What is being done to control and eliminate them?
7. Determine the nature, extent and adequacy of the food control program in your community. Who is responsible for it? What is the training of the personnel? Are food handlers required to be examined?

Suggested Reading

1. JACOBSON, ALVIN R.: *A Bookshelf on Environmental Health,* Am. J. Public Health, 52:559, 1962.
2. *A Strategy for a Livable Environment.* A Report to the Secretary of Health, Education, and Welfare by the Task Force on Environmental Health and Related Problems, Washington, D.C., 1967.
3. GIBSON, WILLIAM C.: *The Social Dimension in Environmental Health,* Ann Arbor, Michigan, National Sanitation Foundation, 1961.
4. DUBOS, RENE: *Man Adapting,* New Haven, Yale Univ. Press, 1969.
5. Public Health Service: *Environmental Health Problems,* Washington, Supt. of Documents, 1962.
6. *Public Exposure to Ionizing Radiation,* Am. Pub. Health Assn., 1958.
7. PARRATT, SPENCER: *Housing Code Administration and Enforcement,* Washington, D.C., U.S. Dept. of Health, Education, and Welfare, 1970.
8. HALSEY, MAXWELL, N.: *Accident Prevention,* New York, McGraw-Hill Book Co., Inc., 1961.
9. SCHULZINGER, M. S.: *The Accident Syndrome,* Springfield, Ill., Charles C Thomas, 1956.
10. LIN-FU, JANE S.: *Childhood Lead Poisoning,* Children, 17:1, U.S. Dept. of Health, Education, and Welfare, Jan-Feb. 1970.
11. MAISEL, ALBERT Q.: *The Health of People Who Work,* New York, Nat. Health Council, 1960.

Chapter 6

Mind Over Matter—Mental Health

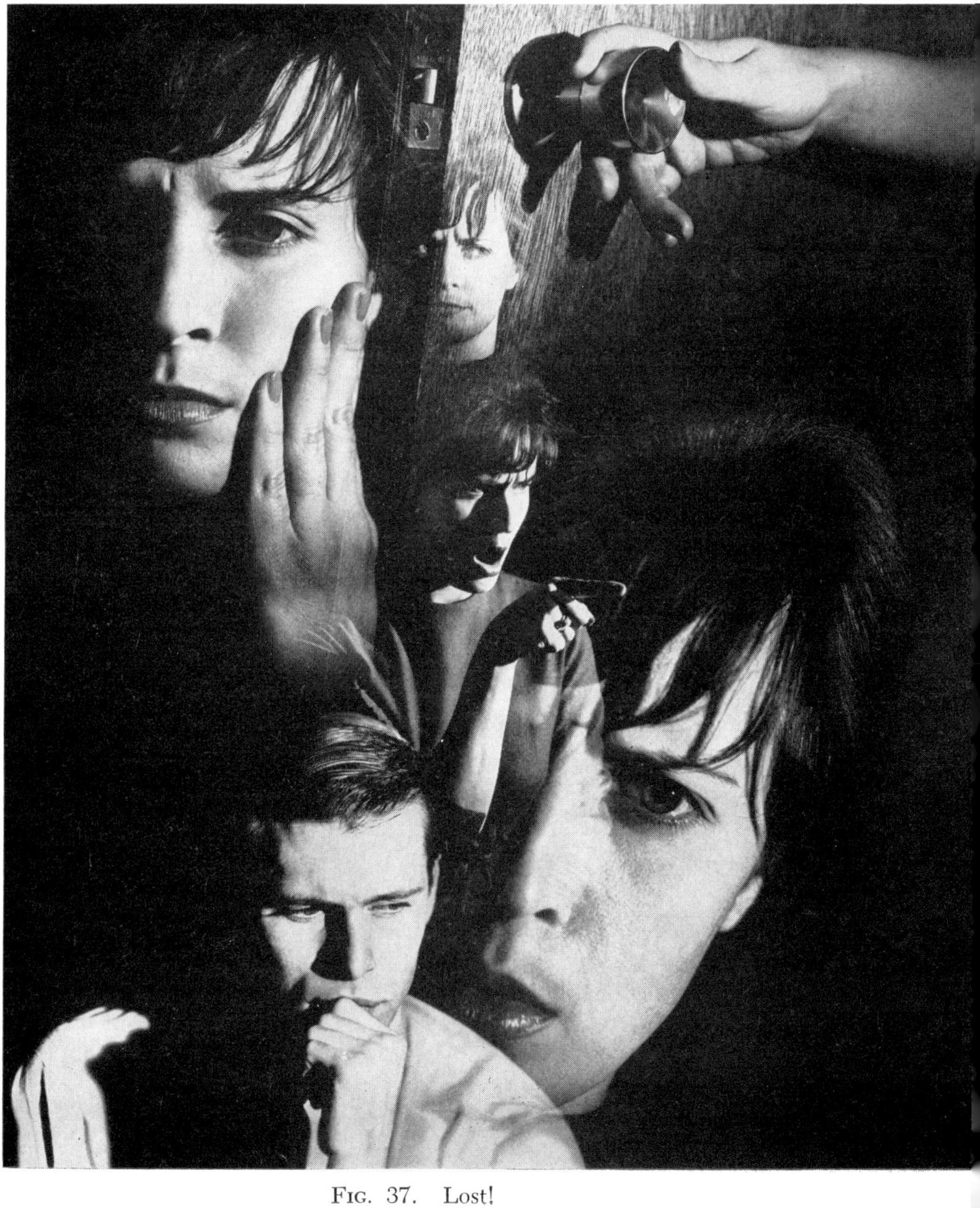

Fig. 37. Lost!

The Development of the Field

The field of mental health is one of the newer frontiers of medicine and community health. A number of factors have served to crystallize the field, and to bring about increased social and community emphasis on it during recent years. As the stresses of urbanized and industrialized living became apparent, there resulted a growing concern about their consequences. The increasing number of those affected, the improved methods for their diagnosis, and the great cost of caring for them, focussed public attention on the problem. Of fundamental importance, of course, was the conceptualization and development of the specialties of psychiatry, psychology, and sociology. Jointly, they brought about a realization that complete health consists of physical, mental and social components. They also led gradually to an awareness of the relationship between mental illness, on the one hand, and of much crime, juvenile delinquency, prostitution, addictions, familial discord and divorce, work inadequacies, many accidents, and a host of other undesirable and costly social phenomena on the other.

Until surprisingly recently, mental illness was regarded as something shameful, to be hidden, an affliction by the devil or other evil spirits which had to be "exorcised," or as a punishment by some higher power for some imagined wrongdoing. Even now it is not uncommon to hear reference to the "criminally insane." Those most markedly affected were usually locked in dark attics or incarcerated in filthy jails or similar institutions, without treatment, and often in company with criminals or diseased persons. They were restrained with chains and straight jackets, cruelly beaten, and exhibited for the amusement of dilettantes and the curious public. About the most humane treatment they received was to be rendered stuporous with drugs.

As is so often the case, both social and scientific impetus came from a few interested and dedicated individuals and groups. Historically, Philippe Pinel may be considered the first great champion of the mentally ill. His efforts to have them regarded as victims of illness met with considerable opposition and ridicule, not only from the French public, but also from the medical profession. He succeeded, however, in having the chains struck off the insane of Paris in 1795, and in having them transferred to hospitals. About a half century was to pass before the efforts of Dorothea Dix began to bring about similar results in the United States.

Meanwhile, the 19th century witnessed the laying of the foundations of modern psychiatry. Contrary to common opinion, the advances involved the efforts and imagination of a remarkably multinational group which included Charcot (French), Pavlov and Korsakov (Russian), Ramon y Cajal (Spanish), Kraepelin (German), Freud and Adler (Austrian), Bleuler and Jung (Swiss), Sherrington and Jones (British), and Meyer (American) to mention only a few. Incidentally, all of those mentioned, did their work since the mid-19th century, and most of it during the first half of the 20th century. The recent origin of psychiatry as a specialty is further emphasized by the fact that most of these pioneers died only within the past third of a century. Gradually, medical schools in the United States, as well as elsewhere, began to add psychiatrists to their staffs, and courses in psychiatry to their curricula. Psychiatric residencies and other forms of specialty training were developed and extended. More recent has been a significant and concerted effort to make practical psychiatry part of the everyday practice of the general or family physician.

The mental health movement as a social force may be considered to date from 1908 when Clifford W. Beers founded the Connecticut Mental Hygiene Association. While a student at Yale, Beers had developed a severe mental illness which required institutionalization for several years. He recovered and wrote a widely read and discussed book entitled *A Mind That Found Itself*.[1] It described the many inadequacies in the care of the mentally ill at that time. The establishment of the Connecticut Association was followed within one year by the formation of the National Committee for Mental Hygiene which later became the American Mental Health Association. Since then, many state and local societies have been formed to educate the public, to assist in professional training, to promote research in mental health, and to perform and promote many other functions and services. Once established firmly in this country, the movement spread to other parts of the world. In 1922, an international organization for mental hygiene came into being, and in 1930 it called the first International Mental Health Congress in Washington.

By the late 1930's a few forward looking local and state health departments, aided usually by certain interested philanthropic foundations, began to introduce a few mental health activities into their programs. For a number of years, these activities were largely exploratory and experimental, and were usually organized and conducted as part of some established and accepted phase of the public health program, such as maternal and child health. The numerous men and women who had to be rejected by military draft and recruitment centers for mental and behavioral reasons during World War II focussed national attention sharply upon the problem. As a result, in 1946 the Congress of the United States passed the National Mental Health Act. This made possible much of the increased thought, action and facilities which have occurred since at all levels of government in this country. The first and most tangible result was the establishment of the National Institute of Mental Health at Bethesda, Maryland, as one of the components of the National

[1] Beers, Clifford W.: *A Mind That Found Itself*, Garden City, Doubleday & Co., 1956.

Institutes of Health of the United States Public Health Service. The National Institute of Mental Health has, since its establishment, provided national leadership of high quality. It has also given extensive encouragement and financial assistance to institutions and organizations throughout the country for training, research and demonstrations in mental health and related fields. It administers large amounts of monies, made available by Congressional appropriations, for grants to individuals and institutions in order that they may carry out worthwhile projects.

One of the most difficult aspects of the problem has been the fact that, because mental health programs until recently concentrated on the diagnosis and treatment of evident mental illness, which involves a lengthy hence costly one to one, patient-psychiatrist relationship, assistance was largely inaccessible to the economically average or disadvantaged person. Recent years have brought about some significant changes in this regard. More psychiatrists and clinical psychologists have been trained and their efforts have been multiplied by the development of a variety of assistants and auxiliaries. More attention has been given to individual and societal prevention of mental illness, early diagnosis and the minimization of progression. In this regard, it is interesting that already a number of psychological and even some biochemical tests have been developed to detect proneness to or precursors of certain mental illnesses such as schizophrenia and mental retardation. Of considerable importance is the great success in the control or elimination of a number of communicable diseases that in the past contributed as complications a significant amount of certain mental illnesses. This gain, however, is unfortunately offset by the undesirable mental consequences of the stresses of crowded urban living and the increased use of alcohol and drugs. Another factor on the positive side of the ledger has been the establishment by many state and local governments of Community Mental Health Boards which have as their chief function the establishment, funding and management, often in company with other organizations, of community or neighborhood mental health clinics. Added to this movement has been the development of an increasing number of diagnostic, treatment and preventive facilities which focus upon certain special mental health problems. Among these are anti-suicide, anti-alcoholism and anti-drug programs, as well as family counselling and marital counselling clinics. Finally, and not to be underestimated are the many excellent articles which appear with increasing frequency in the public press and in popular magazines throughout the nation.

Extent of the Problem

In terms of both magnitude and socio-economic implications, mental illness constitutes one of the greatest problems of modern society. It is estimated that, at any given moment, one person in ten has some form of mental or emotional disorder which merits professional attention. This does not mean, of course, that they all obtain satisfactory, or even any care. In each current year in the United States approximately one million individuals receive treatment in mental institutions. An additional one and one-half million are treated in out-patient departments of hospitals or by private physicians. It is estimated that one-half of all patients seen by private physicians for any reason have some emotional disorder. It has also been estimated that 6 million of the 20 million persons who enter general hospitals throughout the country for physical ailments, have illnesses caused by emotional disorders.

While actually only about 2 per cent of patients admitted to hospitals are admitted for psychiatric disorders, about one half of the hospital beds in the United States are occupied by mental patients. The reason for the discrepancy is the lengthy institutionalization required by the average mentally ill patient. Fortunately, the development in recent years of a number of quite effective pharmaceutics such as tranquilizers and euphoriants has made it possible to make institutionalization of many persons unnecessary or to make earlier hospital discharge possible. Despite this, however, the incidence of mental illness has been increasing. It is still not clear whether the increase is real or apparent. A number of factors must be considered;—the increased stresses of industrialization and urban life, improved diagnosis, increased willingness to suspect mental illness and to seek diagnosis and care, the increase in the population, and the marked increase in average longevity, during the past few generations. Any and probably all of these contribute to the increased number of individuals listed as being mentally ill.

Types of Mental Illnesses

The foregoing raises the question, what is mental illness? In general terms it may be considered to be any disturbance of the thought processes, emotions and behavior. It may vary greatly in degree, from so mild that there is no impairment of living function, to so severe as to be completely disabling. Mental illness may be divided into two general categories, the neuroses and the psychoses.

Neuroses, which are the less serious of the two groups of illnesses, are extremely common. They are emotional disturbances which cause the individual to suffer from marked feelings of anxiety, resentment or hostility which do not prevent him from carrying on an apparently normal life. They do, however, prevent the achievement of a satisfactory and happy existence. While neuroses are bothersome in that they may cause a great deal of unhappiness and inefficiency in those afflicted or in those with whom they associate, they do not constitute a serious medical, social or economic problem. The majority of mild neuroses respond to counselling, guidance or limited psychotherapy by a well-trained physician. The more severe neuroses may require longer treatment involving psychoanalysis. The essential point is that the neurotic person does not lose contact with reality.

Psychoses, on the other hand, cause the patient to be definitely out of touch with reality. He lives in a world apart from that of his fellow men. Often unaware of his identity or that of persons normally close to him, he may similarly be oblivious to his surroundings and environment and be quite unable to control his behavior. He may suffer from illusions, that is, misinterpretation of what he sees or hears; delusions, such as strange fanciful or fantastic ideas; or hallucinations, in which he may see, hear, taste, smell or feel things that do not exist. It is the psychoses that present the truly serious and difficult medical, social and economic problems. Psychoses may result from a number of causes, some quite well understood, others not at all. Among the better understood psychoses are those caused by syphilitic involvement of the brain, chronic intoxication by certain chemicals such as alcohol, certain drugs, lead, and some other heavy metals, the psychoses that sometimes occur at the time of the menopause or change of life, and some of the psychoses related to mental deficiency arising out of the inadequate development of the brain tissue. The two most common and most important psychoses however, are schizophrenia and manic depressive psychosis.

Schizophrenia, or what is commonly referred to as split personality, is by any measure the most important and serious of the mental illnesses. It accounts for over one-fifth of all admissions to mental hospitals. Even this, however, does not adequately depict its importance. Since it may affect a broad age span from about 15 years to about 35 years of age, since treatment is prolonged, and since recovery is rare especially in the higher ages, cases tend to pile up in institutions. As a result, more than 45 per cent of all patients in mental hospitals are sufferers from schizophrenia. Schizophrenics tend to be unduly preoccupied with the functions of the body and show hypochondriacal concern over various imagined symptoms. They may complain of burning sensations that pass over the body or of an object moving inside the head. Abnormal thought processes, such as inability to concentrate, or irrationality as well as pseudo-intellectuality, may become evident. They tend to be highly suspicious or paranoid, and commonly withdraw into themselves. They are very prone to daydreaming, delusions, and hallucinations.

Manic depressive psychosis causes a personality and behavior which typically swings from one extreme to the other. During the manic phase, the individual is highly elated and enthusiastic with many plans, projects and ambitions, few if any of which, however, ever see fulfillment. During this stage nothing can beat him. He is on top of the world. Nothing is impossible. From this, he passes into a period of deep depression during which he withdraws from the world about him. Everything is wrong, nothing counts, what's the use! The depressive stage is dangerous because of a tendency toward suicide. The two extreme stages may be separated by intervals during which the individual is quite lucid. While manic depression accounts for only a little more than 4 per cent of admissions to mental hospitals, the low recovery rate, therefore long hospitalization, causes them to account for almost 8 per cent of those hospitalized for mental illness. The possibility of violent action aimed at either themselves or toward others makes this a peculiarly important condition.

Senile psychosis, or mental disease of the senium, which involves essentially elderly senile persons and individuals with hardening of the arteries of the brain, might ordinarily be expected to represent an important component of the mental health problem because of the numbers of such patients admitted to hospitals. However, because of the advanced average age of these patients, hence their tendency to die soon after admission, they account for only 12 per cent of the population of mental hospitals.

The Risk of Mental Illness

The incidence of the various types of mental illness varies considerably according to a number of factors. For most types, the roots are in early childhood, with the greatest manifestation of the illness during the ordinarily productive adult years. (Table 6) It should be noted, however, that a number of mental illnesses, especially schizophrenia are being diagnosed with increasing frequency in children. (Table 7) The significance of this is not yet clear.

Signs of mental deficiency, epilepsy, personality disorders and schizophrenia usually appear early. Alcoholic and manic-depressive psychoses tend to be concentrated in the middle years of life. As indicated by their names, involutional psychosis appears during the menopause and senile psychoses during the later years of life. The incidence of mental illness varies by sex in a number of interesting ways. In general, mental illness appears to occur somewhat more frequently among females than among males. Thus, about 50 per cent more females than males are admitted to hospitals for both schizophrenia and manic depressive psychosis. Involutional psychosis is almost 3 times as common in women as in men. While psychoneuroses are twice as common in females as in males, the reverse is true with regard to personality disorders. Alcoholic

Table 6. Age at First Hospitalization for Mental Illnesses, United States

Age Group	*Per Cent of First Admissions*
under 15 years	1.2
15 to 34	27.8
35 to 64	48.1
65 years and over	22.9

Table 7. Hospitalization for Mental Illness, by Age and Sex

Condition	*Usual age at First Admission*	*% of first admissions*			*% of hospitalized mental patients*	*chances of recovery*
		Men	*Women*	*Both*		
schizophrenia	16–35	18.6	26.8	22.6	45.6	poor after 50 yr. long hosp.
manic-depressive psychosis	35–50	3.1	5.3	4.2	7.6	poor, long hosp.
psychosis with mental deficiency	15–44	2.7	1.8	2.3	6.0	poor, long hosp.
alcoholic psychosis	25–54	21.8	5.2	13.7	3.0	fair, short hosp.
involutional psychosis	48–58	3.0	8.3	5.6	3.0	poor, die soon short hosp.
senile psychosis	60 and over	21.1	20.5	20.8	12.2	poor, die soon short hosp.
personality disorders (non-alcoholic)	15–34	7.2	3.9	5.6	4.0	fair, short hosp.
psychoneurotic reactions	25–44	6.3	12.4	9.3	6.0	fair, short hosp.
other disorders, each of low incidence	all ages	16.2	15.8	15.9	12.6	generally poor, long hosp.

Table 8. Prevalence of Mental Illness by Socio-economic Status, U.S. (age-adjusted rates per 100,000 persons in each group)

Socio-economic groups*	Neuroses		Psychoses	
	Male	Female	Male	Female
1	381	349	202	176
2	224	250	231	347
3	181	114	474	559
4	235	97	1,814	1,218

*1. wealthy, professional and top managerial
2. small proprietors, white collar and skilled workers
3. semiskilled and unskilled, some secondary education
4. unskilled and semiskilled, less education

psychosis is also much more common (4 or 5 times) among men than women. As would be expected, no significant difference between the sexes appears to exist as to the incidence of mental deficiency or senile psychoses. These variations are presented in Table 7 which lists the conditions in the order of their general ultimate importance, taking into consideration numbers of people involved, length of hospitalization and duration of the illness, cost of care, and chances of recovery.

Interesting variations in the incidence of mental illness exist in relation to socio-economic groups. Of all types of mental illnesses, neuroses occur about twice as frequently as do the more severe psychoses among the wealthy, professional and top managerial groups. This is in marked contrast with the situation among the semi-skilled and unskilled laboring groups of the population where psychoses are many times as frequent as are neuroses (Table 8). Examining this from another dimension, it is noted that neuroses appear to be about twice as common in the higher as in the lower socio-economic groups, while very much the reverse is true with regard to psychoses of greater severity. These discrepancies may be due in part to a greater awareness of neuroses by those in the higher socio-economic groups and their greater tendency and financial ability to seek medical attention for such conditions. On the other hand, people in the lower socio-economic groups may be so overwhelmed in the relative sense by more serious conditions including psychoses that they do not regard neuroses as illness.

The Cost of Mental Illness

The actual cost of mental illness to society is very difficult, if not impossible, to determine. The average cost of treating a patient with mental illness is approximately $1650 per year, or about $4.50 per day. For the United States, the total bill may be estimated to be about five and one half billion dollars per year. Rough estimates in millions of dollars for certain aspects of the annual bill for mental illness are as follows:

	In Millions
Loss in patients earnings and federal income tax revenue	$2,400
Public mental hospital maintenance	800
Care of mentally ill in general hospitals	40
Care of mentally ill in veterans' hospitals	280
Compensation and pensions to mentally ill veterans	350
Public assistance for mentally ill and defective persons	23
Hospital care of mentally defective and epileptic patients	190
Care of senile and aged psychotic patients in nursing homes	335
Treatment of mentally ill in out patient clinics	28
Earnings of psychiatrists in private practice	110
Construction and renovation of state mental hospital facilities	1,000

In addition to frank mental illnesses and deficiencies, it is known that many medical conditions may have a psychological component. Among those that might be listed are a variety of gastrointestinal disturbances varying from vague diarrhea or chronic constipation to gastric ulcers, asthma and a number of skin conditions. In addition, there may be added a number of seemingly unrelated social problems or aberrations including chronic alcoholism, drug addictions, many juvenile and adult delinquencies, some of the prostitution problem and many home, industrial and highway accidents. It is impossible, of course, to set definitive limits on the extents to which such phenomena have their roots in mental problems of a temporary or long-term nature. It can be said, however, the ultimate total cost to society, just of the proportion of these phenomena that is psychologically related, is enormous. It has been estimated, for example, that American industry each year loses the equivalent of about ten billion dollars due to absenteeism related to illnesses with a mental component.

What Can Be Done

The picture is not all dark, however. As has been indicated previously, society and medicine have made a number of notable advances in recent years. Possibly most important is an increasing readiness to accept and discuss the realities of mental illness. In this, teachers and their schools have played and will continue to play a most important role. While the number of psychiatrists, psychiatric nurses, psychiatric social workers, and psychologists fall far short of what the nation needs, their numbers are gradually increasing, thanks in part to career guidance in many of the schools and colleges of the nation. Facilities for diagnosis and treatment, especially on an outpatient basis are also becoming increasingly common.

In relation to methods of treatment, psychotherapy, while not always curative in the true sense, does ameliorate many neuroses and psychoses. Shock therapy, either by means of electricity or insulin, is still valuable in relieving overwhelming tensions and morbid depression, and for the treatment of many schizophrenics. In addition, lobotomy, that is, the operative cutting of certain nerve tracts in the brain, has been used increasingly in the transformation of certain unusually agitated or depressed patients into more adaptable individuals. A most important breakthrough has resulted from the amazing recent developments in psychopharmacology. Beginning in the mid-1950's, there began to appear a series of new drugs commonly referred to as ataraxics or tranquilizers. These medications have already revolutionized the outlook for much of the mental health problem. While they do not get at the root of the individual's problem, they do, by relieving anxiety, depression and confusion, make psychotherapy possible and more effective in a large number of cases for whom this was formerly not possible. These and other drugs may even eventually make unnecessary such drastic treatments as shock therapy and lobotomy.

Of particular significance is the fact that since 1956, while admissions to mental hospitals have continued to increase in number, the mental hospital population has finally levelled off and, in fact, begun to decrease because the new therapies make a much shorter hospital stay possible. Large numbers of patients can now be treated successfully in a shorter period of time and discharged from the mental hospital back to their families and society, many of them to gainful occupations. In addition to their great value in the treatment of the frankly mentally ill, these drugs have also been used widely in the prevention or minimizing of the effects of minor neuroses and psychoses in a large number of individuals who never require the services of a mental institution.

Community Mental Health Programs

As has been mentioned, mental health is still very much a new area of activity for community health organizations and much of what is done is still essentially in the nature of exploration, trial and demonstration. The immediate approach has been well stated by Lemkau to consist of two general dimensions or goals.

1. The vertical or categorical dimension—early diagnosis and treatment
   (*a*) to prevent the development of more serious and handicapping mental illnesses
   (*b*) to remove the sources of stress from family and social environments
   (*c*) to make available specialized services to broaden the horizontal aims
2. The horizontal dimension or goal—long range prevention
   (*a*) to influence every member of voluntary and official community health organizations and of school personnel with sound mental hygienic principles. The essential purpose here is prevention which in the final analysis depends upon the provision of a

satisfactory psychological environment for children in general, and on helping the emotionally disturbed child as early as possible. It has been stated with good reason that mental health is important both at home and in the school, for there lies the fertile soil in which all kinds of mental illnesses may take root.

Since community mental health programs are still in the developmental stage, the types of activities which may be observed vary considerably from nothing to a wide variety of services. Among the activities and services that have been engaged in are the following:

1. The development and maintenance of a roster of mental health facilities,
2. The gathering of reports or data on mental health needs and problems,
3. Development of and assistance to lay and professional education programs,
4. The direct operation of mental health outpatient clinics,
5. The promulgation of rules and regulations relating to mental health,
6. The promulgation of qualifications for personnel and standards for facilities in relation to mental health,
7. Financial assistance to local organizations and institutions such as private diagnostic and therapeutic clinics and hospitals,
8. Promotional, supervisory and consultative services to local, voluntary and official agencies and institutions,
9. Special surveys and research.

In addition to the foregoing general activities, certain specialized programs such as the following may be observed:

10. Anti-suicide programs,
11. Programs aimed at addictive diseases such as alcoholism and drug addiction,
12. Combination health, welfare and recreation programs aimed at the so-called pre-delinquent especially in urban slum areas,
13. Programs for the prevention of senility in the aging population such as senior citizen health and recreation centers.

Mention should also be made of the influence of programs for the improvement of nutrition and for the reduction of certain diseases, such as syphilis, in the prevention of specific types of mental illness.

The School's Role in Mental Health

Because it affords such a long continuing and vital experience spread throughout twelve of the most impressionable years of life, the school may be considered to rank next to the family as the most important determinant of the child's mental health. Thus, upon the school rests a grave share of the responsibility for the mental health of the community. This responsibility is two-fold: (*a*) the provision of a school environment psychologically favorable to the development of sound mental health on the part of each child; and (*b*) the early discovery of the emotionally disturbed or retarded child, and the initiation of adequate follow-up procedures and therapeutic measures for those in need of assistance.

The Total School Environment

Many persons and many factors contribute to the creation of a school environment psychologically favorable to mental health. With regard to mental health, all with whom the child has contact, his interactions with them, and in fact his total school experience, constitute the child's environment. Therefore, the primary consideration of the school system should be the appointment of administrators, teachers, and other school personnel so constituted as to exert a psychologically favorable influence upon this broad environment. This implies the selection of healthy, well-adjusted persons who meet the qualifications established by their respective professions. In addition, each should possess personal qualifications consistent with sound mental health, a genuine liking for children, an understanding of child development and human psychology, and a mastery of skills necessary for the creation of a desirable teaching-learning atmosphere. Since the teacher is the person who is with the child most constantly, she must carry the major responsibility for creating a psychologically favorable school environment. Her specific role will be discussed in detail in a later section.

An emotional climate conducive to mental health implies sound administrator-teacher-pupil relationships based upon respect for the individual. Children respond to such an atmosphere and conversely are sensitively aware of tensions in relationships even though they themselves are not directly involved. Happy interrelations are built upon consideration for others, cooperative thinking in decision making, and a democratic approach to school matters with the children participating actively whenever possible.

Contributing significantly to the emotional climate of the classroom and the school is the prevailing philosophy concerning discipline. In order to make its most effective contribution to mental health, it must be founded upon respect for the individual and have as its ultimate goal self-discipline, or the building of inner controls on the part of each child. Necessary guidelines can often be arrived at through classroom discussion. To succeed, such guidelines need to be clearly stated, based upon sound and equitable reasons, and understood by all concerned. Moreover, there should be consistency from day to day and from grade to grade. Guidelines or discipline patterns developed along these lines foster feelings of security on the part of both the young child and the adolescent. At the same time, through their own participation, they are learning the lessons of freedom and democracy.

Emphasis upon a well-balanced daily routine and time schedule for the school can reduce friction and tensions, and prevent undue striving among staff members, pupils, grades, classes, or homerooms for special privileges.

School mores and customs based upon sound values should be encouraged. School pride and a sense of belonging are important in providing positive motivation. Unfortunately, there have been many instances in which these incentives have been used unwisely by faculty and administrators with overemphasis, based upon false values, particularly in regard to scholastic and athletic achievements.

The school should affirm its deep concern for mental health by emphasis upon curriculum experiences and teaching-learning methods and procedures based upon sound principles of child development and psychology. Individual differences in the needs of children should be given due consideration in providing developmental tasks designed not just for the average but also for the gifted, the mentally retarded, and the slow learner.

The school curriculum should include the teaching of mental health at all levels, using a positive approach, and with content, experiences, and techniques adapted to the maturity of the children. This might well be a full unit in the health course with additional emphasis in other related units and in other subject courses. Units on sex education, family life, addictive diseases, and many other subjects present opportunities for mental health emphasis.

It is the responsibility of the school to extend in-service education in mental health to its teachers and other personnel. School administrators should encourage teachers and nurses to utilize the excellent materials available from local and state departments of health and from various voluntary agencies for their own personal enrichment and for use in their classes at appropriate levels and in parent education.

School Design for Mental Health

A well-planned, sanitary school plant holds many implications for mental health. Here again, responsibility for its maintenance falls upon the school system itself. Classrooms and activity rooms should be free from conditions which foster ill health, such as poor lighting which may cause eye strain, undue noise, and other tension creating features. Children from all types of homes respond to the order, cleanliness, and beauty of the school plant. A sense of pride in the classroom and the school should be fostered, and set a desirable example for the home. It is important that buildings and grounds be free from conditions which might invite undesirable behavior or delinquency. Nooks and corners cannot be readily supervised; poor lighting and unwisely located lavatories invite difficulties.

Adequate space for "big muscle" activity and a sound recreational program, both outdoor and indoor, is a mental health requirement for every school plant. Provision for individual differences in interests implies diversified equipment in sufficient amount to offer a wide range of suitable activities which meet the physical and mental needs of children the year round and during after-school hours. Wholesome expression through art, music, crafts and dramatics is to be encouraged, and space and facilities must be planned for them.

Mental Health Services in the School

Guidance and counseling services in proportion to the school enrollment are a necessity in each school. On the elementary level it is important that the emotionally disturbed or retarded child be discovered as early as possible, and dealt with wisely. Insecurity, undue anxieties, fears, and tensions are all too common problems. Often they can be resolved satisfactorily at this early point in the individual's life. If not, they are likely to persist and increase from year to year so that by the time the pupil reaches junior high school, the same problem, sometimes in different guise, has reached serious dimensions.

At the secondary school level, a ratio of 250 pupils per counselor is usually considered a full load. Counseling at this level often centers about personal problems relating to maturing, vocational guidance, disciplinary problems, and subject failures or difficulties. Careful study often indicates that most problems appear in clusters, many of them actually arising from a single basic health problem.

Guidance should not be regarded as the sole responsibility of the guidance counselor. An effective guidance program permeates every part of the school and involves every teacher. A child is most likely to seek help from someone he knows well and in whom he has confidence. From the standpoint of convenience and frequency of contact, this person is likely to be his teacher, or on secondary level, his homeroom teacher or one of his subject teachers. The guidance counselor should strive to help the entire staff understand this and should indicate his willingness to work cooperatively with them. He should encourage them to make useful pupil observations and to write meaningful anecdotal reports.

Psychological services should be available in all school systems. Large systems usually maintain their own, but even in smaller systems arrangements can usually be made to share community facilities and services. A regular testing program should be planned to reach all pupils. Tests should be selected wisely, administered at designated grade levels in a program planned to extend throughout the child's school life, and the results carefully recorded on the cumulative record of each child. The testing program should be evaluated periodically, and significant findings utilized in the improvement and re-direction of procedures and services.

Provision should be made for the detailed testing of emotionally disturbed or retarded children discovered during the screening or health appraisal, and for those referred at other times by the school physician or guidance counselor. Some school systems arrange and conduct their own case conferences, while others affiliate with an appropriate community agency. It is important for all schools to maintain close liaison with community mental health agencies, clinics, facilities, and services, and to utilize them to best advantage in seeking appropriate means toward the solution of the emotional problems of the school child. This same close cooperation in follow-up procedures should extend also to children in day-care centers and in schools for the mentally retarded. Each child needs to be encouraged to use his own powers to their fullest capacity and to become to the greatest extent possible a self-supporting citizen.

The school might well assume responsibility for encouraging parent education along mental health lines. This can be done through Parent-Teacher Associations or other adult organizations and community groups. In the junior and senior high school, education for family life assumes particular significance in view of the low age at which so many marriages occur today, and also in view of the rise in delinquency and venereal disease rates among youth. In budgeting for trained personnel in psychology and guidance, these educational needs deserve earnest consideration by school administration officials as part of the program for prevention of mental illness.

The Teacher's Personality and Mental Health

As indicated above, from the mental health point of view, next to the child's parents the classroom teacher usually plays the most important role in the child's environment.

The teacher's role in mental health encompasses much that is "caught rather than taught." Actually, her example conveys convincing mental health overtones. Children understand the role of "mother" and "father" through constant observation of their parents' individual practices, attitudes, and relations with each other and with the other members of the family. The role of the teacher is learned in the same way. Moreover, the children tend to identify with her emotionally. There is nothing more revealing and sobering for a teacher than to watch her kindergarteners or first graders "play school," and, through their eyes, to see herself in action.

The teacher's own personality sets the emotional tone of the classroom. One likes to think of the ideal teacher as a warm, happy person who herself experiences happy family relations; a secure person who accepts herself honestly and objectively as to her own limitations; a healthy person with a lively sense of humor. This teacher can relate easily with people of all kinds and enjoy doing so. She accepts people as they are and is free as possible from prejudices and biases. Above all, she is genuinely fond of children.

Her pre-professional preparation should have helped her gain a sound understanding of her mental health responsibilities and opportunities as a classroom teacher. Included should be courses in child psychology and child development; health courses pertaining to personal, family, community and school health; sociology including group work, family life and behavioral science; and biological sciences. There should also be provided opportunities for first-hand observation and experiences with children, and contacts with community agencies. The teacher's professional security stems from such sound preparation and is tied in with her own "teacher image," *i.e.* her concept of her own role as a contributing citizen worthy of significant community status and acceptance. Her teaching load should be scaled to allow genuine satisfaction from her work and to permit her to lead a balanced personal life with time for work, recreation, and rest.

As the teacher approaches her task, she should appreciate the importance of keeping constantly in mind certain basic truths concerning child growth and development. She should recognize the influences of heredity and environment, and the effects of the family and family relations upon the child. She must remember that each child is unique, and strive to recognize his characteristics and the various stages of his development as they appear at successive periods. She should be alert to individual differences among the children in her group and strive to adapt her teaching methods accordingly.

As time and experience go on, the teacher should try to become more and more sensitive to the mental health needs of her children. Her task as teacher is to help the child progress educationally from year to year—a vertical progression. But she must also strive to help each child develop his own personality to its maximum potential—a horizontal development. Discovery of the importance of this horizontal development has not been truly appreciated in the past. The teacher's understanding and skill in bringing these two dimensions of growth into sound relationship is fundamental to helping her pupils achieve a high level of mental health and life fulfillment.

The Child and His Mental Health Needs

Experts in mental health agree that there is constant interaction between the child and his environment, and that his personality development appears to follow certain inner biological laws or patterns. The way a child feels about his experiences determines the quality and degree of his mental health. Erickson[2] alludes to eight successive stages of development which appear to be universal and to embrace one's entire life. Each stage has a central problem to be solved, temporarily at least, if the child is to move successfully to the next. The failure to solve the problem, particularly during the child's critical years, leaves a wake of emotional difficulties which may interfere seriously with his personality development. The struggle to maintain a healthy personality is continuous throughout life. It can never be completely and finally settled. Experts agree that every child has certain emotional needs with which the adult can help best through the simple process of sincere and genuine love, encouragement, and guidance. Obviously, a teacher cannot possibly love and understand all children equally. Reactions vary with each child's uniqueness. However, the teacher can strive to have each child realize that she accepts him as he is, that she is not shocked by unexpected behavior, and that she is always willing to try to understand the underlying motive of the behavior. The child needs to learn to recognize his inner feelings and emotions, to realize that certain of them are undesirable, and to find constructive ways of coping with them. Through discussion, the teacher can help children to examine these inner feelings and understand them better. Often children can help other children very effectively. The perceptive teacher will create situations in which this can happen.

In this respect, the school child's desire to grow is a powerful motivation which continues throughout childhood and adolescence. This striving must be given every practical chance to proceed without the development of emotional blocks caused by the failure of the child to realize his own potentialities. The child needs to realize that he is both an individual and a member of a group. The teacher can help him gain this feeling by providing ample opportunity to work and play with a group and to contribute to its progress and success by drawing upon any special talent or skill he may possess as an individual. Deep within every youngster is the need to "belong." Status in a peer group is paramount, particularly at adolescence. Group work frequently provides this supportive feeling of status. In a small group both the shy child and the aggressive one are likely to find status satisfaction.

Children need to learn to cooperate happily and successfully not only within their peer groups, but also with adults. Cooperative teacher-pupil planning can provide valuable experiences which may result in practical plans, standards, and regulations to which all agree. By having a voice in developing and establishing them, the rules or plans become clearer and more acceptable to the pupil and there develops a feeling of responsi-

[2] Erickson, Erik H.: *Childhood and Society*. 2nd ed. New York: W. Norton & Co., Inc., 1964. See also, Witmer, Helen Deland and Kotinsky, Ruth, Ed., *Personality in the Making*: the Fact-finding Report of the Midcentury White House Conference on Children and Youth. New York: Harper & Brothers, 1952, Chap. I: p. 3.

bility for their ultimate implementation. Democratic action as well as good mental health is thus learned through practice.

The perceptive teacher is able to develop an alertness for detecting deviations from the usual physical and emotional behavior of the children in her class. At the same time, she needs to bear in mind that a basic emotion or feeling may manifest itself overtly in different ways, in different children, and at various developmental stages. Some common behavioral signs which should arrest her attention include shyness, thumb-sucking, nail-biting, stammering, stuttering, tic, tension, self-play, frequent day-dreaming, aggressive or withdrawn behavior, and temper tantrums. It is important that early signs of emotional disturbances be detected. The classroom teacher can observe the child in all sorts of situations and peer relationships throughout the day. Home visits, conversations with other children, and conferences with the child's other or former teachers often shed significant sidelights on problems. The school nurse and other members of the health team, the special teachers, and the guidance counselor may also contribute to the total picture. The child's cumulative records may furnish important pertinent data. A plan for the systematic observation of her pupils early in the term proves valuable in helping the teacher discover possible significant deviations.

The skillful teacher can often handle a behavioral crisis or a suspected emotional disturbance in a sort of first-aid fashion. Thus, she may arrange a work or play situation in which the child's attention is diverted so that the undesirable behavior is interrupted and the tension released. However, if the undesirable behavioral manifestation should occur repeatedly, and a tendency or pattern appear to be developing, the teacher should promptly consult the school nurse or the school physician, the parent, the guidance counselor, or the principal according to the policy of the school. The important thing is to initiate appropriate diagnostic and remedial measures as soon as possible. The procedure which the classroom teacher should follow upon finding a child with observable symptoms should be set forth in the school's health service handbook or the teacher's guide. In the elementary school the child is likely to be referred to the school physician or the nurse, then after parent consultation, to the child's physician or to the school psychologist for testing. Eventually the community resources may be drawn into the diagnostic or therapeutic procedures. Each child must be handled as an individual case and the procedures used should be the best available and the most appropriate for that case.

The Teacher as Catalyst

In addition to the early detection of emotional disturbances, the teacher meets many other opportunities for emphasizing a positive approach to mental health. On both elementary and secondary levels the teacher needs to keep in mind that hostility, although apparently directed at the teacher, may actually be the result of difficulties with a parent or some other adult authority. The feeling of hostility may be simply extended to the teacher as another adult. One tends to meet hostility with hostility. This fans the flame even higher. It is important that the child should learn early in life to handle his hostility before his resentment can mount to explosive size.

On the secondary level the opportunities for the subject teacher to promote mental health are legion. The student talented in music, for example, shares a common vital interest and feels a close kinship with his music teacher. The teacher needs to understand how to guide the pupil's interest more deeply into music, even causing this engrossing interest to serve as an effective step toward fostering a wider range of interest in his studies. The arts afford endless opportunities for the expression of individuality in extremely satisfying ways.

Because all students participate in the program, physical education seems even more replete with opportunities for observation of behavior patterns and personality difficulties. The teacher has the best possible observation point from which to study the student's behavior and relationships in a variety of informal free situations: the playfield, the gymnasium, the swimming pool, the locker room, and other natural situations. Winning and losing, the constantly changing situation in competitive sports and games, the learning of a new skill, and many other kinds of circumstances encountered in the physical education program abound in tests of emotional stability as well as of physical stamina and skills.

The student unable to handle abstract material frequently finds his success in sports. A wise teacher can often help such a student to use this as a stepping stone to successes in other areas. The shy or withdrawn student may find success in an individual type of sport and gradually find himself participating comfortably in group games. The aggressive person can frequently work off his emotions in the combat type of sport. The physical education teacher with some background in and understanding of mental health can often contribute at a case conference and aid in the readjustment of a student with an emotional problem.

The teacher of the adolescent needs to realize his responsibility for the wise handling of a pupil's crush. He needs to remember that the crush may indicate a lack of parental affection and a great emotional void in the life of the student. A crush needs to be handled without inflicting deeper wounds or injuring the student's self-esteem. Attempting to center the student's interest in a group or an activity, giving him a responsibility and due praise for accomplishing it and tactfully including other students in every teacher-pupil contact, are some ways of helping the student to gain emotional satisfaction and maturity.

The lack of parental affection or societal recognition are frequently at the root of sex delinquency, destructiveness, bizarre dress and other reactionary behavior. Often, teachers need to cooperate with the social worker or others concerned with the working out of a family readjustment program for the benefit of the pupil.

Educational Procedures and Mental Health

The central purposes of education and the procedures for attaining them are consistent with desirable life values from the mental health point of view. Included in the usual list of desired mutual goals are the following:

1. Helping the child get along well with others,
2. Learning to work successfully as a member of a group,
3. Establishing goals for himself and working toward their realization,
4. Developing self-discipline and a desirable value system,
5. Learning to lead others with skill and to follow the leadership of others creditably,
6. Recognizing problems and trying to solve them, thereby developing judgment, and experience in decision making,
7. Seeing a task through to completion,
8. Learning to evaluate objectively.

Certainly such goals are sound from the mental health point of view. If the procedures used by the teacher to achieve these goals are conducive to desirable emotional experiences and attitudes on the part of the child, the educational process can be said to contribute effectively to mental health.

It is hoped that the foregoing convincingly indicates that the school can contribute effectively to the success of the total community mental health program through the maintenance of a psychologically sound environment, the provision of adequate physical and mental health instruction, and the early discovery and follow-up of the emotionally disturbed child.

It is only realistic to recognize some urgent needs for the improvement of the situation in the decade ahead. Included are the following:

1. More guidance counselors, psychologists, and psychiatric social workers in schools,
2. More mental health education for prospective teachers and other staff personnel,
3. More research studies:
   (*a*) to understand more adequately emotions, attitudes, motivations, and teaching-learning procedures which would bring greater contributions to mental health,

(*b*) to discover more effective ways of teaching mental health at all school levels,

(*c*) to secure close cooperation among all the mental health resources in a community.

Addictions and Habituations

Addictive diseases, habituations and drug misuse constitute a specialized aspect of the mental health problem. Recent years have witnessed a number of changes in the attitude toward and management of these conditions. There is more general recognition of the growing magnitude of the problem, especially among the young, people are more willing to read, think and speak about it, the medical profession now looks upon it as an illness usually with an underlying socio-psychic base, and not a matter of mere degeneracy, and a number of new approaches to therapy have been developed. It is appropriate to ask, "What is an addiction or habituation?" In simple terms, it is an unreasoned compulsive consumption of certain chemical substances, some of which occur in nature and some man-made, to the ultimate physical, psychic and social detriment of the user. The chemical substances involved fall into four groups: (*a*) alcohol, (*b*) naturally occurring narcotizing alkaloids, (*c*) naturally occurring substances such as marijuana and mescaline which, while non-narcotizing and actually non-addicting, do have the potential to produce various abnormal and deleterious mental effects and aberrations, and (*d*) certain synthetic therapeutic pharmaceuticals. The last of these constitutes a relatively new and increasingly important group, including the barbiturates and other "sleeping pills," amphetamine or benzadrine (pep pills), tranquilizers, euphoriants, and other ataraxics.

Alcohol, narcotics and "mind-expanding" drugs such as lysergic acid diethylamide (LSD) have played a long and diverse role throughout the history of mankind. They have been used as important adjuncts to social intercourse, religious ceremonies, political activities, witchcraft and medicine. Repeated references to their use may be found in the literature of most civilizations. From time immemorial they have been used at festivals to celebrate the harvest or other cyclical natural events, to release the spirit, to provide courage or carelessness to warriors and assassins. In fact, the last word is derived from hashish, the Middle Eastern name for Indian hemp. In some cultures their use has been restricted variously to chieftains, the priesthood, or the medicine man.

Alcoholism

Many people drink alcoholic beverages. In the United States, for example, the number is estimated at about 70 million persons. For most of these, however, no difficulty arises. Only about four and a half million may be regarded as problem drinkers. However, this represents 2.4 per cent of the total population or 7 per cent of those who drink. Furthermore, since six out of seven problem drinkers are adult males, this means a prevalence of 7.5 per cent in the male population over 20 years of age.

Contrary to a frequently held opinion, problem drinking has little relationship to "skid row." The residents of "skid rows" are found there usually for quite different reasons. Not all of them are alcoholics, and those who are usually have alcoholism only as an incidental to other social and behavioral problems. About 80 per cent of problem drinkers are regularly employed, that is up to the point where they may become disabled by their addiction. About three quarters of them are executives in large and small businesses, professional men, salesmen, and skilled laborers. The implication of this in relation to social, economic and professional productivity and morale are obvious.

Fundamentally, there are two types of problem drinkers. The first is an individual who is maladjusted to begin with. Typically he is a neurotic with what is referred to as a constitutional psychoneurotic inferiority which usually stems from early childhood. It is manifest by vague but constant feelings of uncertainty, anxiety, apprehension, inadequacy and inferiority. He feels he is "licked before he starts." As a result he tends to predetermine failure in school, work, love and society. He fears situations which will put him to the test, and wants to avoid them. Alcohol provides a sense of release, some measure of confidence, so why not repeat it? When the effect of alcohol wears off, the problem is compounded because of new feelings of fear, guilt, and rejection, leaving the individual worse off than before. The basic problem is clearly mental, and without psychiatric help the chances of recovery are poor.

The second type of alcoholic is an apparently well-adjusted individual, often somewhat of an extrovert, whose social life and business get him involved in overdrinking. While his action is not compulsive, he begins to let things slide, and begins to lose his sense of responsibility and proportion. This begins to affect his relationships at home and at work. He worries, becomes defensive, then offensive, this causing him to drink more. At first, his family, friends and employers are usually tolerant, but eventually become impatient. He then tends to blame his problems on hard luck and lack of understanding by others. The only thing that restores his ego is more alcohol. As in the first type of case, a vicious cycle is now established. The largest proportion of problem drinkers are in this group. The chances of recovery are much better because the excessive use of alcohol is not superimposed upon a deep-seated basic mental inferiority.

The total cost of alcoholism or problem drinking is difficult or impossible to determine. It has been estimated at about one and one-half billion dollars per year in the United States. This takes into consideration job absenteeism; high spoilage rates of trained individuals; decreased productivity; job turnover; part of the costs of police, jails, hospitals, medical care, social, charitable and welfare agencies; domestic relations organizations and the like. Even less tangible are the ultimate costs to others—children, spouses, parents, friends, and fellow workers.

A factor of particular significance is the relationship of alcohol to accidents. An extensive study of 1,370,000 alcoholics in industry listed 1500 fatal accidents at work and 2850 fatal accidents at home, in public places and in traffic. The total of 4350 represents a death rate from accidents of 321 per 100,000 individuals per year, or twice the rate for non-alcoholic workers. As far as automobile driving is concerned, there is a clearly consistent increase in the probability of accident with an increase in the amount of alcohol in the blood. As little as 0.03 per cent of alcohol in the blood reduces driving skill. The risk at 0.10 per cent is twice that at 0.05 per cent and at 0.15 per cent the risk is increased ten-fold. Studies of traffic deaths in a number of localities have indicated that approximately 50 per cent of automobile-related (driver, passenger, or pedestrian) deaths involved significant blood alcohol levels.

An increasing number of health agencies have established programs to combat this serious and difficult problem. The most effective involve a multidisciplinary approach using medical internists, psychiatrists, social case workers, religious groups and Alcoholics Anonymous. As with all diseases, early diagnosis or recognition is important. This is followed by intensive medical treatment and hospitalization if in an acute stage, psychiatric counselling, group therapy, social and vocational rehabilitation, and religious counselling. One large program involving a university medical center and an extensive manufacturing company achieved the rehabilitation of 70 per cent of problem drinkers by using these approaches intensively.

Drug and Narcotic Addictions

While these conditions are much less common than alcoholism, they represent a most difficult and growing problem. It is important to distinguish between drug habituation and drug addiction. The former results from repeated consumption of a drug, characterized by a desire but not a compulsion to take it, little if any tendency to increase the amount, some degree of psychic but no physical dependence upon it, and by few if any detrimental effects which if they occur involve the habitue alone. Most affinities for the so-called "mind-expanders" and for synthetic drugs are habituations. Drug addiction, on the other hand, is a state of periodic or chronic intoxication produced by the repeated excessive consumption of drugs, usually narcotizing alkaloids, and characterized by an overpowering compulsion and need to obtain and take the drug by any means and regardless of consequence, a tendency to increase the dose, the development of psychic and usually physical dependence upon the effects of the drugs, and detrimental effects on both the individual and society.

About 35,000 narcotic addicts are known and an additional 25,000 are estimated to exist at present in this country. This is a rate of 1 in 3,500 persons in the population. It represents, however, a significant decrease from the rate of 1 in 400 persons in 1914. This is in contrast with the marked increase in the amount of "mind-expanders" and synthetic drugs consumed in the United States. The annual consumption of barbiturates for example, is over 300 tons, or an average of 24 doses of 0.1 gram, per capita in the population! The amount of marijuana currently used is unknown but certainly is increasing significantly. One of the many unfortunate facts concerning narcotic addiction is the age group affected. Fifteen to 25 years of age is the most susceptible period. It is more common in males than in females, but the difference is not as great as with alcoholism. Most addicts are in the upper and lower socio-economic groups, the middle third tending to be spared. Those addicted live for the most part in large cities convenient to illicit supplies of narcotics and 77 per cent are in the four states of New York (45 per cent), Illinois (14 per cent), California (13 per cent) and Michigan (5 per cent).

There is a marked uniformity in the personalities and backgrounds of boys who become addicted to narcotics. Typically, they are non-aggressive, and passive, giving a false appearance of ease and poise. Their interpersonal relationships are weak and superficial with the notable exception of their relationship with their mother, which is very close. They tend to have many acquaintances but few friends. Often they were their mother's favorite. Many choose domestic occupations such as cooking or tailoring.

Narcotic addicts may be considered in four categories depending upon the reasons for addiction. The first and largest group consists of neurotics who resort to drugs in order to overcome their feelings of fear, inadequacy and inferiority. The second are psychopaths who take drugs as part of their deliberate and determined search for thrills or "kicks." This is probably the smallest group. Third, is a group of relatively normal individuals, usually adolescents, who succumb to urging to "try" the drug, to be one of the group, or to regard it as a manifestation of protest against the real or imagined restraints and errors of parents and society. The size of this group varies through time and place, depending upon cultural mores, fluctuations in group behavior, fads, law enforcement, availability of supplies and other factors. Finally, there is a small group of emotionally well-adjusted persons who take or are administered narcotics for pain and who may, if treatment is prolonged, become addicted. From the standpoints of addiction-proneness, and low rehabilitation potential, the first two groups, neurotics and psychopaths, are the most difficult and serious.

Treatment and rehabilitation of the true narcotic addict is difficult and discouraging. Withdrawal is a very painful and sometimes dangerous process. Two things are certain: (*a*) prevention offers the only successful long-term approach, and (*b*) the place for an existing narcotic addict is in a hospital, not in a prison. The Public Health Service operates two large federally supported hospitals for narcotic addicts at Lexington, Kentucky and at Fort Worth, Texas. Every practical approach to treatment is used, medical and psychiatric therapy, nursing care, social case work, education, vocational rehabilitation and religious counselling. Many, however, cannot be rehabilitated, and of those who are, 3 out of 4 relapse and are readmitted subsequently. When cure is accomplished, it usually follows several relapses.

Prevention involves several factors, a desirable parent-child relationship, good education by competent alert and understanding teachers, and vigilant customs and law enforcement. Great Britain has achieved some success by attempting to attack the economic base of the illicit narcotic trade which keeps the fires of addiction smoldering. The method has been simply to make narcotics available to addicts under a controlled program. An individual, under the law, may declare himself an addict to a physician who registers him as such. This entitles him to an adequate maintenance supply of a narcotic at minimal or no cost. The goal is to reduce or eliminate the profit potential from the illicit drug "racket," and to put an end to efforts to "hook" susceptible young people. While the theory and logic of this approach seem sound, for a variety of reasons, the incidence of new drug addictions has actually increased.

What the Teacher Can Do

Children need to be fortified with sound facts before they encounter the problem of depressants and stimulants so that they may be prepared to act wisely in situations which otherwise they might not even recognize as dangerous. It has been rather generally recognized that because of the sharp rise in drug abuse, education needs to begin early and extend from kindergarten through grade 12. As a result of viewing television at home, even small children have been exposed to constant glimpses of commercials for various types of pharmaceuticals. The school, therefore, has an obligation to incorporate in the curriculum at appropriate levels, the teaching of scientific facts concerning the various depressants and stimulants, their immediate and long-range effects, and the inherent and related dangers. School personnel need to see this problem in its community setting, to know what is being done by the other agencies concerned, and to understand the role of the school in the total picture.

The teacher needs to be alert for early signs of emotional patterns which are characteristic of frank or incipient alcoholic and drug addiction: inability to handle frustrations and conflicts, loneliness, inability to relate to people, excessive shyness, habitual use of escape and withdrawal mechanisms, or extreme immaturity for the age level. It is important that teachers realize the potential seriousness of these behavior patterns and draw such children into social situations which will encourage and help them to establish sound mental health habits.

About the time of adolescence, the peer group becomes all-important to the child and, as a determinant of behavior, frequently supersedes the influence of the parent and the school. Curiosity becomes intensified, the tendency to protest, dissension and even rebellion become greater, the desire for adventure grows keener, and leads to eager experimentation, characteristics which peddlers of drugs count upon. For experimentation this age group turns most often to tobacco, alcohol, and marijuana, and sometimes barbiturates and heroin. Students tend to follow the example of their elders in the use of coffee, tea, and cola drinks. Aspirin is widely used, and sometimes so-called "pep pills," especially at examination time and at parties. These tendencies indicate the teacher's special responsibility to stress in health courses and in other related subjects or situations in which they might fit naturally, the following areas of information:

1. The names of commonly known depressants and stimulants, their contents or classification, dangers, and in some cases, legitimate uses and sources
2. The reasons why people use depressants and stimulants
3. The progression from experimentation to habituation, addiction, and dependence
4. The true nature of addiction
5. The nature and extent of illicit and anti-social traffic in depressants and stimulants, and methods of involving young people
6. The importance of reading labels on patent medicines to discover alcoholic and narcotic content (cough remedies, tonics, and others)
7. The dangers of self-medication, including the danger of deadening pain without removing the cause
8. The psychological, social, and economic effects upon the individual, the family, and the community.

It is most important that the teaching-learning atmosphere be kept objective and that the pupils' questions be answered as fully as possible and in ways that are emotionally satifying. Teachers responsible for school social events, athletic affairs, and other occasions, which draw crowds of non-school persons, need to plan carefully to offset possible experimentation with depressants or stimulants, or situations which could make it possible. The teacher should know the signs and symptoms associated with the most common narcotics and report possible suspects to the appropriate school person.

Along with the information concerning addictive diseases, the teacher needs to emphasize positive ways of coping with the underlying mental and emotional problems, particularly recreational interests such as scouting, sports participation, hobbies, church activities, and other community affairs. On the preventive side, in many places parent-teacher organizations have faced the social situation in company with the children and have evolved social codes which have proved effective means of setting conduct standards and a common social code for the area. The whole problem of addictive diseases with its many ramifications should be recognized as a community concern and responsibility. The teacher should use every opportunity to encourage other agencies and community leaders to participate in a joint approach toward solution. The teacher needs to cooperate with the home, the social worker, the school nurse, and other persons responsible for the follow-up of the individual pupil in preventive and rehabilitative measures.

Questions for Discussion

1. What facilities in the form of hospitals, out-patient clinics, and the like are there in your community for the treatment of the mentally ill?
2. What phases of the public health program of your community contribute to the prevention and promotion of mental illness?
3. Is there a voluntary agency primarily concerned with the problem of mental illness and/or addictions? What types of activities does it engage in?
4. Is there an alcoholism program in your community? What does it consist of, and how extensively is it used?
5. What is the attitude in your community toward problems such as mental illness, alcoholism, and addictions?
6. Does the school system of your community provide special facilities and classes for children who are handicapped by various types of mental problems?
7. What do you consider to be the teacher's role in mental health?
8. Contrast the narcotics control program of Great Britain with that of the U.S. Which do you think has the greater chance of success in the long run?
9. Do you consider there is any relationship between mental health and juvenile delinquency?

Suggested Reading

1. SANDERS, D. S.: *A Bookshelf on Mental Health,* Am. J. Pub. Health 55:502, 1965.
2. *What Are the Facts About Mental Illness in the United States,* Washington, D.C., National Committee Against Mental Illness, 1957.
3. RIDENOUR, NINA: *Mental Health in the United States,* Cambridge, Harvard University Press, 1961.
4. PASAMANICK, BENJAMIN, (Ed.): *Epidemiology of Mental Disorder,* Washington, Am. Assn. for Advmt. of Science, 1959:
5. *National Action to Combat Mental Retardation, Report of President's Panel on Mental Retardation,* Washington, U.S. Supt. of Documents, 1962.
6. HIMWICK, HAROLD E.: *Alcoholism,* Washington, Am. Assn. Advmt. of Science, 1957.
7. HAGGARD, HOWARD W. AND JELLINEK, E. M.: *Alcohol Explored,* Garden City, Doubleday & Co., Inc., 1954.

8. McCarthy, Raymond G.: *Teenagers and Alcohol,* New Haven, Yale Center for Alcohol Studies, 1956.
9. Winick, C.: *The Narcotic Addiction Problem,* New York, Amer. Social Hygiene Assn, 1964.
10. Tolalay, P. and Minagham, J. H.: *Drugs in Our Society,* Baltimore, The Johns Hopkins Press, 1964.
11. *Mental Disorders: A Guide to Control Methods,* New York, Amer. Pub. Health Assn., 1962.
12. Jahoda, Marie: *Current Concepts of Positive Mental Health,* New York, Basic Books, Inc., 1958.
13. Kotinsky, R. and Witmer, H. L. (Eds.): *Community Programs for Mental Health,* Cambridge, Harvard University Press, 1955.
14. Allinsmith, W. and Goethals, J. E.: *The Role of the Schools in Mental Health,* (A Report of the Joint Commission on Mental Illness and Health), New York, Basic Books, 1961.
15. *Fostering Mental Health in Schools,* 1950 Yearbook: Association for Supervision and Curriculum Development, Washington, D.C., National Education Association, 1950.
16. Farnsworth, Dana L.: *Mental Health in College and University,* Cambridge, Harvard University Press, 1957.
17. Erikson, Erik H.: *Childhood and Society.* 2nd Ed. New York, W. W. Norton & Co., Inc., 1964.

Chapter 7

Silent Saboteurs—
The Chronic Diseases

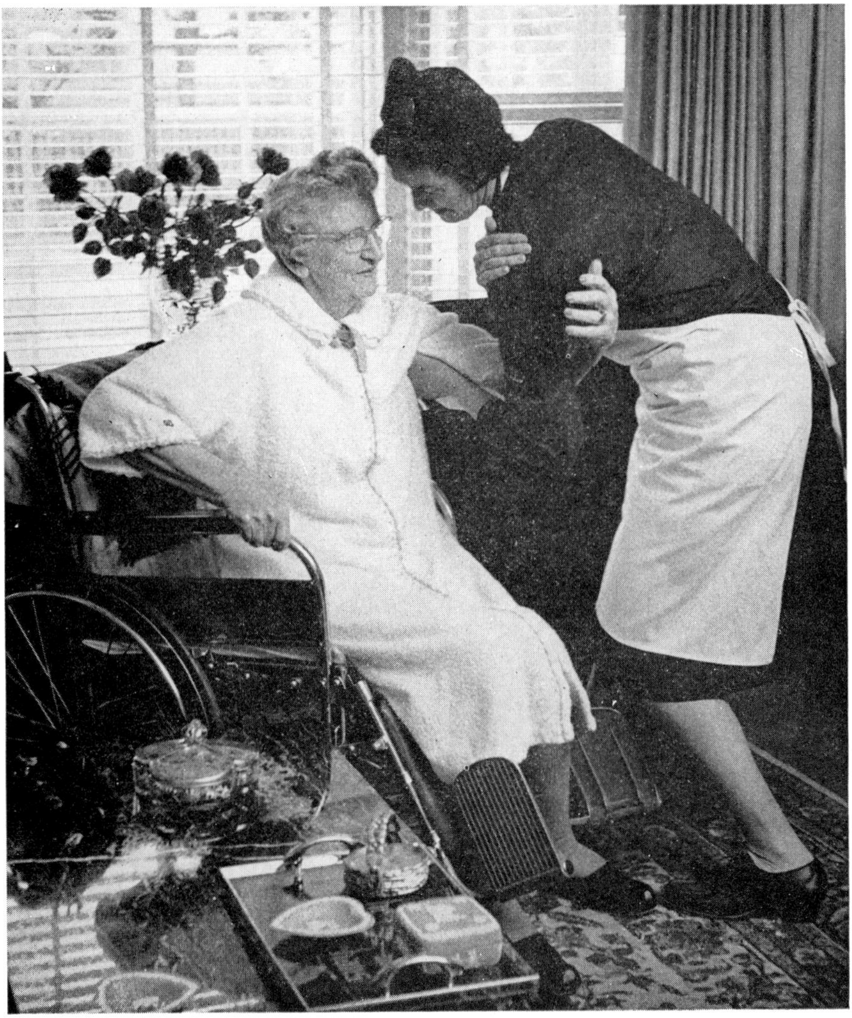

Fig. 38. Victim!

The Problem Appears

One of the consequences of success is often the development of new problems. This has been true in the case of improved public health and medical care. Elsewhere there has been described the remarkable decrease in the incidence of most of the acute communicable diseases, many of the chronic communicable diseases, notably tuberculosis, as well as deaths related to child bearing and the early months and years of life. In 1900, about 40 out of each 100 persons who died were less than 25 years of age. The corresponding proportion now is less than 10 out of every 100 persons. Whereas at the beginning of this century 61 per cent of deaths in the United States were caused by infectious and parasitic diseases, by now only about 6 per cent of deaths are attributable to such causes. Conversely, during the same period of time, the proportionate importance of chronic and degenerative diseases as causes of death has increased from 28 to 80 per cent. Another consequence of the conquest of the great killers of the early part of life has been the cutting of the crude or general death rate in the United States in half, from 17.8 per 1000 population in 1900 to 9.5 in 1969, and the adding of from 20 to 25 years to the average expectancy of life at birth, from 47 years in 1900 to an average of over 70 years in 1969.

Unfortunately, these benefits have not been uniform throughout the population. With regard to age, the percentage decline in the death rate has been much greater in the younger than in the older age groups. In other words, the older population has not benefitted to the extent observed in the younger part of the population (Fig. 39).

Nevertheless, as a result of these forces, certain dramatic changes have taken place in the age distribution of the over-all population. Many people, who otherwise would have died in childhood or early

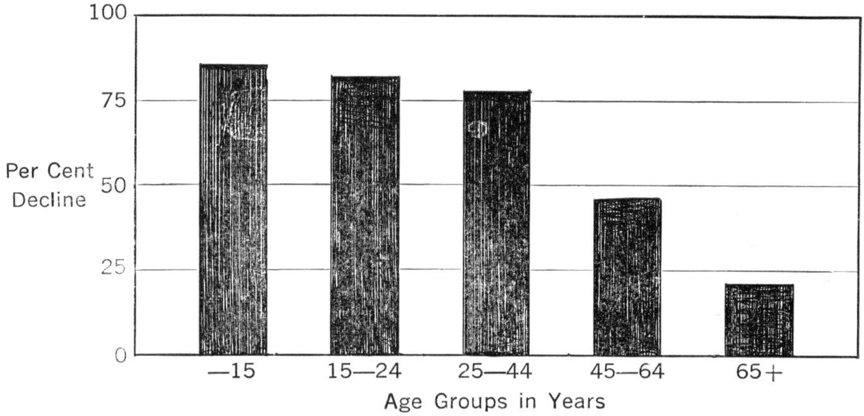

FIG. 39. Proportionate decline in death rates by age United States, 1900 to 1969

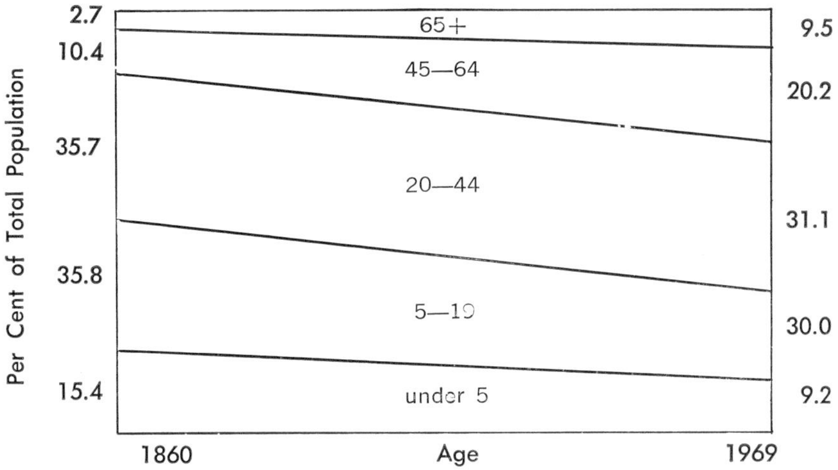

FIG. 40. Change in age distribution, United States, 1860 to 1969.

adulthood, have been allowed to achieve advanced adulthood or old age. This is emphasized by the fact that while the population of the United States has doubled since 1900, the number of persons 65 years or more of age has increased sixfold from 3,080,000 or 4.1 per cent of the population to 19,130,000 or 9.5 per cent of the population in 1969 (Fig. 40). In terms of this rate of change it is estimated that by 1980, about 25,000,000 or more than 1 out of every 10 citizens will be 65 years or older. One of the effects of these changes is to increase the so-called dependency ratio (proportion of the population under 20 and over 65 years). In 1940 there were in the United States about 70 dependents for each 100 individuals of working age. By 1980 it is estimated that the ratio will reach 100, meaning that each average worker will be supporting at least one non-productive person.

Because of the discrepancy in the death rates by sex, for each 100 older men there will be 138 older women. This has far reaching sociological and economic consequences. It means an increasing number of older women left alone, and it also means an already significant concentration of the national wealth in the hands of the female component of the population. Undoubtedly, as many have pointed out, the difference in life expectancy between men and women is attributable not so much to the "frail male" as to the apparently increased cultural pressures and expectations placed upon the average urban American male. Similar discrepancies exist with relation to the races, the non-white population lagging behind the white component of the population in improvement of death rates and life expectancy, hence, degree of shift to the older ages. However, this discrepancy has been narrowing during recent years (Table 9).

Table 9. Life Expectancy at Specific Ages by Sex and Race United States, 1967

Years of Age	*0*	*5*	*15*	*25*	*35*	*45*	*55*	*65*	*75*
white female	75.1	71.5	61.7	52.1	42.5	33.2	24.5	16.5	9.9
white male	67.8	64.6	54.9	45.7	36.4	27.4	19.5	13.0	8.2
non-white female	68.2	65.8	56.1	46.6	37.7	29.4	21.9	15.8	12.0
non-white male	61.1	59.0	49.4	40.5	32.2	24.6	18.0	12.7	10.3

The Price of Longer Life

Prolonged survival, however, brings its handicaps and problems. The majority of the increasing number who are now reaching advanced ages are by no means in good health. On the one hand, they reap the delayed consequences of now more evident illnesses and injuries that occurred during their youth and young adulthood. On the other hand, they have added the burden of a wide array of conditions which are

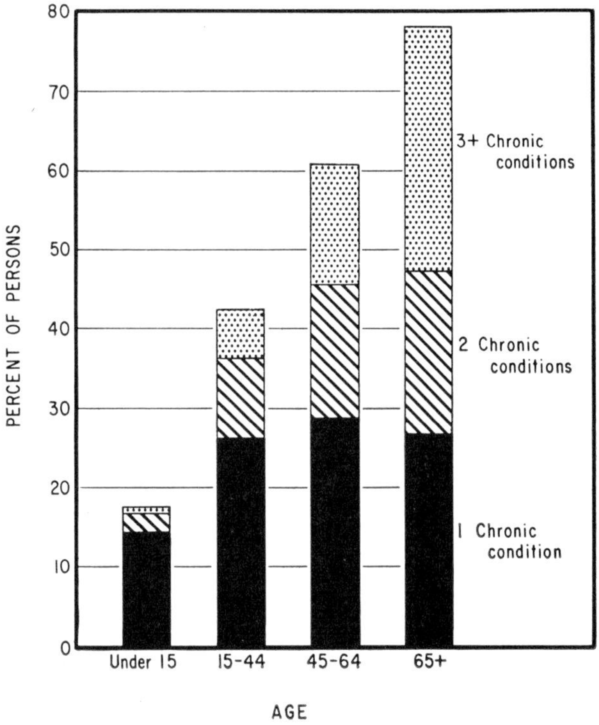

FIG. 41. Percentage of persons with chronic conditions according to age. (Health Statistics, National Health Survey, Series B-11, Pub. Health Service Publ. No. 584-B-11, p. 2, Washington, July 1959.)

more or less peculiar to advancing years. This is illustrated in Figure 41, which presents the increase in the amount of chronic illness as one becomes older. It should be noted that a surprising 17 per cent of children under 15 years of age have some chronic illness which actually or potentially requires medical care or is disabling, although only 1.4 per cent actually limit activity. A much greater cause for concern and ultimate consequence is the 42 per cent of those between the ages of 15 and 44 years, supposedly the healthy young-adult period of early productive life, who have some chronic illness. From here the figures jump to 61 per cent in the age group 44 to 64 years, and to more than 78 per cent of persons 65 years or older. Only 22 per cent of those in this higher age group do not suffer from a chronic illness. Furthermore, the majority of those affected are decidedly limited in mobility and activity (Fig. 42). Undoubtedly, if greater attention were given to healthy living and to the prevention of physical and mental insults during childhood and young adulthood, there would be less tendency for the advanced years of life to be synonymous with senility.

The extent to which chronic non-communicable diseases assume the dominant role in the older population may be appreciated by a consid-

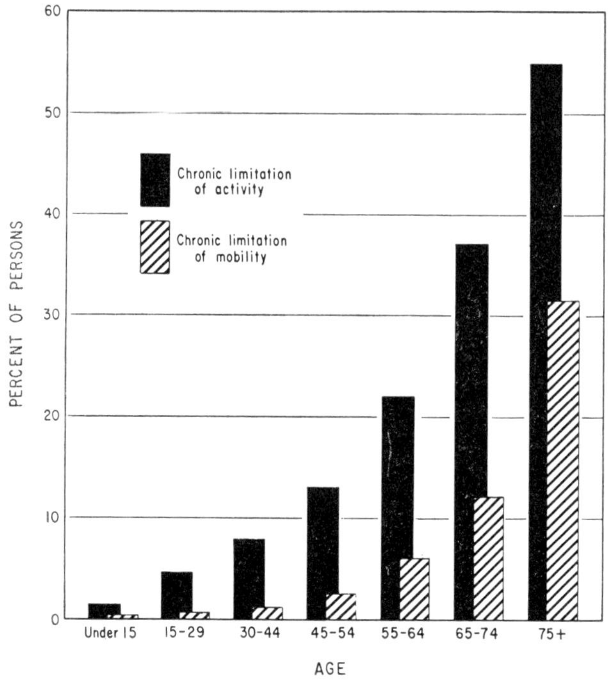

FIG. 42. Percentage of persons with any degree of chronic limitation of activity and mobility according to age. (Health Statistics, National Health Survey, Series B-11, Public Health Service Publ. No. 584-B-11, p., 1, Washington, July 1959.)

eration of their illnesses. Surveys have shown that about 30 per cent of those over 65 years of age suffer a day or more from a respiratory disease during the course of a year. This incidence is less than found in the general population. However, almost one-quarter had a degenerative disease which incapacitated for at least a day, and about one-eighth were ill at some time from a digestive condition. Six per cent suffered from a rheumatic or related condition, 3 per cent from a skin disease and 2 per cent from a nervous disease. More than 8 per cent were incapacitated for a day or more because of accidental injuries. In addition, but not included above, are a considerable frequency of foot ailments and visual defects which limit ambulation and promote accidents, as well as many hearing defects and a great amount of dental difficulty which affects mastication, hence diet and nutrition. These most common illnesses, however, are not prominent as causes of death in the elderly. Death, as already indicated, is usually caused by what may be called "silent saboteurs," conditions the seeds of which were usually planted may years before and which develop quietly and insidiously. Table 10 presents, for example, the ten leading causes of death between the ages of 65 and 74 years. They account for almost 90 per cent of deaths in that age perod. From the list one can sense for the most part, the surrender of worn and abused cells, tissues and organs.

Where Does the Problem Begin?

This leads to a recognition of one of the difficulties encountered in considering the problem of chronic diseases. There is an unfortunate tendency to regard them as unique to the older component of the population, almost as if they suddenly developed *de novo*. This error in judgment is compounded by a further inclination to evaluate the relative importance of chronic conditions essentially in terms of the frequency with which they cause the ultimate demise of individuals.

Table 10. The Ten Leading Causes of Death, 65 to 74 Years United States, 1967

Rank	*Cause of Death*	*Deaths per 100,000 Pop.*
1.	Heart disease	2,229.8
2.	Malignant neoplasms	768.8
3.	Vascular lesions of central nervous system	412.6
4.	Diabetes mellitus	94.2
5.	Accidents	91.2
6.	Influenza and pneumonia	85.2
7.	General arteriosclerosis	48.4
8.	Cirrhosis of liver	41.1
9.	Symptoms, senility, and ill-defined conditions	37.8
10.	Ulcer of stomach	22.3

This raises the question for serious consideration—which, in the final analysis, is the more important, the quality of living or the nature of death?

Reexamination of Figure 41 brings out the fact that, while chronic conditions are most frequent in the elderly, a significant number and proportion of the younger part of the population are affected by them. Indeed, it is quite clear that there is a relationship between these two facts, the one contributing or leading to the other. Thus, chronic illness in school children obviously is of immediate concern in relation to interference with education. Similarly, chronic illness in the young adult has attracted national attention because of the large proportion of young men found to be ineligible for service in the armed forces (Table 11). However, there is a much more important reason for concern over the prevalence of chronic conditions in both of these younger age groups. It is the extent to which they contribute to serious and irreparable impairment later on in life.

In addition to the chronic metabolic diseases, such as obesity and diabetes, and the chronic degenerative diseases, such as cardio-vascular-renal conditions, cancer and the like, all of which occur to some extent early in life and gradually increase in seriousness and may kill, there are various other chronic conditions which impair or limit one's function and living activity. For the most part, these too appear to affect young persons minimally, only to increase rapidly in prevalence as years are added to life. Figure 43 presents this visually for a number of these conditions.

Table 11. Medical Reasons for Selective Service Rejection 1953–1958*

Diagnostic Category	*Prevalence per 1000 Examinees*
Disorders of bones and organs of movement	25.4
Psychiatric disorders	21.1
Diseases of circulatory system	19.1
Eye diseases and defects	18.3
Anthropometric reasons (mostly obesity)	11.5
Diseases and defects of ear and mastoid	10.0
Diseases of digestive system	9.2
Allergic disorders	8.6
Infective and parasitic diseases	7.1
Neurologic diseases	7.1
Congenital defects	6.2
All other reasons	25.1
Total	168.7

*Karpinos, B.D.: Qualification of American Youths for Military Service, Medical Statistics Division, Office of the Surgeon General, Dept. of the Army, 1962.

What Can be Done?

Until rather recently, the problem of chronic illness and disability was surrounded by an aura of fatalism and defeatism. Fortunately this has been shifting rapidly during the past two decades to an attitude of determination based upon an increasing number of scientific and philosophic advances. Already it is well recognized that much

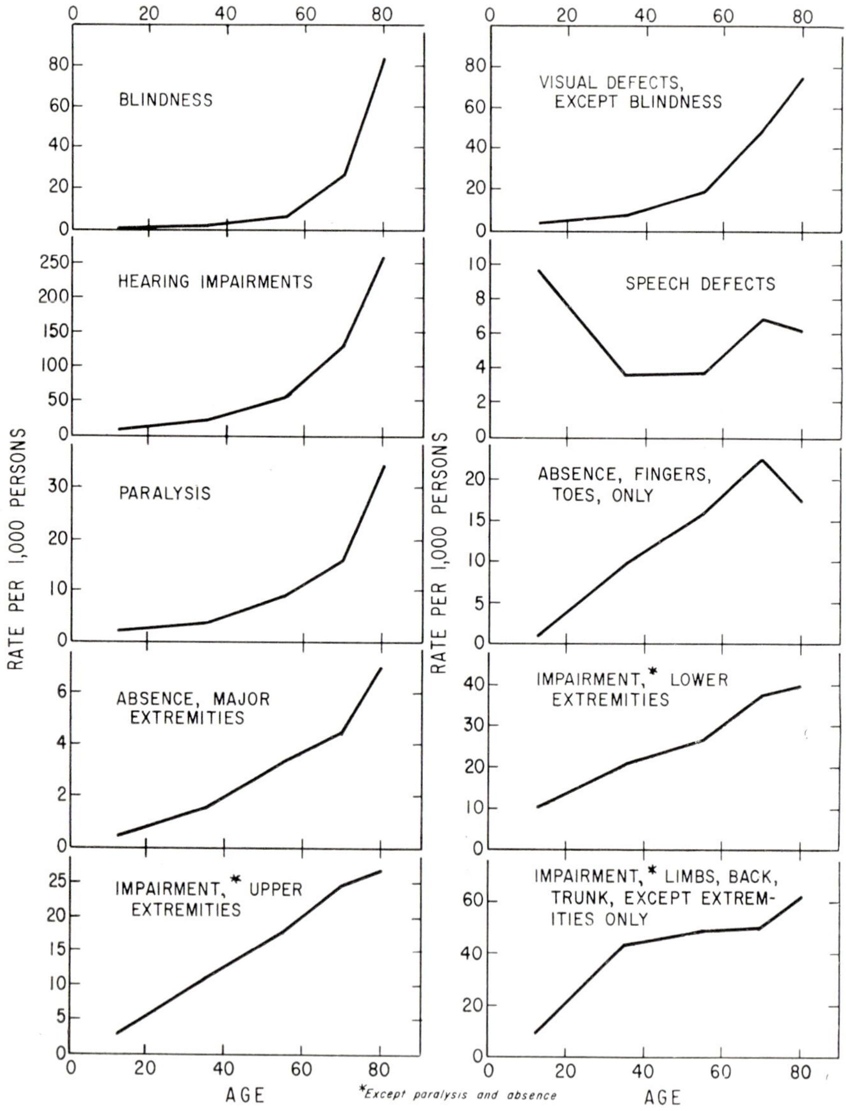

FIG. 43. Number of impairments per 1000 persons according to type of impairment by age. (Health Statistics, National Health Survey, Series B-9, Public Health Service Publ. N. 584-B-9, p. 3, Washington, April, 1959.)

may be accomplished even within the limitations of existing knowledge. As a result, chronic illness and disability which previously were regarded as indvidual and private matters are now considered to be within the province of general public or social concern. This does not mean that the solution of the problem and the meeting of all needs must necessarily become the exclusive responsibility of governmental or social agencies. To the contrary, it emphasizes the necessity to bring to bear all of the many and varied private and public resources to the end of solving a problem of both private and public concern. This involves the individual citizen, private medical and paramedical practitioners, clinics, hospitals and health centers, official and voluntary health agencies, a wide variety of social agencies, and very importantly the schools, to mention but a few of those who have a contribution to make and a role to play. If ever, in the field of health and well being, a true partnership was needed, it is here.

A complete program for attack upon the massive problem of chronic disease is necessarily multifaceted. It should involve at least the following six steps:

1. *Health Protection and Promotion.* This includes the best possible care of expectant mothers, their proper delivery, and complete infant, preschool and school health services. Attention should be given to nutrition, physical fitness and all such positive protective and promotive activities. These activities are considered in more detail elsewhere in this book.
2. *Hygienic Education.* The goal is the development in every individual of a fund of practical, scientifically correct information about daily living, physical and mental development, health and disease, diet, and the formation of desirable hygienic habits. These are also dealt with more extensively in other parts of this book.
3. *Primary Prevention.* This is aimed at the avoidance of the actual occurrence of disease. Included should be a comprehensive immunization program, the avoidance of chronic disease-forming habits such as alcoholism and smoking, the prophylactic use of antibiotics where indicated, the use of fluoride either in water or directly on the teeth, driver education, and the like.
4. *Secondary Prevention.* Because of their insidious nature, many chronic diseases cannot be prevented from occurring. Their effects may be minimized, however, by means of earliest possible diagnosis and treatment thereby preventing their progression to an irreparable or even fatal extent. Certain self-observation and examination procedures are useful here, augmented either by periodic medical examinations or at least screening tests.

With regard to comprehensive medical examinations, the following schedule is recommended:

Prenatal—as early in pregnancy as possible and as often as the obstetrician advises
Infant—immediately after birth and at least three times during first year of life
Preschool—at least once
Primary school—on admission and at least once more during the first six grades
Secondary school—on admission and before graduation
20–39 years—at least once
40–49 years—at least twice
50–59 years—at least thrice
60 years and thereafter—every year

To supplement periodic comprehensive medical examinations, there are now available a number of very useful screening tests, by means of which a large proportion of possible chronic conditions may be found early before they have progressed too far. Included among these are the following:

Ailment	***Test***
Tuberculosis	Chest x ray
Syphilis	Blood test
Diabetes	Blood and urine sugar tests
Visual loss and some other eye defects	Visual field acuity
Glaucoma	Tonometry and visual field
Hearing loss	Audiometry
Dental caries and periodontal disease	Dental examination and x-ray
Heart disease	Electrocardiogram and chest x-ray
Hypertension	Blood pressure determination
Kidney disease	Urine tests for albumin
Obesity	Height and weight measurements
Cancer of the breast	Palpation and mammography
Cancer of the uterus	Papanicolaou smear test

It is anticipated that through time additional screening tests will be added to this list.

5. *Prevention and Control of Disability.* This is essentially the assurance of the earliest possible and most intensive medical care of whatever conditions are definitively diagnosed. The intent is prevention of progression of the disease or disability. This may require physicians, surgeons, dentists, nurses, social case workers, physical and occupational therapists, home nursing services, homemakers services, and individuals from many other fields. Often it will necessitate provision of care in hospitals and other institutions specializing in post hospital or custodial care.

6. *Rehabilitation.* This so-called "fourth phase of medicine" is designed to serve those who are already disabled by birth, disease or accident. Ideally it involves complete medical, social, psychological and vocational evaluation. On the basis of these, goals are set and corrective measures designed to minimize the limitations of the particular condition and to maximize the usefulness in daily living of the facilities which the afflicted individual possesses.

The Chronically Ill or Disabled Child

In the case of a child with a chronic disability, the primary responsibility of the school is to cooperate in every way possible with the program of treatment prescribed by the family physician. It is the duty

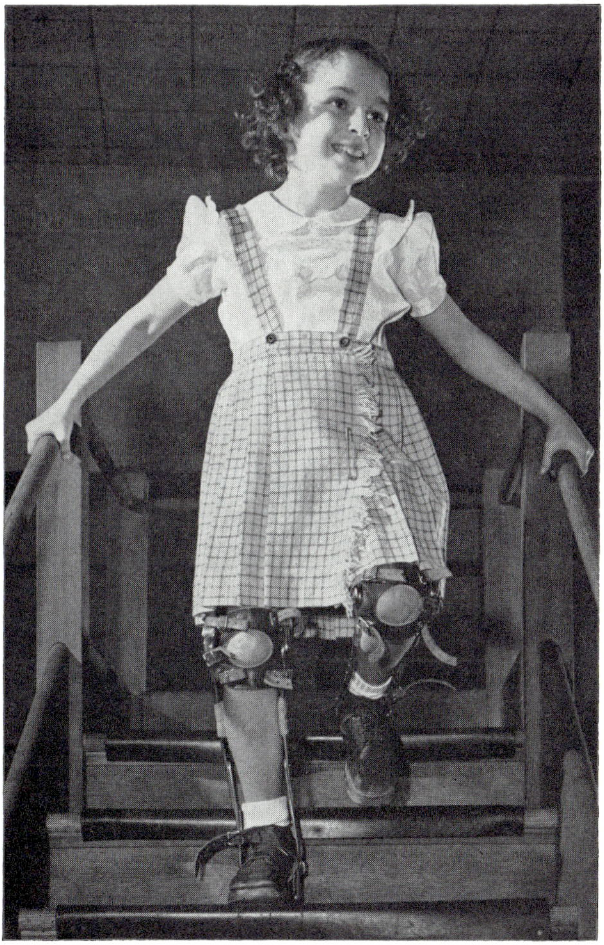

FIG. 44. I too want to play.

of the school physician or nurse to obtain pertinent information from the parent and family physician and to plan with the school staff the best possible daily school routine for the child. The child should be studied from every angle and the decision as to the most suitable educational program should be determined cooperatively.

A large proportion of children with a chronic disease or disability are able to attend regular class and carry a regular schedule. As an indication of what can be done in this regard, Table 12 presents the experience of 98 cities with populations over 100,000 in relation to almost 300,000 handicapped children.

For the sake of his emotional and social development, it is highly desirable that the child be permitted to be with his peer group. The details of the individual child's daily routine can be arranged through the cooperation of the school nurse, the principal, the guidance counselor, and the classroom or homeroom teacher. According to his special health and physical needs, rest periods, supplementary feedings, limited or adapted exercise periods, an elevator pass, a duplicate set of books, transportation to and from school or other ameliorative measures might be instituted.

In some instances, it may seem desirable to have the child assigned to a small special class whose daily routine is centered around health matters with individual attention to each child's problem. For the child whose physical activity is greatly restricted, or whose frequent absence from school is definitely anticipated, or whose physical limitation is known to be merely temporary, this might be a wise decision. However, the child's condition and his reactions should be carefully studied before such assignment is made. If the special class is located within a regular school building, it is sometimes possible to have the child participate in certain classes in company with his regular group. At the

Table 12. Educational Services Provided for Handicapped Children*

Handicap	*Number of Children*	*% in Regular Classes*	*% in Special Classes*	*% in other Placement*†
Cleft palate	678	82	17	1
Epilepsy	1,746	79	9	12
Speech defect	157,392	74	24	2
Rheumatic fever, heart disease	6,174	66	8	26
Hard of hearing	5,109	53	40	7
Orthopedic	18,437	21	13	66
Partially sighted	4,653	14	76	10
Mentally retarded	85,649	13	81	6
Emotionally disturbed	11,231	11	31	58
Blind	1,227	5	74	21
Deaf	3,700	4	40	56

* Wallace, H. M. and Starr, H. M., APHA Conference Report, Pub. Health Rep., *74*, 256, 1959.

† Includes special schools, home or hospital instruction.

time of assignment to a special class of this type, provision should be made for future periodic reviews of the child's health progress, with the possibility of his ultimate restoration to regular class.

Under some circumstances, such as tedious travel to and from school, lack of elevator service, or similar problems, it might be best for the child with a chronic disease or disability to remain at home. Most school districts provide a visiting teacher for individual instruction of the homebound. Naturally this plan of scheduling definite hours each week calls for complete cooperation on the part of the parent. Today, in some communities, it is possible to arrange for home instruction by telephone. This gives the child the opportunity to receive instruction directly from the regular teacher, to hear class discussion, and upon signal, to ask questions. Instruction by closed television circuit is also a possibility in some places. A hospitalized child is sometimes able to attend a school conducted on the premises by a qualified teacher. In other instances the school district may provide individual instruction during the child's hospital stay.

In all of these plans, the school nurse is likely to serve as the coordinator of the efforts of the health team concerned with the child, to keep accurate, cumulative records of the child's progress, and to stimulate periodic re-evaluation.

The Teacher and the Handicapped Child*

The classroom teacher can help the child immeasurably in his personal adjustment to life with the special limitations imposed by his chronic disease or disability, and in guiding his education toward the achievement of realistic goals. The child's foremost problem is to learn to accept himself with his limitations, and to learn to live with them as happily and effectively as possible. During his illness he has perhaps found himself the center of anxious attention in the home or in the hospital. As a result, he may appear unduly self-centered or even spoiled, expecting immediate response to his least whim. Often he is worried, anxious, tense, and insecure. Sometimes he is spoiled, demanding, stubborn or overbearing.

It is important that the teacher accept the child as he is and try to understand the causes which underlie his behavior. In fact, understanding of his physical condition and the regimen outlined by his physician are imperative in order that the teacher may cooperate intelligently within the framework of the total program. Through careful planning, she should strive to help the child establish some realizable goals so that he may win the successes so necessary to building up feelings of security and self-confidence.

*This important subject is discussed in more detail in Chapter 12.

Since his illness has probably curtailed the child's usual opportunities for social development, the teacher needs to provide work and play experiences in small groups and thus help him to increase his ability to relate to others. These experiences will lead to his eventual acceptance by the class and by the school. Moreover, he will gradually realize that his acceptance is related to his own participation and contribution to the group. Classroom activities might well include some emphasis upon leisure time skills and interests, for these too lead to friendships and social development. The teacher can overcome signs of apathy and resignation by interesting the child in noting his own progress by means of self-evaluations.

The child needs to be encouraged to become a productive member of his family group and to contribute in some way to the family's daily routine. Through school experiences it is possible to help him build good work habits. The teacher should encourage him to be realistic and, to adjust to the idea of the world of work, especially at the secondary school level. The child with a chronic condition often has to adjust his vocational sights to the realities of his condition. The parent too, may need help in readjusting his own ambition for his child. The teacher is in a position to aid both.

Often the teacher can help the parent realize that the child, particularly the adolescent, needs to gain a feeling of independence, despite the existence of a serious or chronic illness or disability. Activity or food restrictions at this age level can be embarrassing, but careful planning can minimize these feelings. Through their joint approach to such problems, the parent will gradually appreciate the need for consistency in the child's environment and seek the teacher's aid in order to assure it.

During fire drills, civilian defense drills, field trips, and other special events, the teacher may need to make special provision for the chronically ill or disabled child. However, her plans must conform with the policy of the school and the school district.

Special Problems of Chronically Ill Children

Diabetes. Today most diabetics are taught to take responsibility for their own routine and receive careful instructions from the physician or clinic nurse. The teacher needs to cooperate with the policies and wishes of the child's physician in every respect and follow his instructions in case of signs of insulin shock or coma. The teacher of a very young diabetic child needs to be watchful about his adherence to his special diet during snack or lunch time, and particularly at a school party or picnic.

Rheumatic Heart Conditions. In the case of rheumatic heart disease, the school nurse should inform the teacher about restrictions necessary in the child's daily regimen as relayed to her by the parent and the family physician. Usually, the two main areas for teacher concern are the avoidance of re-infection, and the limitation of physical activity. The teacher should be familiar with early or suspicious signs or symptoms of rheumatic heart disease and realize that chronic fatigue, infection, so-called growing pains, and other unusual conditions should be reported to the nurse promptly. With other cardiac conditions, the nurse and the teacher should cooperate with the recommendations of the family physician.

Allergies. The parent and the school nurse should inform the teacher about the child who has significant allergies such as asthma, hay fever, skin reactions, and the causes if they are known. This is important, for the teacher may be able to protect the child from exposure to the irritant. Since fatigue and psychological disturbances are often considered as contributory causes of an attack, the teacher can perhaps reduce the possibility by recognizing the need for rest and relaxation, by setting goals within the reasonable reach of the child, and the maintenance of a calm friendly atmosphere. In the case of asthma, the teacher may need some specific instruction as to what to do to help the child in his struggle for breath should an attack happen in school.

Epilepsy. With today's wide use of special efficacious drugs, the epileptic child is not so likely to have a seizure in school. However, the teacher needs to be informed about specific ways in which she may cooperate with the child who is aware of warnings (aura) of an impending attack. If a seizure of grand mal should occur in school, the teacher needs to be prepared to care for the child in an approved first aid manner. But her task also involves the calming of the other children and in helping them view the attack as an illness and to accept the child as an ill child without attaching stigma.

In case of petit mal, the teacher can tactfully steer the attention of the class away from the affected pupil. If the child's attacks should intensify or occur more frequently, the teacher should inform the school nurse.

Summary. Regardless of the nature of the chronic illness, the teacher can help the child merely by easing pressures, by regulating the amount of homework, and by giving assignments far in advance. Frequently she can minimize tension through individual help and direction in study periods. All efforts of the school health team should be geared toward the total health of the total child, with the intent of helping him become to the greatest degree possible, a happy, self-accepting individual and a self-supporting, contributing citizen.

Questions for Discussion

1. What is the age distribution of the population in your community? Has it been changing during recent decades? How?

2. If there is a general hospital in your community, determine the percentage of people who are admitted to the out-patient clinics and to the in-patient facilities for chronic, non-communicable illnesses. What are the predominant conditions?
3. Is there a program in your community for the home care of the sick? What agency or agencies are involved in it?
4. What facilities or programs are there for the promotion of good health among the older population of your community? Does your community have any special housing facilities for people of advanced years?
5. What is the status of nursing homes for the elderly in your community? Are conditions in them supervised by any agency?
6. Determine the program of your school system in relation to children with various physical handicaps. Do you think it is adequate?
7. Does the health department or any other agency in your community conduct programs for the early detection of any of the chronic diseases such as cancer, diabetes, glaucoma and the like?
8. How can the individual help his physician in the early detection and treatment of specific chronic diseases?

Suggested Reading

1. *Control of Chronic Diseases in Man,* New York, Am. Pub. Health Assn. 1966.
2. *National Health Forum on Chronic Illness* (Summary), Pub. Health Repts., 71:675, 1956.
3. Commission on Chronic Illness: *Prevention of Chronic Illness,* Cambridge, Harvard University Press, 1957.
4. *Chronic Disease and Rehabilitation, A Program Guide for State and Local Health Departments,* New York, Am. Pub. Health Assn., 1960.
5. Allan, W. S.: *Rehabilitation, A Community Challenge,* New York, Wiley & Sons, 1958.
6. Shock, Nathan W., (Ed.): *Aging, Some Social and Biological Aspects,* Washington, Am. Assn. Advmt. Science, 1960.
7. *Development of Community Programs for the Chronically Ill,* Washington, D.C., Public Health Service, 1967.
8. *Report of the President's Commission on Heart Disease, Cancer and Stroke,* Washington, D.C., U.S. Govt. Printing Office, 1964.

Chapter 8

Medical Care

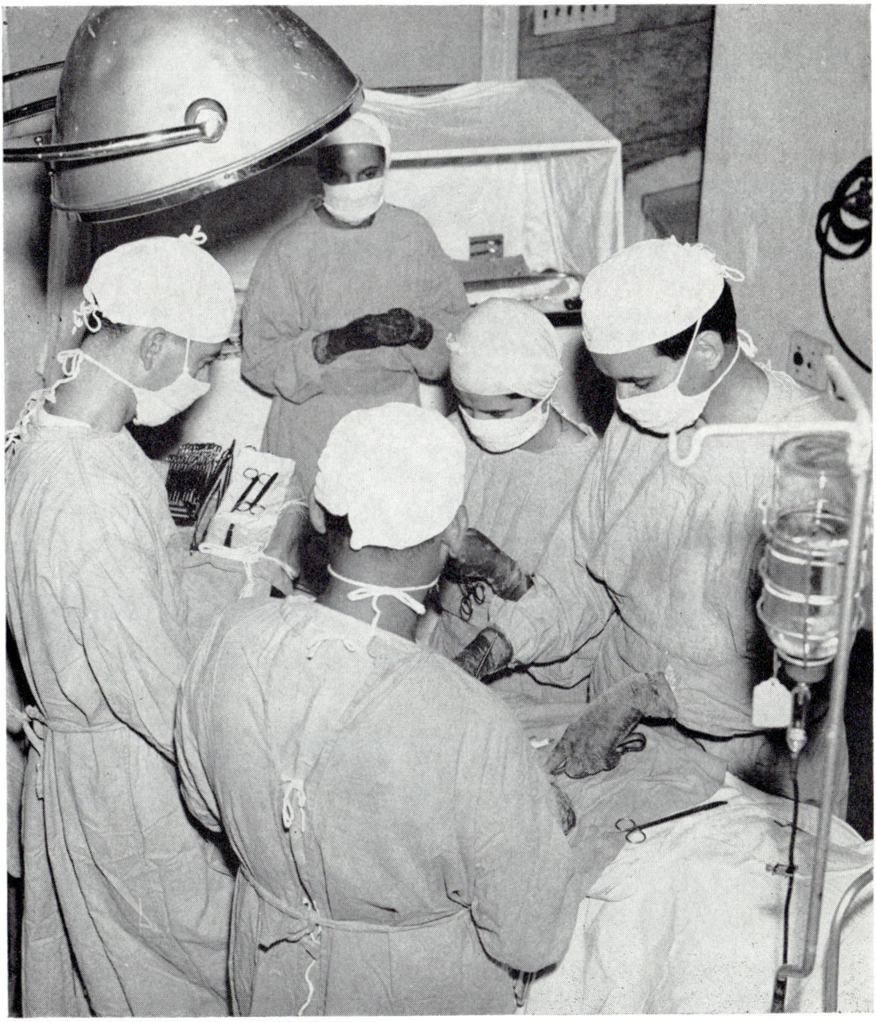

FIG. 45. Drama under the lights.

Background of the Problem

The health of a community or nation is inevitably and intimately a reflection of the amount and quality of the medical resources available. At best, health and medical care represents one of society's greatest problems and its costs are enormous. It currently costs the United States of America an estimated $55 billion each year. About 95 per cent of this is required for personal medical care in private offices, clinics, and hospitals, one-fifth of it under governmental auspices. There should be added to this the value of the average of 7 working days lost each year by the average wage earner because of sickness, and the very great capital investment value that may be placed upon the lives lost due to illnesses that are currently preventable.

Who are the people who require medical or hospital care and for what reasons do they seek it? Many studies of the subject have been made which indicate a fairly consistent pattern as far as our society is concerned. The frequency of visits to physicians is highest for children under 5 years and for adults over 65 years of age. Females in all age groups seek the services of physicians more frequently than do males. Sixty-nine per cent of patients go to the doctor for diagnosis and treatment of some existing condition. Two-thirds of such visits are related to chronic illnesses. Ten per cent go for a general checkup, 7 per cent for immunizations, 4 per cent for prenatal care, and 10 per cent go for other purposes. For cultural as well as medical reasons, pregnancy is the most frequent cause of hospitalization in America, accounting for about one-sixth of hospital admissions. It is followed in order of importance by digestive disorders, respiratory illnesses, genitourinary conditions, illnesses involving the heart and circulatory system, neoplasms (both benign and malignant), and accidents (Table 13).

Table 13. Reasons for Hospitalization United States*

Diagnosis	*Per Cent of Admissions to General Hospitals*
Pregnancy	17.4
Digestive disorders	16.6
Respiratory illnesses	12.0
Genitourinary conditions	11.4
Circulatory conditions	9.9
Neoplasms	9.3
Accidents	5.3
Nervous system and sensory organs	4.5
Bone conditions	2.9
Allergic and endocrine conditions	2.8
Skin conditions	2.1
All other reasons	5.8

*McCabe, J. L. and Robertson, H.: Modern Hospital, *94*:99, 1960.

It should be noted, as pointed out elsewhere however, that mental illnesses require about one-half of the hospital beds in the country. This is because of the accumulation of conditions that require long-term care.

Social and Economic Factors

One of the most difficult aspects of the medical care problem is the unpredictability of illnesses and accidents. While the average person in this country suffers an illness or injury about two and one-half times a year, there are many who go through a year safely, while the experience of others greatly exceeds the average expectation. Thus, in a typical year, of each one million people, 470,000 will suffer no serious illness or injury, 320,000 will experience one, 140,000 will experience two, 50,000 will experience three, and 20,000 will experience four or more illnesses or injuries. More than chance is involved in these variations. Individual, family and regional economics, ways of living and working, and education are three of the factors that play significant roles. It is known that the lower the individual is on the economic scale, the more apt he is to experience one or a number of serious illnesses or injuries each year. The national health survey showed, for example, that the annual frequency of acute and chronic illnesses which disabled for one week or more, per 1,000 persons, was 232 in families on relief as compared with 146 in families with incomes of $5,000 or more. As would be expected, persons in families not on relief but with low incomes also had high rates. Complicating this is the fact that, since lower income families experience more illness, they necessarily must and do spend a higher proportion of their incomes for medical and hospital care. As an example, a national study showed that families with incomes under $2,000 a year spent 13 per cent of their income for medical care; families with incomes between $3,500 and $5,000 per year spend about 6.4 per cent of their incomes, whereas families with incomes of over $7,500 a year had to spend only about 4 per cent of their incomes for this purpose.[1]

Returning to the factor of unpredictability, while the average family can somehow manage relatively minor illnesses and injuries, a medical problem of major seriousness can be economically catastrophic. This is particularly true if the family member affected is the wage earner. This is one of the strongest arguments in favor of prepaid medical care insurance, whether privately or governmentally sponsored.

Distribution of Resources

The same factors that affect the variations in the incidence of illnesses and injuries also influence the distribution, hence availability, of medical

[1] *Progress in Health Services*, New York, Health Information Foundation, 1959.

care resources. Overall there are in the United States (1968) 325,000 physicians, 100,000 dentists, 700,000 nurses, and 3 million other health workers. In terms of current needs, the nation requires an additional 50,000 physicians, 10,000 dentists, 150,000 nurses, and many thousands of all other kinds of health workers. One of the most significant problems is that the less economically favored and the more rural parts of the nation typically have been unable to attract and support sufficient numbers of adequately qualified medical and medically related personnel and their auxiliary physical facilities such as hospitals and accredited nursing homes. The more affluent New England, Middle Atlantic and Far Western States are quite well supplied with physicians, dentists and hospitals in contrast to the southeastern and southwestern states which have only about one-half as many physicians and dentists per unit of population. If one examines further in terms of average quality of personnel and facilities, average age and extent of specialization, the discrepancies become even more marked. This is illustrated in Figure 46 which presents the distribution of different types of physicians by state. Ignoring the District of Columbia, more than 100 per cent discrepancy will be noted both in the over-all availability of physicians and in the proportion with advanced specialized training and hospital affiliation. In line with this, and as would be expected, rural areas fare the worst. Figure 47 emphasizes this, by showing that the metropolitan areas have 3 times as favorable a physician-population ratio as do rural areas, and that very few of the physicians in rural areas have advanced specialized training. One bright spot is that the situation with regard to the availability of adequate hospitals and hospital beds has been undergoing significant equalization in recent years as a result of Federal support of hospital construction.

How Much Does it Cost?

As previously indicated, if medical, dental and hospital care are considered together, about $55 billion are spent on them annually. This represents 7 cents out of every dollar the public spends. While this may seem high, it is interesting to note that the same amount is spent on recreation, that about one-half of this amount is spent on alcoholic beverages, and about one third that much is spent on tobacco. For further comparison, about twice the amount is spent on the family car.

While many people are understandably concerned with the increasing costs of medical and related care, it is important to emphasize that the significant increases that have been occurring have not been related to the personal service aspects of medical care such as fees to physicians and dentists or to the cost of drugs. Rather, most of the increase is accounted for by the increasing costs of hospitalization. By now (1969) the average total cost of a day's hospitalization in the U.S. is about $68. The pro-

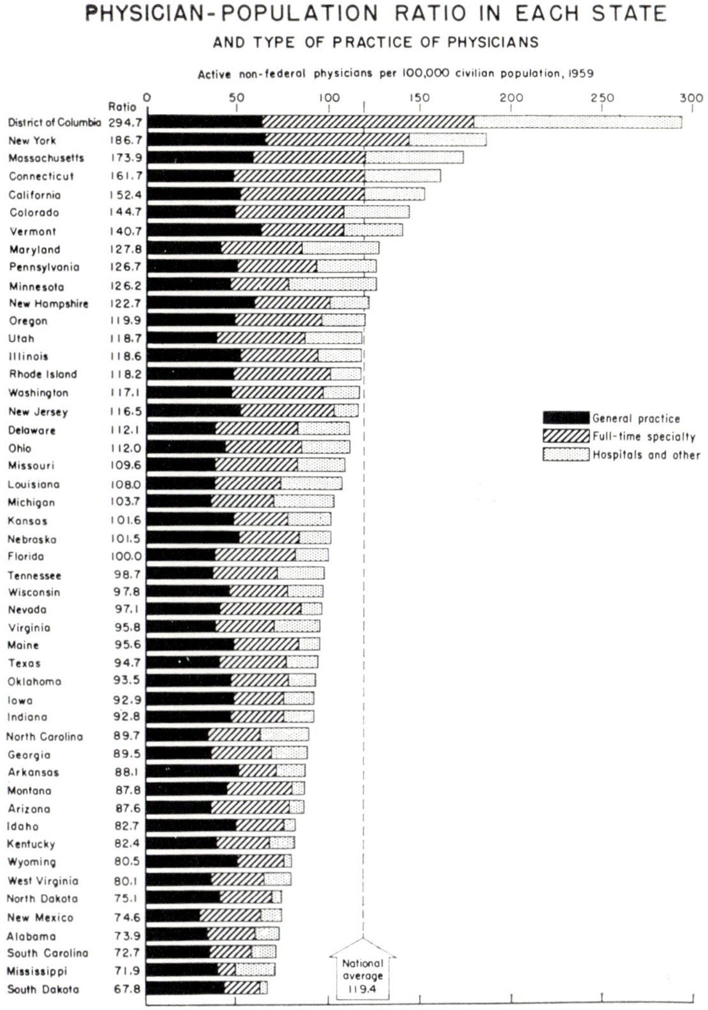

FIG. 46.

Source: Public Health Service, Department of Health, Education and Welfare

portion of the medical dollar devoted to hospital costs has risen from 18 per cent in 1940 to about 30 per cent in 1969. This is in contrast with a decline in the proportion of the medical dollar paid to physicians from 30 per cent in 1940 to 27 per cent in 1969. The proportion of the medical dollar which is paid to dentists has also decreased significantly during the past 30 years from 14 per cent in 1940 to 10 per cent in 1967, while the proportionate amount for drugs has also dropped from 21 per cent of the medical dollar to 17.5 per cent. Actually, while medical care costs have gone up 85 per cent during the past 30 years, this is less

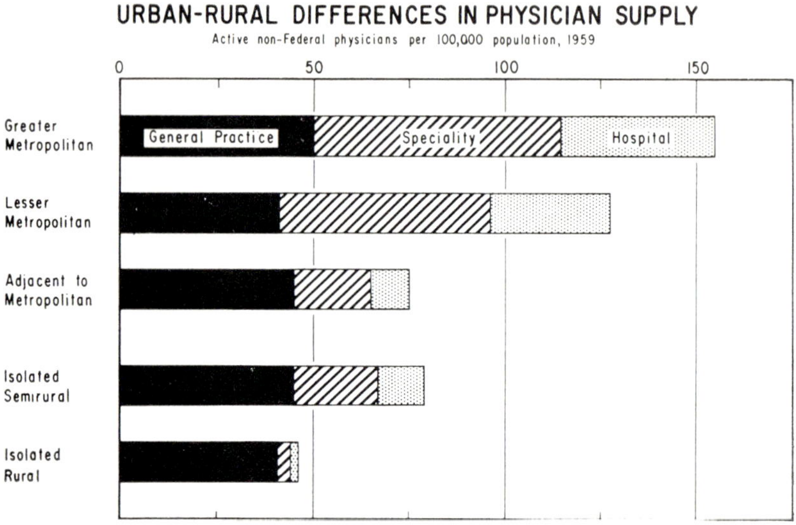

FIG. 47.
Source: Public Health Service, Department of Health, Education and Welfare

than the increases in the costs of food, housing, personal care and wearing apparel, or of transportation. As far as hospital costs are concerned, it must be realized that much of the increase is attributable to the introduction of many new life saving techniques and types of equipment and also to increasing demands for more comforts and services by patients, personal services which are not always necessary to adequate care and treatment.

How Medical Care is Obtained

Historically, until very recently, illness and injury were regarded more or less as a personal or private concern. This was particularly true during the many generations of man's existence when some such events were even considered a form of punishment by the gods. For most of man's existence he felt no compulsion or responsibility to be his brother's keeper. During the Middle Ages and subsequently, there developed a number of charity and religious nursing orders that built hospices and similar havens for the poor and the diseased. Out of these there eventually developed the modern hospital, for which other private groups and more recently government began to accept a share of the responsibility. Meanwhile, as part of the Age of Enlightenment and more recently the scientific and technological revolutions, the practice of medicine was placed on a much sounder basis. In place of journeymen physicians, many of them self-designated and most of them very poorly trained, there came about the establishment of an increasing number of centers of medical education, and physicians adopted the pattern of settling down in a community. Thus, the concept of the private physician and the family physician came about. This had the great advantage of providing a much needed time dimension to the care of the health needs of the individual and his family. The medical profession and the increasing number of other related professions which developed began to organize into professional societies for the purposes of establishment of standards and qualifications, the greater protection of communities, and for continued education and professional intercourse.

Many of these professional organizations, especially those of physicians, achieved positions of considerable social and political importance and influence. Initially and until recently, official medical policy was in favor of little else than individual private practice. As time went by, however, considerable changes in official attitudes have taken place, including the favoring and support of official as well as voluntary health agencies, the establishment of group medical practices, and the promotion of voluntary hospital and medical insurance plans. By now the medical profession is one of the strongest advocates of adequate, well-qualified health departments and a large and ever increasing number of physicians are coming together to form efficient group medical practices. By now (1969), about 85 per cent of the population is included in some form of voluntary health insurance plan. While practically all of the 85 per cent insured carry hospitalization insurance (78 per cent), only 77 per cent of the population carry surgical insurance and only about 68 per cent carry medical insurance. Dental care insurance is still in its infancy with only about 3 per cent of the population covered. Another difficulty is that benefits vary considerably. Hospital insurance on the average meets approximately 80 per cent of hospitalization costs. In contrast, medical and surgical insurance plans on the average provide for less than 25 per cent of the total bill for private medical care, including the costs of physician's services, nursing care, drugs and appliances. Another problem is that voluntary plans for the most part are limited to groups, and because of this, in addition to their increasing cost, rule out many who are in the greatest need for coverage because of age, income or chronicity of condition. This is well documented by Table 14 which shows the per cent of persons under 65 years of age, in different income groups, who have some hospital insurance coverage.

Government and Medical Care

Since the period of economic depression of the 1930's, there has been ever increasing consideration given to the entrance of the federal government into the field of medical insurance in order to provide for the economic protection of all citizens in the event of illness. All

Table 14. Per Cent of Persons Under 65 Years of Age with Hospital Insurance Coverage by Family Income, U.S., 1968

Family Income	Per Cent in Group With Hospital Coverage
under $3,000	36.3
$3,000—4,999	56.8
5,000—6,999	78.5
7,000—9,999	89.3
10,000 and over	92.3

Vital Statistics Report, Nat. Center for Health Statistics *18*, No. 11, Feb. 2, 1970.

such measures have met with strong opposition from organized medicine and a number of other groups in our society for fear that it might result in undue governmental interference in, or control of the scientific and professional aspects of medical practice. Actually, as the years have gone by, the two extreme poles represented by organized medicine on the one hand and by governmental, social and economic planners on the other have been gradually, though slowly, approaching each other. The concept of governmentally underwritten, sponsored and operated social insurance systems and specifically those relating to medical care is by no means new. Some type of such plans exists in the majority of countries in the world. The first compulsory health insurance plan applied to the entire population of a nation was established in Germany in 1883 by Bismarck.

Many people in the United States have tended to consider the very idea of prepaid medical care insurance as foreign to our social and political tradition. Interestingly enough, the first medical insurance plan in the world was developed in this country. It was established by the young American Congress in June, 1798. This new country recognized from the beginning that its future depended upon international trade, and that an extensive merchant marine should be encouraged. The businessman of Boston, the farmer of Carolina and the tradesman of Philadelphia had roots they could fall back upon in case of illness or other calamities. The merchant seaman, however, had none. He was apt to get sick at any time and at any place, and when he did he was left at the nearest port to shift for himself. Because of the importance of this growing group of individuals to the nation, the Congress established a program which authorized the President to appoint physicians in each port in order to render medical and hospital care for sick and disabled seamen. At first it was financed by a levy of 20 cents a month deducted from the pay of each seaman. Later, this was supplemented and eventually replaced by a tonnage tax paid by ship owners. This in turn was supplemented by federal appropriations.

Before long, the need grew to the point where first full-time physicians, then government owned hospitals became practical. The physicians eventually formed the basis of the Commissioned Corps of the Public Health Service, and the hospitals became known as Marine Hospitals and more recently Public Health Service Hospitals. As time passed, a number of groups in addition to the merchant seamen became eligible for care through this mechanism—personnel of the United States Coast Guard, the United States Lighthouse Service, the United States Coast and Geodetic Survey, the United States Public Health Service, Federal employees under the supervision of the Bureau of Employment Compensation, American Indians and Eskimos, and persons afflicted with leprosy, certain mental conditions, and drug addiction.

Not too much opposition was voiced as long as the beneficiaries were federal employees or federal charges. However, when during and since the depression, attempts were made to expand the concept to the general citizenry, or even to special groups such as the aged, considerable and continuing opposition has been voiced. It would seem inevitable that some type of governmentally sponsored, comprehensive medical, surgical and hospital insurance plan will be developed. An increasing proportion of the population has expressed a wish for it in one form or another, and a number of groups, notably organized labor, are strongly in favor of such a move. It should be possible, on the basis of good faith and careful mutual study, negotiations and planning, for the various proponents of a national medical and hospital insurance plan and those concerned with protecting the interests and finest characteristics of medicine, dentistry and hospital administration to work out a system which will be economically sound, which will provide for the needs of all of the people of the nation, and which will protect the interests of all professions which participate.

The federal government is already active to a significant degree in many other aspects of medical care. It is now the largest single sponsor and underwriter of medical and other health researches through the National Institutes of Health and the various research grant programs of the N.I.H. and the Public Health Service in general. It has already gone far toward the solution of the inequities that exist in the distribution of hospitals and hospital beds by means of the Hospital Survey and Construction Act. It is active in many aspects of professional education. In this area it has played a particularly significant role in the nurse recruitment and training efforts across the nation, as well as assisting in the training of many ancillary health professionals and technicians. In most states, state governments are already assisting in the financing of private as well as public medical schools and the federal government is increasingly attempting to assist in the solution of the problems of these educational institutions. Because of the present and increasing shortage of physicians, the Congress is giving careful consideration to the provision of long-term, low-interest loans as well as fellowships to medical students.

A great step forward was taken on July 30, 1965 when Public Law

89-97 was enacted. Title 18 of the Act established the Medicare program which provided, after a $40 deduction, hospital care, nursing home care, home visits by health personnel and most of the cost of diagnostic tests. The cost of the program was covered by raising the taxable wage base of the Social Security Program. Another section of the Act, Title 19 or Medicaid, extended eligibility to all persons eligible for federally aided public assistance—the aged, blind, disabled and families receiving Aid to Dependent Children assistance. Medicaid allows states to pay for any deductibles and for the voluntary medical insurance premiums for the elderly. As of this writing the Congress is considering further amendments which if passed would provide comprehensive health care (preventive, therapeutic, nursing, and rehabilitative) to all of the people on a tax-supported basis.

Needs

The dramatic increase in the population of this as well as other countries is well known. Its consequences are far reaching and involve among other things the proportionate supply of medical care personnel and facilities. If the present rate of training of physicians continues, the ratio of physicians to population which is already beginning to drop will by 1980 be far below the nation's needs and demands. Merely to maintain the inadequate 1955 ratio of 132 physicians per 100,000 population will require the formation of an additional 20 new medical schools during the next decade. During the past few years several new medical schools have been established and many existing schools have enlarged their classes. There is a point, however, beyond which the latter cannot practically be pursued.

With regard to hospital beds, despite the progress that has been made, it is estimated that there now exists only about 60 per cent of the number needed in the nation. There are now about 1,200,000 acceptable hospital beds in the country. It is estimated that approximately 850,000 additional are needed. The greatest shortage is for chronic disease hospitals exclusive of mental illness and tuberculosis. Existing acceptable beds for chronic disease total only about 17 per cent of the number needed. In the face of ever increasing hospital operation costs, increased governmental support appears to be here to stay. The situation has been summarized by one of us elsewhere as follows:

> It must be recognized that a tax-supported plan for medical care is certain to have both advantages and disadvantages, potential dangers as well as benefits. Undoubtedly the outstanding advantages of such a plan would be the equalization of geographic and economic differences among states and regions, and among the citizens of a community and the nation. This

equalization would manifest itself, among other ways, in a more equitable distribution of medical personnel and facilities. Furthermore, and perhaps of greatest importance would be the equalization through time of the costs to an individual of medical diagnosis and care. Against these advantages are the potential dangers of political influence on the selection of patients, the appointment of administrative and professional personnel, and the methods of institutional management. Physicians and others might in some instances be poorly selected or poorly trained and practice under inadequate or no supervision. It may be pointed out, however, that in the complete absence of a plan, these same poorly selected or trained persons would be engaged as they now may be in private practice with no supervision. Similarly the cry is often heard that a publicly or governmentally sponsored medical care program will cause the quality of care to suffer. Objections on these grounds imply that all present physicians would be disenfranchised and an altogether new group would move in. It should be realized that the aim of all proposals up to the present has been control of the economic risks of illness and not of the manner in which those illnesses are treated. If under any plan, private or public, the quality of the care rendered decreased, the fault could be attributed only to those who render the service, and not to the manner in which they received payment. Much depends of course, on the structure of a plan and the manner in which it is administered. A tax-supported medical care program must involve some degree of governmental administration and supervision, but this does not necessarily imply governmental control over technical and professional procedures and personal relationships.[2]

Questions for Discussion

1. Study the adequacy of the supply of practicing physicians, hospitals and hospital beds, nursing and other medical care facilities in relation to the population of your community. Compare it with the State and the country as a whole.
2. Are there any medical specialties that are lacking in your community? What recourse do the citizens have when they need certain types of medical or surgical care that is not locally available?
3. How much did your family spend for medical care last year? Divide it into expenditures for medical care, hospitalization, dental care, medicines and drugs, *etc.* What proportion of it was for preventive and promotive health in contrast with treatment after something went wrong?
4. What percent of the families in the community might be considered medically indigent? What do they do when they need medical care, hospitalization, dental care?

[2] Hanlon, John J.: *Principles of Public Health Administration,* 5th ed., St. Louis, C. V. Mosby Co., 1969, p. 482.

5. Does your health department or any other governmental organization operate treatment facilities? Do you think they should?
6. Are there in your community voluntary medical, surgical, and hospital care pre-payment or insurance plans? How adequate do you consider them to be? Do you belong to one? What is the extent of its coverage?
7. How do you account for the remarkable growth of Blue Cross and Blue Shield medical and hospital care prepayment plans?
8. What are the arguments for and against government sponsored as opposed to private or voluntary health insurance plans?

Suggested Reading

1. WINSLOW, C.-E. A.: *The Cost of Sickness and the Price of Health,* WHO Monograph Series #7, Geneva, 1951.
2. WEISBROD, B. A.: *The Economics of Public Health,* Philadelphia, University of Pennsylvania Press, 1961.
3. RICHARDSON, HENRY B.: *Patients have Families,* New York, Commonwealth Fund, 1945.
4. APPLE, DORRIAN (Ed.): *Sociological Studies of Health and Sickness,* New York, McGraw-Hill Book Co., Inc., 1960.
5. *Health for the American People, A Symposium,* Boston, Little, Brown & Co., 1956.
6. *Readings in Medical Care,* Chapel Hill, University of North Carolina Press, 1958.
7. SOMERS, H. M., AND SOMERS, A. R.: *Doctors, Patients, and Health Insurance,* Washington D.C., The Brookings Institute, 1961.
8. *National Conference on Medical Costs,—Chart Book,* Washington D.C., U.S. Dept. of Health, Education, and Welfare, 1967.
9. *To Improve Medical Care—A Guide to Federal Financial Aid for the Development of Medical Care,* Washington, D.C., U.S. Dept of Health, Education, and Welfare, 1966.
10. CUNNINGHAM, R. M.: *The Blue Cross Story,* New York, Pub. Affairs Pamphlet, 1958.
11. CUNNINGHAM, R. M.: *The Story of Blue Shield,* New York, Pub. Affairs Pamphlet, 1954.
12. *The Evolution of Medicare,* Washington, D.C., U.S. Dept. of Health, Education, and Welfare, 1969.
13. *Comprehensive Health Care—A Challenge to American Communities,* Washington, D.C., Public Affairs Press, 1967.

PART III

The Players: People

A play must have a cast. The cast of our play is very large. It includes all of us and we each have our role. The lead parts necessarily are assigned to the children who depend upon the rest for guidance and help. It is for them that the play is written and presented, and upon them that all future performances depend. Of great importance are those to whom the supporting roles of our play have been assigned—those who will teach the children. Without them, the main thesis of the play could not be developed properly if at all. In the background and in the wings is a great multitude of different kinds of people who constitute the supporting cast—parents, physicians, health workers, industrialists, laborers, economists and numerous others. It is only by each performing his respective role that this play on life's stage may be brought to a successful conclusion.

Chapter 9

The Formative Years

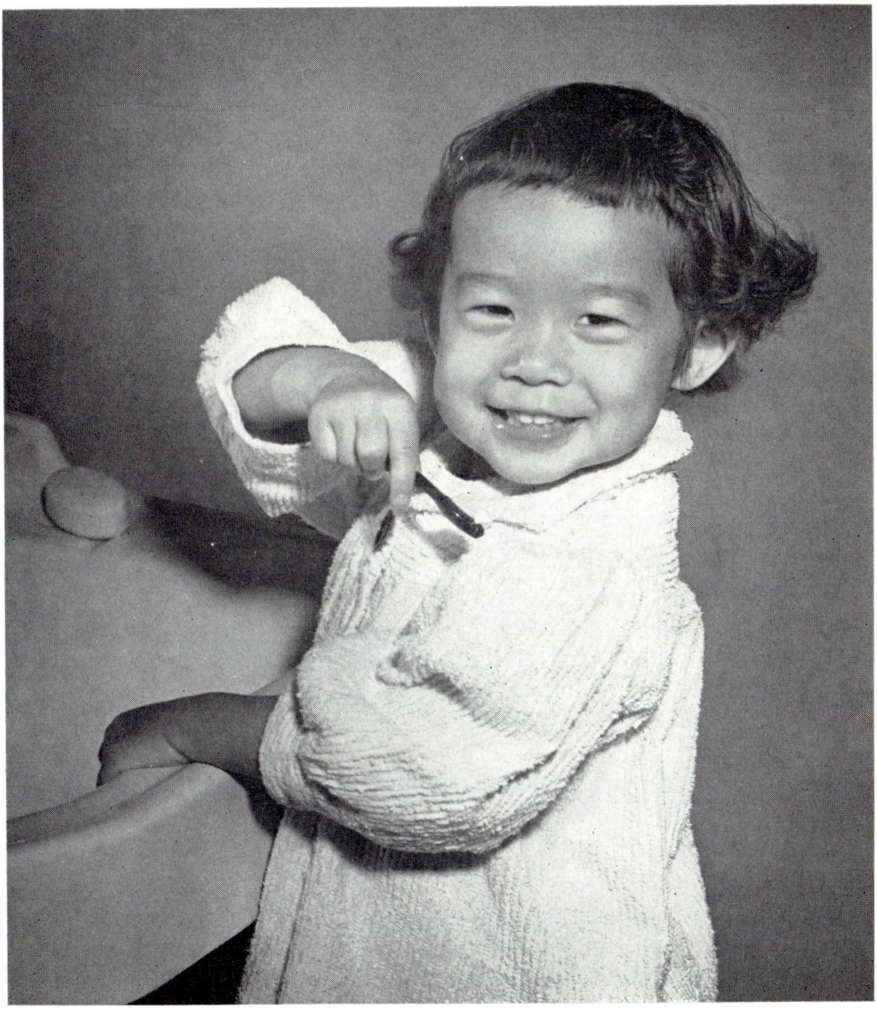

Fig. 48. On the way.

Introduction

Community health programs traditionally have placed special emphasis upon activities that relate to the health and protection of expectant mothers and young children. There are several reasons for this. A woman is subject to certain unique stresses and potential illnesses during the periods of her pregnancy and delivery. If anything undesirable happens to her, not only is she placed at risk, but also are her unborn child, and indeed any other children she may already have who are dependent upon her. A dominant concern, therefore, is the unborn child she is carrying. It has its entire life before it, and every care must be taken to assure that nothing happens to it while in the mother's womb that will limit its chances of being born alive and healthy and of living an unimpaired and fruitful life. Some of the greatest successes of public health and medicine have been in this area of endeavor.

The Mother

During the last half century in the United States, maternal mortality has declined remarkably from more than 600 maternal deaths per 100,000 live births in 1915 to 28.0 in 1967, while infant mortality has declined from about 100 infant deaths per thousand live births in 1915 to 22 in 1967. Whereas not so long ago childbearing was approached with fear, the American woman can now anticipate it with confidence. These remarkable gains have been due to many factors: improvement of obstetrical, pediatric and hospital standards and practice; the rise in the average standard of living including improved nutrition; the sanitation of food, milk and water; the development of an impressive array of new diagnostic technics as well as biological and pharmaceutical agents for the effective prevention and treatment of many diseases; the widespread establishment of prenatal and well-child supervisory services in physicians' offices and health department clinics; the reduction in incidence of a number of diseases such as tuberculosis, puerperal sepsis, syphilis and others which formerly affected many mothers and infants; and cutting across all of these a considerable improvement through education in the general health knowledge and practices of the average person.

Dramatic as have been the improvements, gross figures can be somewhat misleading. Progress has not been uniform. Thus the maternal mortality for non-white women in the United States is about four times that of white women, although the rate of improvement is almost the same for both groups. Given equal economic status, education and health practices, there is no reason to expect any difference. These discrepancies tend to parallel to some extent the differences that may be observed among the states of the union. Generally speaking, the eco-

Table 15. Maternal Mortality by Age of Mother, United States, 1967 (per 100,000 live births in specified group)

age in years	*under 20*	*20-24*	*25-29*	*30-34*	*35-39*	*40-44*	*45 and over*
maternal mortality	22.1	16.6	20.4	43.9	72.6	131.2	312.7

nomically less favored states, particularly in the southeast, have higher maternal mortality (and infant mortality as well as general mortality) rates than do the northern states. However, an equalization appears to be under way. At the present time (1967), maternal mortality rates vary from a low of 4.2 per 100,000 live births in Vermont to a high of 69.4 in Mississippi. Again, it must be emphasized that the variations observed are not attributable to anything intrinsic to race or geography. Extensive studies have pointed, as might be anticipated, to the significant roles of economic status and standard of living, availability and utilization of adequate medical and hospital facilities, and similar factors.

Another area of variation relates to the age of the mother. The risk of death during pregnancy and delivery is greatest among the youngest and oldest age groups. At present, for example, the maternal mortality rate per 100,000 live births is 22.1 for females under 20 years of age, it declines to 16.6 for women between 20 and 24 years, then gradually increases to a high of 312.7 in women over 45 years of age (Table 15).

The slightly higher rate in the early ages may be the result of physical immaturity, small pelvis, and possibly induced abortions. In the higher ages, complicating diseases probably account for most of the increased risk. It is of interest that while maternal mortality rates have improved at all ages, the decrease in young girls between 10 and 14 years has been only 40 per cent and in women over 45 years only 66 per cent in contrast with a 90 per cent improvement in the intervening young adult groups.

Most maternal deaths occur during or soon after delivery or abortion. Thus about 60 per cent occur during or soon after delivery, 18 per cent during or soon after abortion, 13 per cent before delivery and about 4 per cent are related to ectopic pregnancy, (development of the fetus in the tube or abdomen instead of in the uterus). Table 16 shows the causes of maternal deaths at the present time. Many of these are still subject to considerable decrease on the basis of existing knowledge, obstetrical techniques and antibiotics. As is so often the case, the single greatest deterrent is the factor of human behavior.

Early and consistant medical supervision during the prenatal period, proper diet, avoidance of infections of all types, and careful delivery in a suitable hospital by qualified personnel are the greatest safeguards to the life of the expectant mother.

Table 16. Causes of Maternal Deaths, United States, 1967

Cause	*Per cent of deaths*
Toxemias of pregnancy	19.2
Hemorrhage of pregnancy and childbirth	14.4
Sepsis of pregnancy and childbirth	12.9
Ectopic pregnancy	6.7
Abortion with sepsis	10.5
Abortion with toxemia	0.3
Abortion, sepsis or toxemia not mentioned	5.3
All other reasons	30.7
Total	100.0

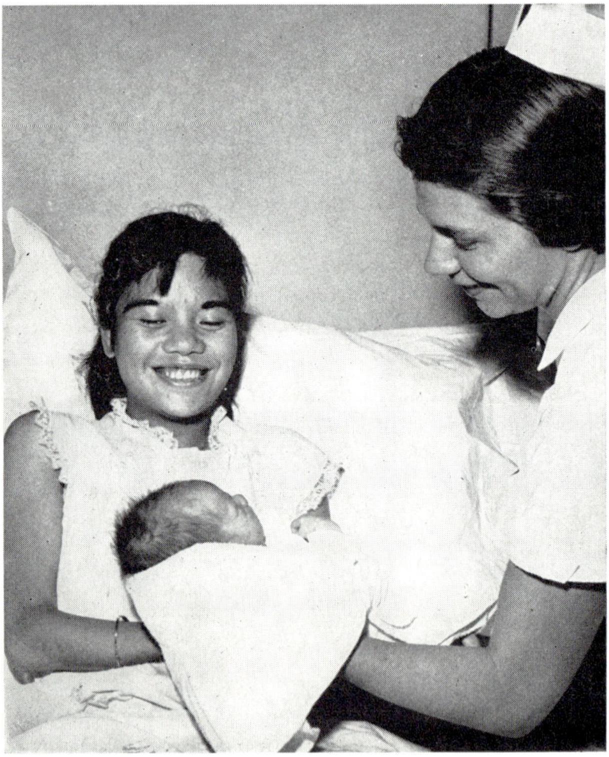

FIG. 49. Happy Moment

The Maternal Health Program

To wait until a woman is pregnant is much too late for an adequate maternal health program. It should begin much earlier, before the child is conceived and even before the expectant mother herself, and her mate, have reached physiological maturity and marriage. During this period the teacher and the school should play a most important role. Much education is required with high school and even elementary school girls and boys. Scientifically correct and socially acceptable facts must be presented to them concerning many aspects of physical and social hygiene: anatomy and physiology of reproduction; the dangers of abortions, venereal and other infections; the significance of courtship; the desirability of premarital examinations; the importance of medical supervision before, during and after delivery; and the proper care of the infant and other responsibilities of parenthood. If the schools, in company with parents and the medical profession, would do a better job on these than frequently has been the case, fewer young couples would approach marriage and parenthood in blissful but confused ignorance, and less physical and emotional harm would be done to themselves, each other and their offspring.

As has been indicated, the prenatal or antepartum period of pregnancy is of great consequence in relation to the well being of both mother and child. It is most important that a woman place herself under the supervision of a qualified physician as early as possible in her pregnancy in order that he may watch her general health and nutrition, protect her and her unborn child against any actual or potential threats, perform whatever tests are necessary and be prepared for the time of delivery.

A good plan of prenatal care includes visits which begin within the first 3 months of pregnancy, and, for the usual patient, are repeated monthly through the 7th month, every 2 weeks during the 8th month, and weekly during the 9th month. At the first visit, a history is taken including medical, obstetrical, family, and social considerations. The woman receives a complete physical examination including a pelvic examination, and her height, weight, and blood pressure are measured. Laboratory tests including a serological test for syphilis, hemoglobin, Rh type and ABO group, urinalysis, and chest x-ray are performed. Immunization levels against poliomyelitis, and in high incidence years influenza, are brought up-to-date. Advice and counseling are given on nutrition, dental health, prenatal hygiene, common problems of pregnancy, and the danger signs of complications of pregnancy.

At subsequent visits, the patient's interval history and concerns are discussed, repeated physical examinations (including an estimation of the size, presentation, position, and heart rate of the fetus) are performed, and weight, blood pressure, and urine protein and glucose are determined. A test for syphilis and hemoglobin should be repeated late in pregnancy. Social service, dental care, medical and obstetrical consultation, and further diagnostic studies should be available and used if needed. In a good program of prenatal care, long before the expected onset of labor, the physiology of pregnancy and of labor should be reviewed and explained, along with what should be done to prepare for delivery, what will happen in the hospital when she enters for delivery (including a visit to the hospital if possible), and the financial aspects of her maternity care. Decisions concerning breast or bottle feeding of the infant and the source of his subsequent medical supervision should be made before delivery, with the advice and help of her obstetrician. Optimally, the husband is involved in these discussions as much as possible.

The health department can assist in a number of ways. Public health nurses may visit the patient's home to render certain services at the direction of the physician, or to remind and encourage patients who have missed prenatal appointments. Incidentally, the nurses, in the course of their rounds for various other reasons, frequently encounter other pregnant women who have not yet sought prenatal care either from a private physician or from a health department clinic. In such instances, the nurse emphasizes the importance of such care and urges that it be sought. Many health departments hold classes for expectant mothers, and sometimes for expectant fathers. If nutritional or social

Local Registrar's No. ______

COMMONWEALTH OF PENNSYLVANIA
DEPARTMENT OF HEALTH
VITAL STATISTICS

State File No.

Primary Dist. No. ______

CERTIFICATE OF LIVE BIRTH

1. PLACE OF BIRTH a. County
b. City, borough, or township
c. Name of hospital or institution

2. MOTHER'S MAILING ADDRESS a. Street address, R.D. or box number
b. Post office, zone, and state

3. Informant

CHILD

4. THIS CHILD'S NAME a. (First) b. (Middle) c. (Last)

5. THIS CHILD'S SEX | 6 a. THIS BIRTH WAS Single ☐ Twin ☐ Triplet ☐ | 6 b. If TWIN or TRIPLET. This child was born: 1st ☐ 2nd ☐ 3rd ☐ | 7. DATE OF BIRTH (Month) (Day) (Year)

FATHER

8. FATHER'S FULL NAME a. (First) b. (Middle) c. (Last) | 9. HIS COLOR OR RACE

10. HIS AGE Years | 11. HIS BIRTHPLACE (State or foreign country) | 12 a. HIS USUAL OCCUPATION | 12 b. KIND OF BUSINESS OR INDUSTRY

MOTHER

13. MOTHER'S FULL MAIDEN NAME a. (First) b. (Middle) c. (Last) | 14. HER RACE OR COLOR

15. HER AGE Years | 16. HER BIRTHPLACE (State or foreign country) | 17. WHERE DOES MOTHER ACTUALLY LIVE? a. State b. County

18. CHILDREN Previously Born to This Mother (DO NOT include this child)
a. How many OTHER children are NOW living? | b. How many OTHER children were born alive but are NOW DEAD? | c. How many were STILLBORN; i.e., delivered dead after sixteen weeks pregnancy?

c. Does Mother Live in a Township? (NOT within the limit of a city or borough)
☐ YES, she lives in ______ Township.
☐ NO, she lives within the actual limits of ______ City or Borough.

19. I hereby certify that this child was born alive on the date stated above at ______ m., E.S.T.
Signed ______ ☐ M.D. ☐ D.O. ☐ Other (Specify) Certifier's Address ______
Date Signed ______

20. DATE RECEIVED FOR FILING | 21. LOCAL REGISTRAR'S SIGNATURE

CONFIDENTIAL medical report below MUST be completed for MEDICAL and HEALTH use

22 a. LENGTH OF PREGNANCY IN ______ COMPLETED WEEKS | 22 b. WEIGHT OF CHILD AT BIRTH ______ grams or ______ lbs. ______ oz. | 23. LEGITIMATE? Yes ☐ No ☐ | 24. SEROLOGIC TEST FOR SYPHILIS ON MOTHER'S BLOOD Yes ☐ No ☐ Date of last test.

25. IN WHAT TRIMESTER WAS FIRST VISIT PRENATAL CARE? 1st ☐ 2nd ☐ 3rd ☐ No visit ☐ Unknown ☐ | 26. DESCRIBE ANY COMPLICATION OF PREGNANCY

27. DESCRIBE ANY CONGENITAL MALFORMATION | 28. DESCRIBE ANY COMPLICATION OF LABOR

29. DESCRIBE ANY BIRTH INJURY | 30. METHOD OF DELIVERY

FIG. 50. Example of a Birth Certificate.

services are needed, arrangements are made to obtain them. Health departments often assist in other ways: by providing free laboratory service for certain important tests, and making immunizing agents and gamma globulin available in case an expectant mother is or might be exposed to certain communicable diseases, such as rubella or German measles, that might affect her child. An important role of the health department, in cooperation with the medical and hospital association, is the establishment of standards and qualifications concerning the individuals and institutions that may play a part in the delivery of the expectant mother. In certain areas where home deliveries may still be done, sterile obstetrical packs and layettes as well as the services of a specially trained nurse may be made available to the private physician at the time of delivery. The purpose here is threefold (*a*) service to the patient and the physician, (*b*) education of the patient, and (*c*) occasionally education of the physician. Another often underestimated function of the health department is the insistence on the filing of a properly completed certificate of birth (Fig. 50). This is of great importance for many reasons: proof of legal existence and citizenship, the right to inherit, to attend school, to get working papers, to vote, to marry, to serve in the armed services, to obtain a passport, and to draw benefits of many kinds.

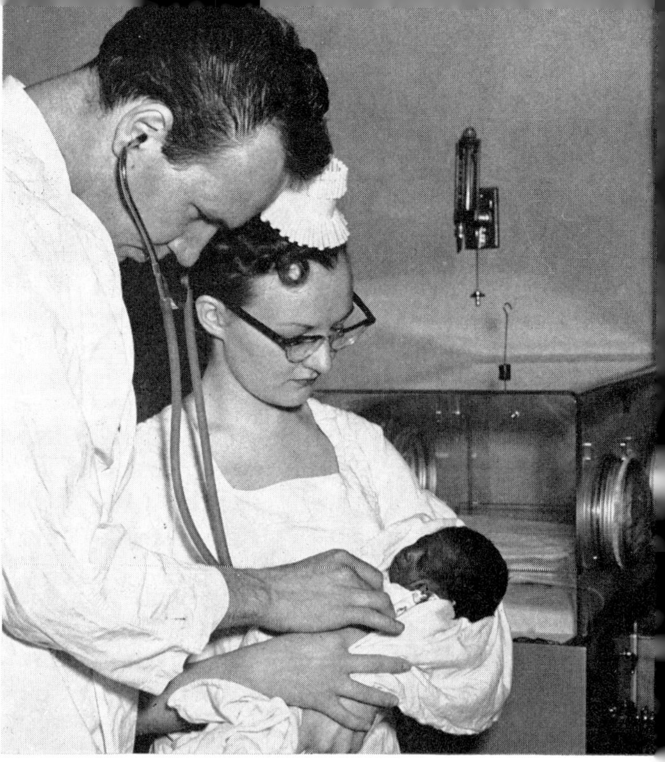

FIG. 51. A "Premie" barely able to live.

Following delivery, the mother and her newborn child require medical and nursing supervision, the former temporarily, the latter for an extended period as described subsequently. The mother should be examined several times to assure that her body and physiology are returning to the normal non-pregnant state, that any cervical tears or other undesirable effects of delivery are properly repaired, and that she is able and competent to care for her infant. In this, the physician, whether in private practice or in a health department or other clinic, has available to him the home visiting services of public health nurses who are trained to render not only personal nursing services, but also competent instruction in the home with regard to the various facets of the needs of the mother, as well as of the infant and the home as a whole.

The Infant

With respect to infant mortality in the United States, while great gains have been accomplished, the situation is only relatively good. It is true that if the rate of 50 years ago still prevailed, about 430,000 babies would die this year instead of about 75,000. However, another way of looking at it is that while throughout the entire period of World War II, 281,000 Americans were killed in action, during the same period of time 430,000 American babies died before reaching their first birthday!

Many of the factors that are involved in maternal mortality also play a role in infant mortality. For example, while the rate of decline in infant mortality has been about the same for all races, non-white babies are still about twice as apt to die within the first year of life as are white babies. Again the same factors are at work: lower standard of living, less adequate education and a tendency on the part of mothers to neglect prenatal care. The geographic discrepancies are also similar, with the poorer states experiencing higher infant mortality rates. (In this connection, the reader is referred to the chapter on Medical Care which points out the marked differences in the quantity and quality of medical personnel and facilities available.)

The commonly used statement that the first day is the most difficult certainly applies to new born. In fact the death rate of newborn babies within the first 2 days of life is about equal to the rate for all of the rest of the first year, and about 80 per cent of the deaths during the first 2 days, occur within the first 24 hours. A consideration of the causes of death of infants leads to certain conclusions. Prematurity is clearly the single most important factor. As indicated in Table 17, by itself it accounts for 24.5 per cent of the deaths during the neonatal period (first month of life). Unquestionably, it also plays an important role in many of the deaths attributed to postnatal asphyxia and atelectasis (imperfect expansion of the lungs at birth) as well as some deaths attributed to nutritional difficulties and pneumonia of the new born.

Table 17. Leading Causes of Neonatal Death, United States, 1967

Cause of Death	*Number*	*Per Cent*
1. Postnatal asphyxia and atelectasis	12,536	24.6
2. Immaturity, unqualified	11,842	21.3
3. Ill defined diseases peculiar to infancy including nutritional problems	9,821	19.3
4. Birth injuries	6,555	12.9
5. Congenital malformations	7,850	15.4
6. Pneumonia of the newborn	2,219	4.4

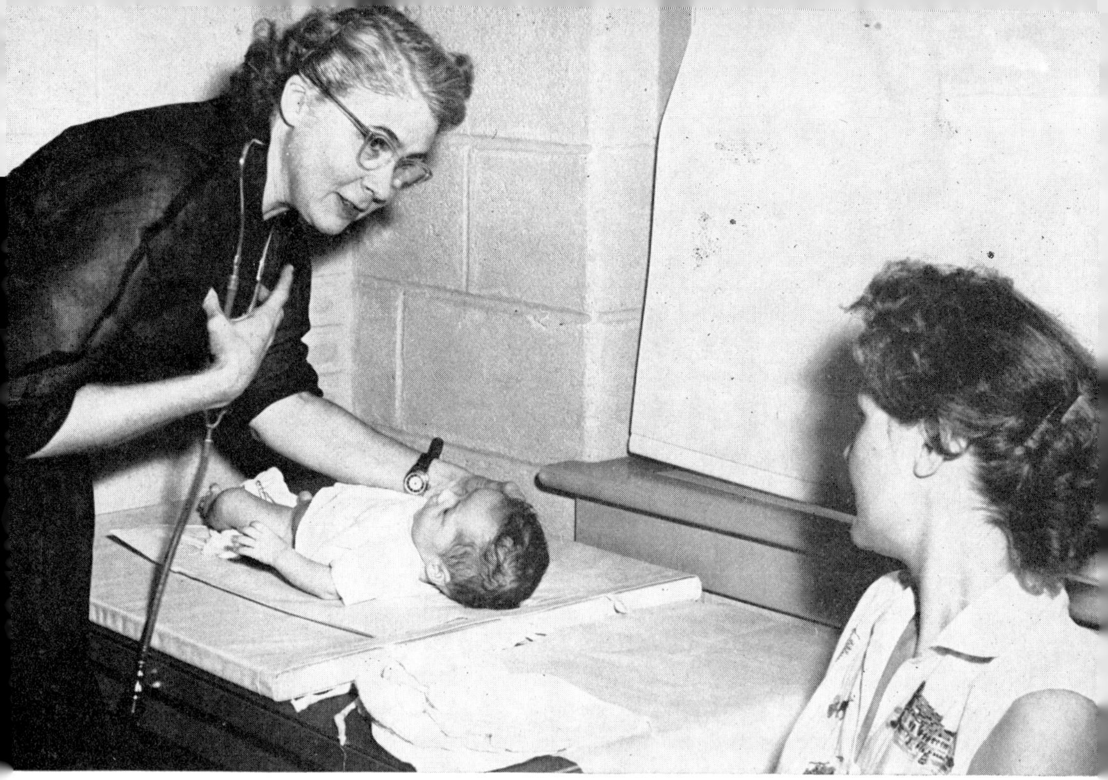

FIG. 52. Well infant examination.

The risk of death within the first month of life is almost 30 times as great for a prematurely born infant (2500 grams or less) than for non-premature infants (2501 grams or more). In fact, in New York City, more than 70 per cent of neonatal deaths of infants of known weight occurred in those who weighed under 2500 grams at birth. Premature infants who weighed less than 1001 grams at birth had the least chance of survival, over 88 per cent dying within the first month of life, most of them during the first day.[1] There is a direct relationship between the amount of prenatal care the mother receives and the chances of her child being born prematurely. Numerous studies of births and infant mortality have indicated that premature births occur twice as frequently in women who have obtained no prenatal care as among those who do. It has also been shown that, as would be expected, the neonatal death rate among babies of mothers without prenatal care is 75 per cent higher than among those whose mothers have been medically supervised.

The Infant Health Program

Given an infant who has been born alive and who has survived the first few risky days of life, there are still many potential threats to well being, and steps that must be taken to circumvent them. The list of the most significant threats to the life of the infant following the neo-

[1]Report of Bureau of Records and Statistics, Dept. of Health, City of New York, June, 1961.

16

natal period includes several items that may surprise many (Table 18). Where formerly, infections of various types predominated, they are now generally in a secondary position. The continued importance of that old hardy perennial, gastroenteritis, should be noted however. More interesting and significant is the important position occupied by accidents during infancy as the fourth leading cause of death (actually in second place after the first month is passed), and the fact that heart disease and malignancies (cancers) must be included this early in life. Actually, there are none of these ten leading causes of death during the first year of life against which some preventive steps cannot be taken, and often these potential steps are substantial.

The infant requires proper and adequate feeding, protection against infections and accidents, correction of any defects that may exist and exposure to a satisfactory emotional environment. In the absence of these, even if the infant achieves his first birthday, he is apt to be affected to some degree later in his childhood, or even in his adult life. Therefore, at the time of discharge from the hospital following delivery, the mother should be given an appointment for her newborn infant's first visit for health supervision. This visit should coincide with his one month birthday and should be repeated monthly during the first 6 months, and every 2 months during the last half of the first year.

At the initial visit to the physician, the family's medical and social history; the mother's prenatal, labor, and delivery history; and the infant's course in the hospital are elicited. At each visit, the infant's progress, current feeding, sleeping and health history are reviewed. Nutritional advice is given, immunization against diphtheria, tetanus, pertussis, poliomyelitis, and smallpox is administered, with immunization against measles, rubella and routine tuberculin testing deferred until the end of the first year. On each occasion, the infant is weighed and measured, his growth and development are reviewed, and the parent is counselled not only regarding problems as they arise, but also in anticipation of future development. The physician performs a complete physical ex-

Table 18. The Ten Leading Causes of Infant Deaths, United States, 1967

Cause of Death	*Deaths per 100,000 Infants*
Diseases of early infancy	1,364
Congenital malformations	329
Influenza and pneumonia (except neonatal)	162
Accidents	78
Bronchitis and other bronchial diseases	43
Gastroenteritis (except neonatal)	29
Meningitis (except meningococcal and tuberculosis)	19
Hernia and intestinal obstruction	19
Heart disease	11
Malignant neoplasms	6

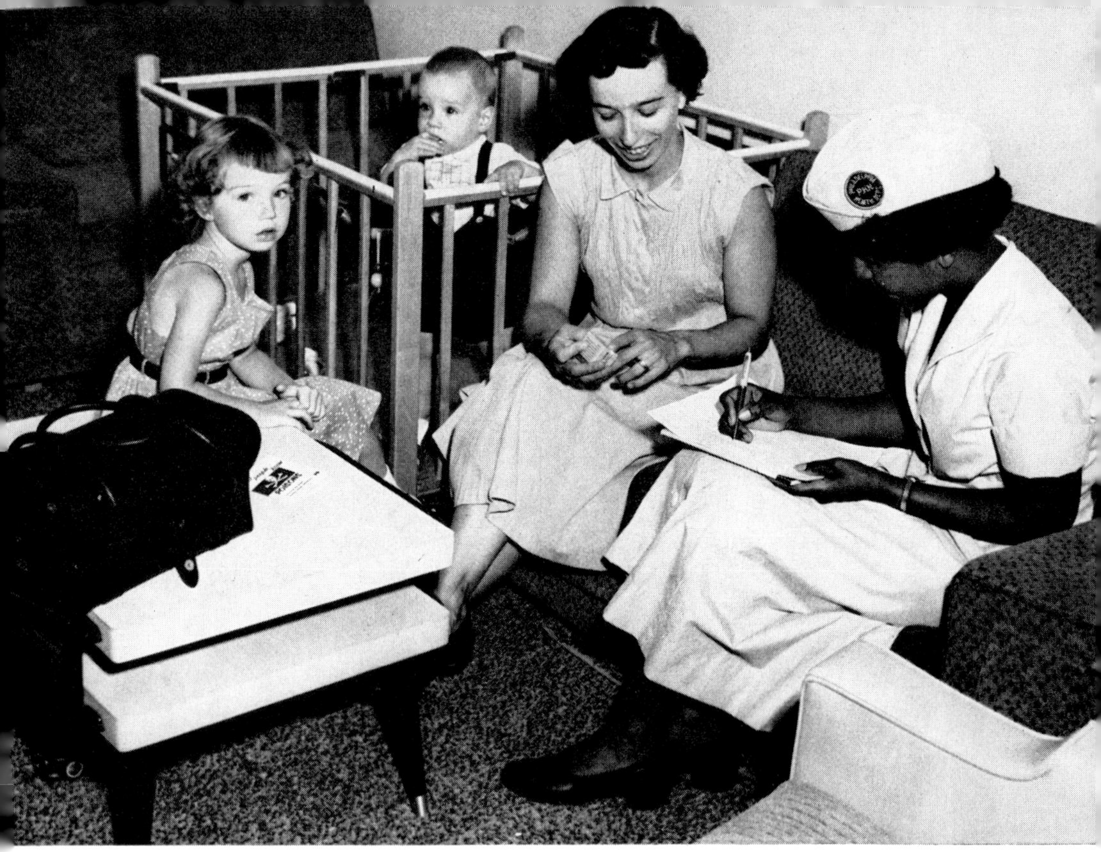

FIG. 53. Protecting the preschool child.

amination every three months, and such additional examinations as is indicated by the child's development. Referral may be made for laboratory studies, special examination, treatment for illness, home nursing, or social services as these needs become apparent.

Concurrently, the public health nurse supplements the work of the physician by means of her visits to the new mother in her home. She begins to watch the general health and nutrition of the mother and child, and to instruct the mother concerning physical and emotional problems, infant feeding, and immunological schedules. She also gives instruction concerning early signs and symptoms of the common communicable and non-communicable conditions that may affect the infant. Wherever possible, the public health nurse works under the general direction of a physician, and reports her findings to him. In instances of handicapped children, the public health nurse works closely with the parents, the physician and others in attempting to bring all pertinent available community resources to bear on the problem in the best ultimate interests of the child.

The Preschool Child

The period between the first birthday and the time of admission to school is often regarded as the most neglected period of life. The novelty

Table 19. The Ten Leading Causes of Death, 1 Through 4 Years United States, 1967

Cause of Death	*Deaths per 100,000 Children*
Accidents	32.4
Congenital malformations	9.7
Influenza and pneumonia	9.2
Malignant neoplasms	8.2
Symptoms, senility and ill-defined	2.4
Bronchitis and other bronchial diseases	2.3
Meningitis (except meningococcal and tuberculosis)	2.0
Gastritis, enteritis	1.9
Meningococcal infections	1.2
Diseases of the heart	1.1

of the young child has worn off. Hence the attention given to him diminishes, and he is left more and more to his own devices. However, he has little or no degree of maturity or experience upon which to base judgment and action. He is often at great risk of being dependent without sufficient regard to his dependency. Too often parents tend to feel that since he survived his infancy, he can be more or less left alone to "grow like a weed." It is true that the death rate during this period of life is low. However, it is still much higher than it need be in view of our present preventive potentials. Furthermore, many non-fatal preventable conditions occur which can adversely affect the quality and quantity of subsequent life. The list of the ten leading causes of death for this age group indicates this readily (Table 19).

Even as early as this period in life, accidents have assumed the dominant place as the leading cause of death, indicating the combination of the natural curiosity of the preschool child, and neglect of him by his parents and others around him. Incidentally, the major proportion of the accidents of the preschool child occurs in and around the home. Malignant neoplasms have moved up dramatically in relative importance and diseases of the heart are still included. During this period of life, various infectious diseases become important considerations. Fortunately, most of these are avoidable through immunization and other means.

Perhaps of greater significance than the relatively low mortality during this age period is the high incidence of illness. The National Health Survey of eighty-three cities showed an annual frequency rate of 251 disabling illnesses per 1000 preschool children. This was only slightly less than the rates for the next age group (5 to 9 years) and for persons 65 years and over. Fortunately, the illnesses of preschoolers, while frequent, tend to be of relatively short duration.

The Preschool Child Health Program

The nutritional and emotional aspects of the life of the preschool child are of particular importance. During this period, the child undergoes rapid physical and mental development. Because of this, things that might appear at the moment to be inconsequential influences of a nutritional, physical, dental, or emotional nature, may have far-reaching cumulative consequences far out of proportion to their initial appearance. It is essentially around such factors that the disease preventive and health promotion programs for the preschool child must be designed.

The mother who has accepted the value of routine health supervision for her infant will also be willing to accept similar supervision for her preschool child. Between the first and second birthday, the toddler should be seen by a physician every 6 months and annually thereafter. At these scheduled visits, a complete interval medical history is taken; the child's growth, development, and current status recorded; and any parental concerns or problems elicted. The child receives a complete physical examination, including blood pressure determination, routine urinalysis, and hemoglobin determination; a yearly tuberculin test; booster immunizations as required; and referrals as necessary for laboratory studies, special examinations, treatment for illness, home nursing or social service. His mother receives counseling regarding her child's diet, help with her current child-rearing concerns, and anticipatory guidance. At least by the time of the third birthday, the child should be referred to the dentist for dental prophylaxis and topical fluoride applications if the drinking water is not fluoridated. Before school entrance, visual and auditory screening tests should be performed and referral for care made if indicated.

Questions for Discussion

1. What is the maternal mortality rate, and the infant mortality rate in your community? How do they compare with those of the state and the nation?
2. Can you determine about what per cent of the women of your community obtain adequate prenatal care during their pregnancy?
3. What facilities exist in your community for prenatal care for those who cannot afford to pay?
4. What are the chief causes of deaths among infants in your community? What specifically is being done about each? Is there a program for prematurely born infants?
5. Do there exist in your community any non-governmental agencies concerned with problems of maternal, infant and child health? What are they? How are they financed? What do they do?
6. Do any agencies in your community conduct programs concerned with preparation for parenthood? Do the schools?
7. Investigate and outline the maternal and child health programs of your local health department—your state health department.
8. Is the school system in your community at all concerned with or involved in health promotional activities relating to the preschool child?

Suggested Reading

1. Schmidt, W. M., and Valadian, I.: *A Bookshelf on Maternal and Child Health,* Am. J. Pub. Health., *54*:551, Apr. 1964.
2. *Standards of Child Health Care,* Evanston, Amer. Acad. of Pediatrics, 1967.
3. Wallace, Helen M.: *Health Services for Mothers and Children,* Philadelphia, W. B. Saunders Co., 1962.
4. Ginsberg, Eli (Ed.): *The Nation's Children,* The 1960 White House Conf., 3 Vols. New York, Columbia University Press, 1960.
5. Harper, Paul A.: *Preventive Pediatrics, Child Health and Development,* New York, Appleton-Century-Crofts, 1962.
6. Watson, Ernest H. and Lowrey, Geo. H.: *Growth and Development of Children,* 4 Ed., Chicago, Yearbook Medical Publishers, Inc., 1962.
7. Children's Bureau: *Your Child from 1 to 6,* Washington, Supt. of Documents, 1962.
8. Jensen, Gordon D.: *The Well Child's Problems,* Chicago, Yearbook Medical Publishers, Inc., 1962.
9. *Health Supervision of Young Children,* Am. Pub. Health Assn., 1960.
10. *Guides to Services for Handicapped Children,* Am. Pub. Health Assn., New York:
    Cerebral Palsy (1955)
    Cleft Lip and Cleft Palate (1955)
    Dentofacial Handicaps (1955)
    Emotional Disturbances (1961)
    Epilepsy (1958)
    Handicapped Children (1955)
    Hearing Impairment (1956)
    Heart Disease and Rheumatic Fever (1960)
    Orthopedic Handicap (1962)
    Vision and Eye Problems (1956)
11. Coleman, James S.: *The Adolescent Society,* Glencoe, Free Press, 1962.
12. Edelston, H.: *Problems of Adolescents,* New York, Philosophical Library, 1956.
13. Sadler, W. S.: *A Doctor Talks to Teenagers,* St. Louis, C. V. Mosby Co., 1948.
14. Gallagher, J. R.: *Medical Care of the Adolescent,* New York, Appleton-Century-Crofts, 1960.

Chapter 10

Guarding the School Child's Health

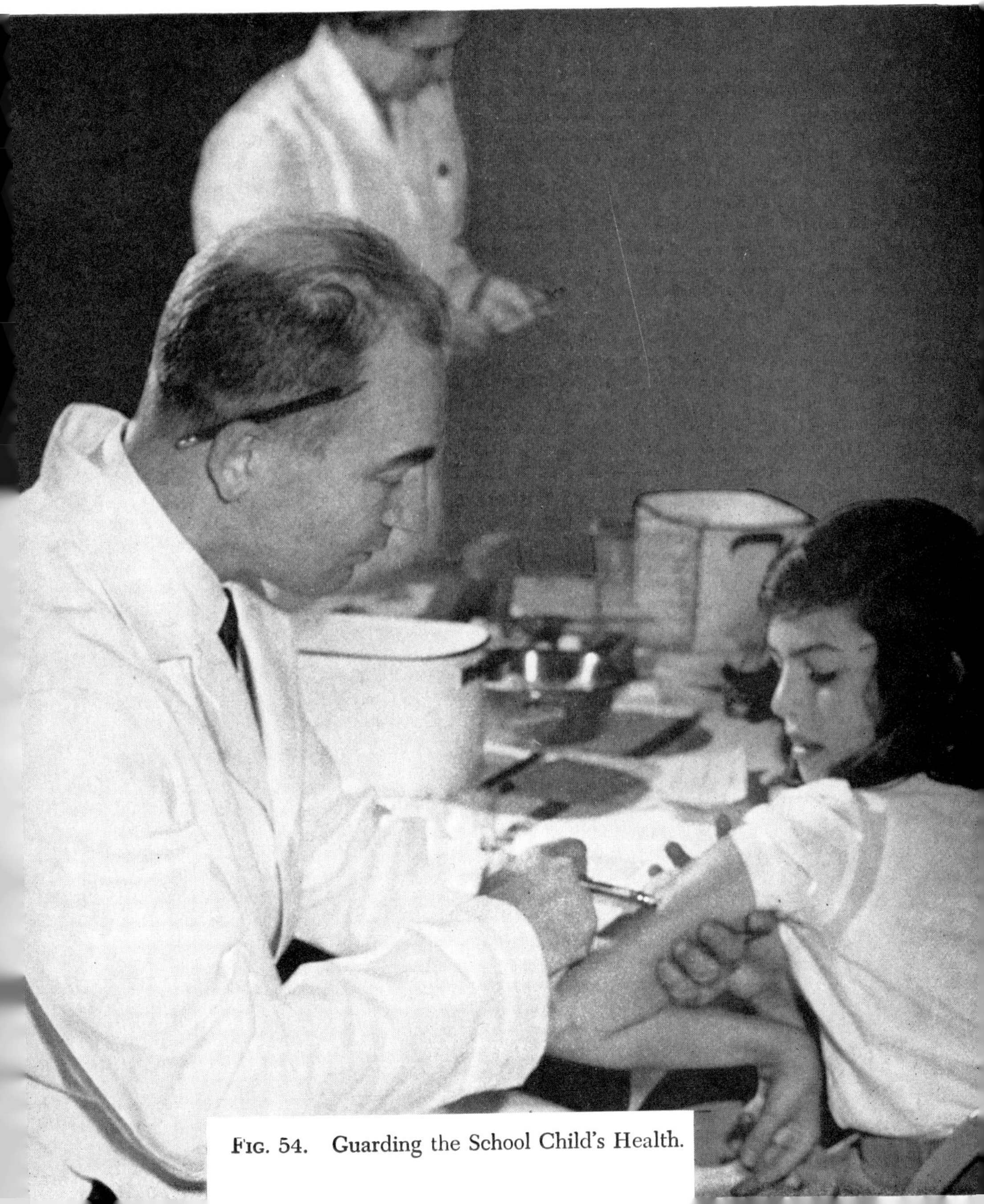

FIG. 54. Guarding the School Child's Health.

Introduction

The past 20 years have witnessed a marked widening of perspective in the area of school health. New patterns have emerged, communication has improved, and certain fundamentals have gained acceptance. Evidence of this increased interest in school health and health education is shown in the current acceleration of research and experimentation encouraged by such national professional organizations as the American School Health Association, the American Association for Health, Physical Education and Recreation, and the School Health Section of the American Public Health Association. Even more convincing has been the recent unprecedented flow of textbooks, pamphlets, periodical literature, and teaching materials designed to meet the needs of students and teachers as well as those engaged in school health services. As a consequence of all these efforts, vast improvements in school health programs, services, practices, skills, facilities and teaching methods can be noted in many localities.

In the face of the vast amount of authoritative detailed material available elsewhere, the purpose here is not to present a detailed, repetitive analysis of everything included today under the now sizeable umbrella of school health. Instead it is proposed to afford the serious student, the mature teacher or health educator the opportunity (*a*) to gain a panoramic over-view with emphasis upon the place of school health in the total community health picture; (*b*) to help him recognize new or different relationships influenced by world change, thought, or recent research; and (*c*) to peer as far as possible into the future in order to trace possible new directions and trends as to what may logically be expected to come into fruition within the lifetime of the reader. Inevitably, in pursuit of these purposes, the well-prepared and seasoned health worker is bound to find some repetition; it could hardly be otherwise. It is hoped, however, that the glimpse of familiar facts in new juxtaposition may suggest new ways of using skills and imagination in the furtherance of a richer, more forward-looking school health program.

The Relation of School Health to Community Health

It has already been pointed out that one's health is usually regarded as a highly personal matter. Only the individual himself can know his true feelings or his inner symptoms and make decisions as to next steps. But the well-known saying of John Donne that "No man is an islande entire to himself" applies very much to health. If an individual's condition or action should endanger the health of others, his health can no longer be regarded as a purely personal affair. Moreover, not infrequently, necessary alleviating or remedial action prescribed by his physician may be a sheer impossibility to carry out unassisted by outside resources. The previous chapters have shown the great extent to which health matters have come to be looked upon as a social responsibility. This concept has been amply substantiated by new knowledge and recent research in human motivation.

Group concern and a high level of education usually go hand in hand. Where these exist in a community, the health department is likely to be forward-looking, alert, and of high quality. Community health programs are concerned with the health of all citizens from the pre-natal stage to the grave. In most cases the home is primarily responsible for the health of the infant and the pre-school child. Nevertheless, efficient support and assistance by the various health resources of the community is absolutely essential to ensure adequate health conditions and care during these critical beginning years of life. The community carries also the responsibility for making the parent aware of available resources and facilities, and of the importance of utilizing them toward the best health interests of the child.

School health focuses upon health matters that involve or affect the school child (*i.e.*, from 5 or 6 years of age to 16 or 18) and that are fostered or initiated by school personnel; matters which may have their inception within the school and reach out into the home and the community, or which may have originated in the community and presently involve the school and school personnel. The school health program has been defined as, "The school procedures that contribute to the understanding, maintenance, and improvement of the health of pupils and school personnel, including health services, health education, and healthful school living."[1]

For convenience, the school health program is usually perceived as consisting of these three main divisions, although actually there is necessarily a great deal of inter-relationship. Each of these divisions possesses a wide scope including important facets of the program as stated here briefly and spelled out in more detailed form in Table 20:

1. *Health Services* include all services related to the health of the pupil and school personnel: the periodic health appraisal, referrals and follow-up; immunizations; provision for planned emergency care of illness and accidents; provision for the exceptional child; the dental program; and other important services.
2. *Healthful School Living* has to do with the establishment and maintenance of a healthful, sanitary, safe school environment—physical, mental, social, and emotional. Included also are such concerns as the daily routine, administrator-teacher-pupil relationships, the school lunch, and other contributory factors.

[1]*Report of the Committee on Terminology in School Health Education.* The Journal of the American Association for Health, Physical Education and Recreation, Vol. 22, No. 7 (September, 1951), p. 14.

Table 20. *Components of the School Health Program*

School Health Service	*Healthful School Living*	*School Health Education*

Health appraisal
  periodic medical examination
  screening examinations
  dental examination
  special examinations:
    school entrance
    referrals
    athletes
    school employees
	Maintenance of a safe sanitary plant:
	  buildings
	  grounds, playfields
	  gymnasiums, swimming pools
	  health service unit
		Planned, direct health teaching

Follow-up procedures: referrals	Seating, lighting, ventilation, heating,
	  sanitation, drinking fountains
		Indirect health education:
		  assembly programs, exhibits, etc.
		Incidental health education

Correction of remediable defects	Safety and accident prevention:
	  protective equipment
	  fire drills
	  general safety
	  civilian defense and disaster
	  safety patrols, traffic safety
	  transportation
	  driver education
		Integrated health education

Care of exceptional children	Administrator-teacher-pupil relationships	Correlated health education:
		  health units in other subject
		  courses

Prevention and control of disease	Recreation program	In-service health education:
		  school personnel
		  planning sessions
		  workshops
		  conferences
		  courses

Planned emergency care:
  illness
  injury
	School luncheon	Parent education

Health counseling	Custodial care	Preparation of health curriculum guides

Health of school personnel	Healthful school day:
	  length
	  class size
	  routine
	  grading and marking procedures
	  promotions
	  classroom procedures
		Utilization of resources:
		  teaching aids
		  textbooks, supplementary books,
		    periodicals
		  community personnel
		  community facilities:
		    museums
		    libraries
		    health centers

Cooperation with community agencies:
  official
  voluntary
  civic
  parent
		Cooperation with community health
		    education efforts:
		  official agencies
		  voluntary agencies

Program coordination		

3. *Health Education* includes planned, direct, indirect and incidental health instruction and experiences as they may pertain to pupils, staff, and parents; integration and correlation with other parts of the curriculum; and relationships with community and world health.

Because of their close relationships and the numerous ramifications having health connotations, many phases of physical education and safety are necessarily considered along with each of these three divisions.

When public school days are over, usually at the age of 16 to 18 years, the youth needs to rely upon the public health department as his main resource in health education in his effort to stay abreast of advances in health knowledge, medicine and care, and hopefully, will continue to do so throughout maturity and old age. Community facilities and programs will need to meet his and his family's health requirements and to take steps to keep him informed as to where they are available.

School health, therefore, may be thought of as a segment of the total community health pattern, concentrating its efforts upon the individual during a specific period of his existence. School health is actually the common concern of the school, the parent, and the community at local, state and national levels. The success and effectiveness of the program depends in large measure upon the common understanding on the part of each group and each individual involved as to (*a*) the precise scope of its sphere of action, (*b*) its role in the total community health picture, and (*c*) the need for consistent cooperation in its implementation. In other words, at its best, it must be a concerted attempt to put into practice for the school-aged child the thought embraced in the Children's Charter, "Every child has the right to be well-born and to attain the best possible quality of health of which it is capable."[2] All community health personnel need to pool their efforts in order to realize this obviously desirable goal to the greatest degree possible.

The Health Needs of School Children

In the autumn, the first grade teacher or the kindergartener meets the children for the first time as a group. Assuming that the children have been born into and dwell in a community with a reasonably advanced and forward-looking health department, alert as to current practices and understandings, more than ninety per cent of these children will be healthy and can look forward to the prospect of surviving childhood and entering young adulthood. Each child will have brought with him to school his own set of personal health understandings and health attitudes, and what is most important, certain health practices which stem largely from the cultural and social group of his origin. The child's parents have

[2] The White House Conference, 1930, New York, The Century Company, 1931, p. 45.

been his health teachers and his health will continue to be their responsibility until he has achieved the status of an independent, income-earning citizen responsible for his own health decisions, usually in the late teens or early twenties. The community, up to the time of school enrollment, has had some indirect share in the home's responsibility, but from now on both the school and the community will have major roles to play.

Infant care consists largely of careful continuing attention to the physical and psychological needs of the child. Thanks to our generally effective pre-parental preparation, pre-natal and infant care programs as has been described previously, certain health habits and practices have probably become well-established on the part of the child by the time he enters school. But the very first day, the observant teacher becomes well aware of the varied backgrounds of health experiences these children have had. Madeline who arrived in a station-wagon driven by her attractive young mother, carries a supply of tissue hankies for the day; David copes with his sniffles by the simple use of his coat sleeve. Jack drinks his mid-morning milk with gusto; Ruth pinches her lips into a straight line and refuses to even taste "school milk." Johnny stares at the wart on his hand whole minutes at a time. "Look, my grandmother buried a Lincoln penny in the ground to make it go away," he tells the children with complete confidence. To the teacher it becomes obvious that each child is surrounded by a defensive armour of faith in the practices, ideas, folk-ways, and traditions of his family. These have already colored the child's attitudes toward food, nutrition, cleanliness, and other so-called basic concerns of child health.

Family attitudes toward health reflect and repeat those of the neighborhood and the social milieu in which the family moves and lives. The migration of thousands of Puerto Ricans mostly to cities in the eastern part of our country has afforded this generation a first-hand opportunity to observe the tenacity with which health habits of a cultural group persist, and how entwined they are with the social structure of the group. Had it not been for the vigilence of health departments and the Public Health Service, adherence in the new environment to homeland customs and ways of living might have led to serious epidemics and health problems affecting many persons.

Economic considerations play a major part in determining the quality of the child's health. The economic status of the family necessarily dictates to a great extent the kind and quality of housing, nutrition, clothing, and medical services possible, and their availability when need arises. The education of the parent significantly affects his recognition of the child's health needs and his knowledge of appropriate action at a crucial time. Involved also are the parent's own attitudes toward health and health practices as determined by his own past experiences and the attitudes of his family and sub-cultural group toward illness, health, and remedies. Religious beliefs and prejudices frequently determine actual practices which vitally affect the child's health and well being.

Thus, it is impossible to think of the school child and his health as disassociated from the setting of his family and cultural group. The warp and woof of cultural beliefs, customs, practices, and attitudes shape the child's health patterns from the beginning of life, sometimes even determining the place, mode, and nature of his entry into the world. The teacher frequently finds herself precipitated into a dilemma. It is her responsibility to help the children form sound health habits consistent with scientific thought and at the same time to learn to understand the underlying reasons. The difficulties arise when these desirable goals differ from the attitudes, teachings, and experiences in the home, or when the family refuses to embrace new procedures and even flouts or ridicules the school's sincere attempts. Nevertheless, the teacher must realize the importance of upholding respect for the parent and the home in the eyes of the child, and is often hard pressed to proceed tactfully.

Preschool Programs

School and governmental authorities and interested citizens have long been concerned about the mounting statistics of children falling below grade level, failing promotion, dropping out of school at the earliest legal age with a large percentage adding immediately to the growing numbers of jobless youth, many of whom proved unemployable because of their failure to have absorbed even the rudiments of an elementary school education. Since World War II the problem has been accelerated by the population explosion, the displacement by automation of agricultural workers in the South and their subsequent migration with their families to the over-crowded cities of the North, the urban problems of inadequate housing and sub-standard living conditions, and the hopelessness caused by the lack of job opportunities for unskilled labor.

Recent research in child development and in the psychology of learning has presented convincing evidence that the lack of certain vital developmental experiences during the important formative preschool years may have deleterious life-long effects upon the child which can never be completely overcome. Along with adequate nutrition and appropriate health care, the preschool child needs the experience of inter-action with his peers and the stimulation of association with adults to help him develop language facility, to establish his concept of self, to awaken his curiosity, to stimulate initiative, to develop the ability to make choices and decisions. The learning of physical skills and coordinations, the extensive use of his various senses, and contacts with the various communication media further enrich his experiences and prepare him for more fruitful elementary school years. With this background of preschool experiences, a child is enabled to learn reading and other basic skills at a speed comparable with children from more advantaged homes and economic levels. But the number of public and private nursery schools, kindergartens, and day care centers in existence in the middle sixties could not possibly cope with the enormity of this nation-wide problem.

The late sixties witnessed a giant step toward improvement of the situation. Under the Office of Economic Opportunity and the Department of Health, Education, and Welfare, the Head Start program was initiated. Begun originally as a summer experiment designed to prepare children for entry into school the following September, the first programs were sponsored in some instances by local school districts, in others by volunteer groups or community agencies with assistance from the school district or nearby universities, or a combination of these.

Head Start proved to be practical and feasible. In some instances the School District extended its health services to include the Head Start program with the idea of discovering remediable health defects and initiating remedial measures immediately, thus establishing continuity of health care along with the child's entry into elementary school. The usual daily Head Start program included emphasis upon the formation of sound health habits and concepts.

In many areas these preschool programs soon passed beyond the experimental stage and became a regular part of the school program. In some of the disadvantaged neighborhoods in large cities it has been found helpful to supplement the gains of the preschool years by means of a tutorial program conducted on a one-to-one basis or in small groups. Such programs have been sponsored in some cases by the schools, in others by volunteers and carried on after school hours in churches or community agencies. Some highly successful ventures have been staffed by high school and college student volunteers working under trained personnel.

There is urgent need for trained personnel to carry on quality preschool programs. The teacher at this level needs by way of professional equipment special education in nursery school or kindergarten work along with keen interest in and aptitude for work with small children. She needs to be a sensitive, alert, imaginative, patient individual with a great empathy for children and people in general, able to work happily with professional and non-professional aides, parents, and community agencies.

The Teacher's Role in Discovering the Child's Health Needs

During his first few years in elementary school, the classroom teacher is the person with whom the child spends most of his day. The teacher therefore, is the logical person to be most immediately concerned with the child and his total needs. His health needs are paramount, health in the current usage of physical, mental, emotional and social health. Even before the child's arrival at school and the opening of the fall term, the alert well-prepared teacher will take the first step toward assembling this total picture. If the teacher is taking a new position, she can obtain information concerning the city, its cultural and social structure, economic conditions, resources, and other pertinent facts from the local Chamber of Commerce. From the local department of public health she can secure community health statistics and information about special health problems of the area, particularly as they may pertain to the neighborhood surrounding the school. A visit to the neighborhood will yield graphic information as to living conditions and probable neighborhood experiences of the school-aged child, standards of markets and shops, and available community agencies and health facilities and resources.

A visit to the school will add to the health picture. The teacher will gain an idea of the school facilities, its health standards, possible hazards, and special health and safety problems so that she may begin to focus upon ways of coping with them. At this time or at least prior to her meetings with the pupils, she should obtain from the principal or the medical division, the handbook or guide to school health and safety policies and procedures so that she may familiarize herself in advance as to ways in which she will be expected to meet emergency situations of various types. A conference with the school nurse will yield information as to the significant health problems of the school and possibly some of the individual health problems of her future pupils. She will also have the opportunity of becoming acquainted with the cumulative health records and learn how they are to be used. Interviews with the guidance counselor, the librarian, the principal and even the school cafeteria director and custodian can all prove fruitful in adding to the prospective teacher's total picture.

The first day of school frequently offers possibilities for contacts with parents and significant observation of parent-child relationships and even glimpses of health attitudes. But when the pupils are actually assembled, the teacher can begin systematic observations. The pre-service preparation of the elementary teacher should include, along with the usual child observation and child development courses, ample training in observation of disease symptoms and conditions. Since the teacher is with the child so many hours each day, she is in a position to note the child's usual appearance and health behavior and, therefore, when they occur, unusual deviations. Actually, her observations are likely to be a valuable supplement to those of the school physician who perhaps sees the child for the first time during a possible fifteen minute examination period.

Other opportunities to determine the child's health needs include observations of the child during free play, his responses during informal discussion periods, his conversation with other children, his reactions during field trips, and discussions at parent conferences and PTA meetings. Through practice, one develops the ability to see what is really significant and to develop deeper insight as to possible causes underlying unusual behavior.

Thus, by piecing together her observations and findings, the teacher will gain a vibrant picture of the child in the setting of his home, his neighborhood, his school, and his community. At the same time, she will find herself growing more sensitive to the child's changing health behavior and therefore will be able to plan better or to create situations wherein it might be possible to meet the child's major health needs. She will gain skill in centering health instruction upon the child's own problems while at the same time, anticipating his future needs.

In the intermediate and upper elementary grades the teacher will wish to acquaint herself prior to the arrival of pupils for the opening of the term, with the course of study or course outlines which she will be expected to implement. She will wish to examine them in the light of her preliminary findings if she is a new teacher, or at least in the context of her observations and the total health picture. She will wish to map out tentative additions and possible deletions, and plan supplementary experiences and resource materials.

After the school term begins, the teacher will continue her observations, and probably refer to previous individual test scores of pupils. Before beginning her teaching she may wish to give a diagnostic knowledge test to determine areas which need special emphasis. She may wish to proceed as many teachers do, to preface each unit with its own pre-test Whatever her procedure, her plans should include provision for adequate appraisal at various advantageous steps along the way, in addition to the time-honored final tests. Each of these plans will help to shed light upon pupil health needs and give direction to her teaching. An alert school health council, the composition and purpose of which are discussed later, will also prove effective in disclosing pupils' health needs, in helping to determine priorities, and, on the secondary level, in aiding to plan an integrated approach involving several departments.

Questions for Discussion

1. What are the minimal requirements pertaining to the school health program as prescribed in your state? Where does the responsibility for their implementation rest?
2. How does the scope of the health program in the public school system in your community compare with the suggestions listed in this chapter?
3. Can you substantiate the following statement: The need for the inclusion of sound health teaching in the school curriculum is greater to-day than it ever has been in the history of the world.

4. Educators, for many years, have termed health the first cardinal principle of education How do you account for the fact that in actual practice the schools have so often failed to give it first attention?

Suggested Readings

1. American Association of School Administrators: *Health In Schools.* 20th Yearbook, 2nd ed. Washington, D.C.: the Association, a department of the National Education Association, 1951.
2. Anderson, Carl L.: *School Health Practice.* 4th ed., St. Louis, The C. V. Mosby Co., 1968.
3. Bucher, Charles A.: *The Administration of School and College Health and Physical Education Programs.* 4th Ed. St. Louis, The C. V. Mosby Co., 1967.
4. National Commission on Community Health Services: *Health is a Community Affair.* Cambridge, Harvard University Press, 1966.
5. National Committee on School Health Policies of the National Education Association and the American Medical Association: *Suggested School Health Policies.* 4th ed. Washington, D.C.: National Education Association, and Chicago, American Medical Association, 1966.
6. Nyswander, Dorothy B.: *Solving School Health Problems.* New York, Commonwealth Fund, 1942.
7. Oberteuffer, Delbert and Beyrer, Mary K.: *School Health Education.* 4th ed., New York, Harper and Row, 1966.
8. Patterson, Raymond S. and Roberts, Beryl J.: *Community Health in Action.* St. Louis, The C. V. Mosby Co., 1951.
9. Schneider, Elsa and McNeeley, Simon A.: *Teachers Contribute to Child Health.* Office of Education, U.S. Department of Health, Education, and Welfare, Bulletin No. 8, Washington, D.C.: U.S. Government Printing Office, 1951.
10. Turner, Clair E.: *Planning for Health Education in Schools*: A Study Undertaken on Behalf of UNESCO and WHO. London, Longmans, 1966.

Chapter 11

The School Health Team

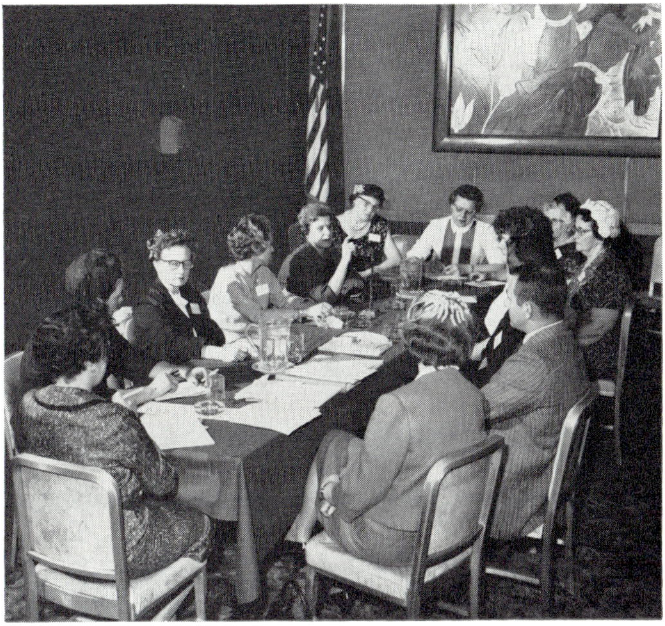

Fig. 55. The School Health Team in Action.

Introduction

The expansion of the school health program and the necessary increase in personnel to conduct it, have emphasized the importance of effective teamwork. With the maze of relationships and interactions involved in working together effectively, it would be impossible to avoid duplication and overlapping of efforts, and waste of funds, without planned cooperation. Each member of the health team must assume certain core responsibilities inherent in his specific task. These responsibilities vary somewhat in different localities and work situations according to the needs of the children, the objectives of the community and school health programs, and the available facilities, funds, and leadership. However, they need to be clearly defined and understood not only by the individual, but also by all other members of the team. Responsibility for decision-making and action plans at various levels must be clearly stated and allocated, and understood by all.

Although the responsibilities and activities of certain members of the team may be centered within one of the main divisions of the school health program, their interests and duties will necessarily extend into other areas. Thus, the school physician, the nurse, the dentist, and the dental hygienist relate primarily to school health services; but these people are also deeply concerned with the maintenance of a healthful school environment and the quality of the health instruction. Similarly, the school administrator, the guidance counselor, and the classroom teacher are naturally intimately concerned and associated with all phases of the health program. A brief look at the roles of some of the key members of the school health team may offer insight into respective duties, work relationships and interactions which may not always be evident to the casual observer, but which underlie effective teamwork and a successful program.

The School Physician

The school physician should be a graduate of an approved medical school and preferably have additional training as a pediatrician or in public health. It is desirable also that he possess some understanding of educational philosophy, organization and procedure. It is essential that he be familiar with state school legislation, the regulations of the State Departments of Health and of Public Instruction relating to the health of the school child, school health services and the school health program. In a small town or county, he would probably be a part-time employee. In a large city system, the chief school physician would be a full-time employee and be assisted by a staff of part-time physicians who also engage in the private practice of medicine.

Usually, the school physician is responsible to the superintendent of public schools, who in turn, serves as liaison with the Board of Education on health matters. The school physician is responsible for the development and conduct of an over-all health service program which meets at least the minimal specifications of the State Department of Health and the State Department of Public Instruction. The program should, of course, be approved by the local Superintendent and the Board of Education. The school physician is also responsible for the selection and recommendation for appointment of qualified personnel for his division and for the preparation of an appropriate budget.

In the school system of a large city, the chief of the dental division and the supervisor of school nurses would be administratively responsible to the school physician. The latter should keep the Superintendent of Schools constantly informed about changing conditions, significant problems which may arise and medical progress that may have bearing upon school services or the health program.

The school physician is responsible for pre-employment health examinations of school personnel and for periodic re-appraisal according to state and local regulations. Standards and supervision comparable to the health requirements for all school personnel should be extended to part-time employees.

The school physician should play an important part in the school physical education and athletic program by providing special examinations of participants in intra-mural and inter-school activities, implementing procedures for the prevention of injuries, screening of all pupils for activities in regular physical education classes, conducting continuous follow-up of those assigned to adapted programs, and cooperating with school camping and outdoor education programs. He should cooperate with the development of the physical fitness program through the encouragement of voluntary participation of pupils and the promotion of parent interest.

The school physician should cooperate actively in local, state, and regional comprehensive health planning. He should aim to make the objectives and goals of the school health services familiar not only to school employees, but to all physicians in the community, and should keep them informed as to progress toward their realization. As a qualified physician he should be a member of his County Medical Society through which he can brief his colleagues on the uses of the school examination forms to be used by all family physicians and secure their cooperation in follow-up and referrals. He should seek the advice of his medical colleagues in the health department in planning immunization procedures and measures to meet emergency situations such as epidemics and disasters, as well as for family education pertaining to new procedures, and special services such as those for the handicapped or exceptional child. The school physician will need to know the community health resources and facilities and seek the best means of utilizing them in the follow-up of defects found by the periodic medical examination. This implies familiarity with programs of official and voluntary health agencies, hospitals, clinics, and other community facilities. In the larger city systems, psychological and guidance services, corrective physical education, speech correction and other special services are often provided within the school system. In rural areas and small towns, these services are more likely to be readily available if a county health unit exists.

In the schools under his supervision, the physician should serve as consultant to the school and community health councils or committees, and as a resource person to teachers and other school personnel, verifying the accuracy of health information introduced into the curriculum and supplying new information as it may appear. Opportunities for in-service education of teachers and maintenance staff can often be arranged through cooperative planning with the school administrator.

The physician should try to make each contact with a pupil an educational experience. For this reason, it is important that time allotment and work conditions be such as to permit an unhurried examination and an opportunity to answer the questions of the children and their parents.

The school physician should assume responsibility for the compilation of a written statement of health policies, procedures, and guidelines (including those pertaining to emergencies) for the school district and secure the approval of the Superintendent and Board of Education for its adoption and implementation. He needs to provide instruction and interpretation for all persons concerned with its implementation and use, for the periodic review and appraisal of the content, and in the light of desirable innovative methods or new information, for re-evaluation and revision.

The School Nurse

Changes in the concept of general health care have greatly influenced the role of the school nurse. In the early days of school nursing, the major portion of the time was devoted to checking on cases of childhood disease, guiding youngsters through their fears of tonsillectomies and dental clinics, and at the close of the year laboriously compiling masses of statistics concerning the numbers and kinds of pupil defects discovered. Typically, these statistics were then deposited at some central point, usually the State Department of Health or of Public Instruction. The process was dutifully repeated the following year. Undoubtedly these accumulations of scores must have generated a frustrating uneasiness in all conscientious pioneering school nurses. Certainly, they struggled gallantly with parents and with existing ignorance of the aims and importance of public health activities.

The role of the school nurse to-day is indeed quite different and much more complex, and eludes succinct and accurate description. A brochure issued by the National League for Nursing describes the present role of the school nurse quite admirably:

> The role of the nurse in the school is to utilize, in collaboration with others, her knowledge and competence in nursing so that it contributes significantly to the achievement of the full health and educational potential of each student. Her ability to serve most adequately within the school setting is dependent upon basic preparation for professional nursing and additional preparation that will enable her to
>
> 1. Utilize concepts of human growth, development and behavior in the milieu of the school health program.
> 2. Recognize developmental and health needs of students especially in relation to prevention, detection, and treatment which must influence educational programing.
> 3. Utilize existing community services for children and youth and spearhead the development of additional services when indicated by the needs of the school health program.

4. Comprehend the nature of the educational setting in which the school nurse works.
5. Select and use processes appropriate to the roles assumed by the school nurse.[1]

The school nurse today wears many hats. Her sensitivity, skill, and discretion as to when to wear which particular hat in large measure determine the degree of her success. Professionally, the school nurse is a public health nurse who works with a limited age group of the population both in the school and in the child's home. This means that in addition to her usual hospital training signified by her R.N., she needs to have a much broader preparation. As a basis for action she must know more about child development, the family and its psychological inter-actions and problems; the community health program and its aims, objectives and facilities; and the place of the school health program in the total community health picture. She needs also to understand the aims of education, the roles of the school administrator, the teacher and the physician in the school, and the inter-relationships and interactions involved in a school health program. It is important that she become an integral part of the school neighborhood efforts toward health in order that she might understand specific neighborhood health problems which affect and determine the lives of the children in the school. Coupled with all of these is the need for familiarity with the facilities and resources immediately accessible to families and to know something of the fears, anxieties and hesitancies attached to them by the people, as well as their ability to use them wisely and appropriately.

Naturally, the duties of the school nurse vary depending upon the circumstances of particular situations. In general, however, the nurse is responsible for assisting the school physician in planning and carrying out procedures pertaining to all phases of the school health services: the health appraisal, the medical examination, the follow-up and referral measures involving home cooperation, the handling of special cases, health counseling, the implementation of protective measures, and the provision of emergency care. She should be alert to the teacher's efforts in health education and regard herself as a resource person for the enrichment of the health instruction. If the nurse is to assume some of the teaching responsibility, it will be necessary for her to conform with state education requirements for a teaching certificate. The pupil load per nurse shows considerable variation in states and communities. Naturally, consideration must be given to the availability of other health workers, to the allocation of duties and responsibilities, the use of aides

[1]*The Preparation and the Role of the Nurse in School Health Programs.* Guidelines for the Use of Administrators, Educators, and Students prepared by Helen Goodale Florentine. National League for Nursing, Department of Baccalaureate and Higher Degree Programs, 10 Columbus Circle, New York 19, New Yark, 1962, p. 7.

and other personnel. There is general agreement among nurses, however, that a nurse's load should never exceed one thousand pupils in urban schools.

Various time studies and re-appraisals of the wide range of duties and responsibilities usually carried by the school nurse have pointed up the need for setting up priorities in order to secure the best utilization of her unique professional competencies. It has been found that many duties such as recording, filing, receptionist duties, and even simple first aid procedures (if performed by a person properly certified by the American Red Cross), can be performed satisfactorily by non-professionals after some preliminary training by the nurse and under her constant supervision. Thus, the school nurse is enabled to devote more time to case-finding, prevention of illness, and promotion of health. She is available for more counseling of students, conferences with teachers, parents, and community health workers, to provide resource services in health education classes, to participate in and arrange for in-service education, and to play a more active role in comprehensive health planning in the community.

In large school districts employing a number of nurses, there is need for a supervisor of school nursing. To qualify for this post, advanced preparation in education is required in addition to the usual school nurse requirements. In New York State, for example, the teacher-nurse plays a very special role. Both the dedicated supervisor of school nursing and the nurse working in a single school need to plan for continuing evaluation of their activities and to cooperate when possible, with on-going related research in the school district and the community. The administrator of the health service division and the supervisor of school nurses should arrange in-service opportunities for the members of their staffs to add to their professional competencies.

In summary, the school nurse occupies a key spot in the school health picture as a catalyst who can really bring together the elements likely to result in specific health action or social change.

The School Dentist

The school dentist should be a graduate of an approved school of dentistry and preferably have experience in children's dentistry or public health dentistry. He should be a member of his local, state and national associations. As with the other members of the school health team, it is desirable also that he have some understanding of education and educational objectives and procedures. In a large city school system, the chief dentist is most likely to be a full-time employee. His assistant dentists will probably be part-time employees with the rest of their time devoted to private practice.

The school dentist or dental division usually functions under the administration of the school physician who is director of the school health services. This appears to be practical in terms of scheduling, budgeting and record keeping. In most states, a periodic dental examination is mandatory.

The school aims to have its dental program foster on the part of parents and children, an appreciation of dental health, an understanding of the need for a continuous life-time program of dental care, and the habit of participating regularly in such a program. Accordingly, its main emphasis is upon having the child receive his periodic dental examination, preventive care, and follow-up service from his family dentist. Public schools, therefore, cooperate with the dental program by excusing the child during school hours if necessary to keep such appointments if they cannot be arranged at other times.

Children who do not have a family dentist should be given an examination by the school dentist using one of the types of examinations suggested by the American Dental Association, or an appraisal by the dental hygienist (who, of course, is not permitted to make diagnosis). Parents should be notified about the results of the examination and the importance of initiating remedial procedures immediately. In the case of an indigent child, most communities provide dental correction free or at a nominal cost. This may be obtained at dental clinics maintained by the local or State departments of health, by hospitals, or voluntary agencies. In numerous instances the local dental society has taken the initiative in working out arrangements for such service, sometimes by utilizing private dentists. In areas where fluoridation of drinking water has not been instituted, the topical application of fluoride is sometimes made available at clinics.

It is important that the dentist be regarded as a member of the school health team. He needs to be able to see his specific professional contribution in the wider perspective of the total health situation. His active participation in school and community health planning groups is conducive to the attainment of the best results for the school program.

The school dentist has an excellent opportunity to serve as a resource person to the classroom teacher and to those responsible for the curriculum. He should be alert to his responsibility for verification and implementation of new information, methods, and procedures in his field and for evaluating materials for use in health education classes. During recent years the dental profession has made a notable contribution through emphasis upon dental safety in sports, through the development of football mouth guards, and by education about dental accident prevention.

Children and parents need to be educated to an appreciation and understanding of the value of a dental program throughout life, the importance of orthodontia, and the prevention and correction of dental and other oral defects. The school dentist is in an admirable position to provide community leadership in this direction.

The Dental Hygienist

The dental hygienist is a graduate of an accredited school of oral or dental hygiene and frequently has a bachelor's or master's degree. In a large city school system, the chief dental hygienist should have at least a master's degree in health education or public health. In addition, she should possess a good understanding of education, its administration, aims, objectives, and methods.

The dental hygienist functions in somewhat the same relationship with the dentist as the nurse with the physician. She assists the dentist with the periodic dental examination, records, and other procedures. She is authorized to give dental prophylaxis to children in schools and in some states is permitted to give topical applications of fluorides. She functions also as a dental health educator and as a resource person to teachers. Her pre-service preparation has provided her with skills in the uses of materials and methods for dental health education. The dental hygienist releases the dentist for more emphasis upon strictly dental professional procedures.

Because of her direct contact with the children, the dental hygienist is in an excellent position to exert positive influence and should be well aware of the potentialities inherent in her position. Her assigned duties should include giving assistance to the classroom teacher in preparing the children for the periodic dental examination by allaying fears and anxieties. She should fully understand her role in relation to the total school health team and to the community.

The School Administrator

A successful school health program involves understanding and leadership by the superintendent in his role of top-ranking coordinator and liaison with the Board of Education and the community. It is highly essential that the professional preparation of the administrator include courses which will prepare him for this part of his responsibility. He must have an understanding of what constitutes a sound school health program, its aims and objectives, approved procedures, standards, and evaluation methods, and a practical grasp of the interactions necessary within the various school segments and among the members of the health team, as well as insight as to ways in which the home, the school, and the community may work together in the interests of the health of the student population. It is important that he perceive the school health program as a segment of the total community health picture and that he realize his obligation for conveying this concept to his staff. In this regard, either he or some other qualified official representative of the schools should participate actively in the over-all community planning for health. The superintendent or his representative should be able to present school needs to such planning bodies and at the same time be able to visualize and utilize opportunities for the fullest application of community health plans and facilities for the furtherance of the health of the school child.

Within the schools, much of the superintendent's operational authority is necessarily delegated to certain members of his staff: to division heads, supervisors, and principals of schools. As already indicated, the chief responsibility for school health services to meet state and local requirements is delegated to the Chief School Physician or Director of School Health Services who in turn delegates specific parts of the work to the various members of his staff.

The superintendent's administrational responsibilities for healthful school living are not quite so simple to delegate. In a large system, for example, a Division of Buildings and Grounds or of School Maintenance carries responsibility for the maintenance of safe and sanitary buildings and grounds. The head of this division might also supervise the janitorial staff and similar personnel. Frequently, the task of the sanitary inspection of buildings falls to the chief physician. However, in many states, the law requires that such inspections be performed by trained sanitarians from the local health department. This is logical since the health department regulations or ordinances concerning water supply, waste disposal, milk, food control, restaurants and food handlers, swimming pools and public buildings apply to schools as well as other parts of the community. Observance of fire laws and traffic safety regulations is another public concern, and involves local fire and safety inspectors and police. Plans for new school buildings must conform to the local building code and to specifications and standards as prescribed by the State Department of Public Instruction.

Since the superintendent is responsible for the entire curriculum, he is concerned with health instruction. This he delegates to the heads of curriculum at various levels who in turn prepare appropriate courses of study to meet the requirements of the State Department of Public Instruction. Supervisors, heads of departments, and teachers then assume responsibility for the implementation of the courses of study. The superintendent, aided by his staff must select and recommend to the Board of Education qualified personnel for the various staff positions. It is therefore important that he and his associates be familiar with the qualifications for the various kinds of health positions as set forth in the standards adopted by their professional organizations. Considering these many involvements, it is obvious that without administrators who possess real understanding of the implications of all phases of the school health program, optimum results would be unattainable. Courses fitting him for his responsibilities for the health program should be considered as part of his professional qualifications.

The Principal

The school principal functions as the administrator within a single school unit. As a result, he naturally is concerned with all three areas of the school health program. His responsibilities in each are similar to those of the superintendent but limited to the confines of his school. For this as well as other things, he is directly responsible to the superintendent of the schools or his deputy.

In a small school, the principal will need to work closely with the school physician and the nurse in planning the implementation of the periodic health appraisal, protective measures such as immunizations, emergency medical care, employee health maintenance, health counseling, provisions for adequate follow-up and referrals of health defects, programs for handicapped pupils, special examinations of athletes, regular nurse services and medical records. He will need to familiarize his staff with the policies and procedures set forth in the health policies handbook for the school system.

A safe and sanitary environment must be maintained constantly. This implies attention to lighting, ventilation, cleanliness, seating, laboratory safety, satisfactory lunchroom and other facilities, fire drills and civilian defense provisions, and many other health-related concerns. Required inspections must be coordinated with the proper authorities and all recommendations must be carried out promptly. To accomplish this, the principal must work closely with his maintenance staff, the Superintendent of Buildings, and representatives of the local Health, Police, and Public Safety Departments. The principal is responsible for suitable school fire-drills and other safety and traffic regulations, and, with his department heads, must assure that safety rules are observed in the laboratory, shop, physical education and recreation activities. In the elementary schools, he will work with classroom teachers for safe school living. The implementation of approved courses of study in health and related subjects is also a concern of the principal.

These are some of the more obvious responsibilities and duties which fall within the province of the principal. Like the superintendent of schools, he will need to participate actively in community and civic planning for health. Certainly he should be familiar with the health problems, facilities and resources of the school neighborhood and those of the wider community, and to know the leaders and their workers. He should be able to marshal the strengths of the Parent-Teacher Association in the furtherance of the school health program. He should foster the formation of a school health council or committee to bring teachers, pupils, and parents to focus upon health matters.

To weave all these elements into a workable structure requires skill, sympathetic insight, and a well-rounded general health background. The principal's professional preparation should be similar to that of the administrator's to insure worthwhile positive results. He should regard himself as one of the health team and seek to meet the demands of the role with due respect to the parts played by the other members of the team. In order to do so, he needs to be familiar with the responsibilities and abilities of each of the members of the school health staff. Because of the complexity of his role and the multiplicity of his duties, the principal sometimes designates a member of his staff to serve as coordinator of school health affairs. In fact, in some states there is a definite trend toward the appointment in each school of a health coordinator specifically trained for the position.

The School Health Coordinator

The school health coordinator should have a master's degree in health education and related subjects and some classroom experience in teaching health. As the title implies, he or she is responsible for the organization and coordination of all health matters within the school. His responsibilities include many of those ascribed above to the principal of the school. In addition, the health coordinator is likely to have complete supervision and coordination of health education. The acceleration of new knowledge in health and medical science and the better understanding of child development awakened professionals to a greater awareness that physical education and health education, although closely related, are two distinct subject areas and call for widely different skills in teaching methods and approaches. During the past decade numerous personal and community health problems have snowballed to such extent that concerned community groups frequently have demanded that the schools strive to meet these problems, and in some instances have even made funds available for necessary associated research and implementation. These developments have led not only to an increasing recognition of health education as a vital segment of a child's curricular experience at all levels, but also to the inadequacy of the time allotment in the curriculum, and the lack of teachers with adequate background and preparation for the new task. The obvious first step, the certification of teachers of health education, has been implemented in some states, accompanied in most instances by provision for in-service education opportunities for the present teachers to meet the new standards within certain time limits. In many situations, however, the Director of Health, Physical Education, and Recreation is still the person responsible for health instruction. Certainly, the health coordinator, because of his involvement with all the health activities of the school, is in a strategic position to effect a high degree of articulation of all health efforts.

One of the more important responsibilities of the school health coordinator would be the chairmanship of the School Health Committee or Council. He should serve as official school representative in various community health enterprises particularly in comprehensive health planning. In-service education of staff and parent education might also logically form part of his assigned duties. Obviously there are many advantages in having this type of leadership in developing a coordinated program, particularly in the secondary school where the school health program so often appears to the staff as hopelessly fragmented.

Some large school districts have instituted a coordinator of health services as well as a coordinator of health education, a plan which should permit expansion of the program and better quality of results.

The Director of Health, Physical Education and Recreation

The responsibilities of the director of health, physical education and recreation in a school system are numerous and varied, so the implications for cooperation and teamwork are correspondingly plentiful. In a large city system his duties are likely to be entirely administrative. He would be assisted by a staff of supervisors who in turn supervise the special teachers of health and physical education in individual schools. In a smaller system, the director often combines some teaching with his administrative and supervisory duties. Usually he is directly responsible to the superintendent of schools who, as indicated, is ultimately responsible for the nature and quality of the entire program.

The director should be prepared by graduation from a college or university with an accredited major department in health, physical education and recreation, supplemented by additional work on the graduate level in one of the three components of his field. It is essential that he possess a broad understanding of education to enable him to see his special field in the perspective of general educational philosophy. In addition he needs to understand the objectives of the school health program and its working details in order to coordinate his own planning accordingly, and to cooperate with the school health personnel in every way possible.

Health service procedures significant to his department include health appraisal of all participants in physical education activities, pre-season examination of athletes including chest x-rays, medical supervision during the playing season, and post-season check-ups, the use of physical fitness tests, the promotion of protective devices such as teeth guards, emergency care, and guidance and counseling in connection with adaptive classes in physical education. The utilization of the best health standards in the conduct of all activities should be paramount throughout his entire division. He needs to work closely with the school physician in the implementation of policies, procedures, and regulations governing first aid techniques and the handling of emergency situations, and to ascertain that his staff members have met the required first aid training qualifications. He should encourage the entire physical education staff to cooperate with the school nurse, physician, and other school health personnel by assisting whenever possible with the weighing, measuring, screening, and preparation for the periodic health appraisal. On the other hand, he should try to familiarize the health service personnel with the activities, needs and problems of his division, and to seek their cooperation in the encouragement of each pupil's participation in a program of physical and recreational activities related to his health needs and interests. Requests to be excused from physical education are seldom a problem when the activity program is sufficiently broad and diversified as to offer opportunity for individual adaptive physical education rosters and a wide variety of activities geared to the many goals and interests of children.

A large part of the direct responsibility for a healthful sanitary school environment falls upon this department. Physical education and recreation programs involve the use of playfields, gymnasia, swimming pools, and many kinds of apparatus and equipment. The director needs to secure the cooperation of his staff in the maintenance of safe and sanitary conditions in the physical education plant, including shower and locker rooms. This requires perpetual vigilance to ensure protection against communicable diseases and accidents for those who use these facilities. This means that the director and his staff must work closely with the Superintendent of Buildings or Physical Plant, the maintenance personnel, and the local Department of Health.

Unless some unusual curriculum pattern is in effect, the Director of Health, Physical Education and Recreation is also responsible for the health instruction. He provides for the preparation and adoption of an adequate, comprehensive course of study which implements the requirements of the State Department of Public Instruction, and is responsible for the quality of the health instruction in secondary schools and sometimes, as in team teaching, in the upper elementary grades. He should serve as a consultant and resource person in health education to his entire staff and to other teachers whose subject may or can include certain health units. He should encourage all of these teachers to utilize health service personnel in this capacity also.

Like other individuals carrying responsibilities in all three divisions of the health program, the Director of Health, Physical Education and Recreation should be familiar with official and voluntary health agencies whose services and activities may impinge upon or contribute to his own program area. He should strive to effect smooth articulation wherever possible, and to utilize to the best advantage their materials and resources for the ultimate health and welfare of the school child.

The Guidance Counselor

Although the guidance counselor's role in knitting together the strands and elements needed for the solution of pupil disciplinary and educational problems has been well recognized, his importance in the area of health is frequently overlooked or not appreciated. Individual discipline and adjustment difficulties and school failures very often have as their true source, a deep-rooted health problem—physical, mental, social, or emotional. In fact, it has been stated frequently by guidance counselors that from sixty to seventy per cent of their problem cases involve some type of health difficulty. Such problems frequently center about appearance, nutrition, a physical defect or handicap, over-participation or disinterest in athletics or other school activities, drug abuse, family relationships or world conditions. Problems of finance may also affect nutrition, clothing, transportation, sleep and rest, time budgeting, or absence from school. In order to cope adequately with such diverse problems, the counselor's preparation needs to include a sound foundation in child development, personal and community health, and school health, as well as the usual preparation for counseling and experience in classroom teaching. Wise referrals and the planning of fruitful case conferences require an understanding of the role of each member of the health team to ensure the best utilization of the resources of the school.

Because of the complex organizational structure of the secondary school, it is obvious that to be effective the guidance system must permeate the entire school and its responsibilities must, in a sense, be shared by all who come into contact with the pupils. In-service education of staff members toward this end is a responsibility of the guidance counselor. On the elementary school level, the main objective of the guidance plan should be the prevention of problems and their early identification and solution before they begin to snowball into difficulties of greater magnitude at the secondary level.

The guidance counselor needs a thorough understanding of the community, its cultural, social, economic, and ethnic patterns, and its developmental trends and directions. He needs to familiarize himself not only with the facets of the school health program but with the community groups and resources including those related to health and welfare.

The Teacher

The classroom teacher is in a unique position to contribute significantly to the total school health program. Actually he or she is cast in the role of most critical and constant observer of the school child. Because of this, she can determine the child's total health problems and needs better than almost anyone else, not infrequently better than the child's parents who see him in a different context, and better than the child's physician who sees him only sporadically and usually when something has gone wrong. Therefore, the teacher's possible contributions to the health service program are manifold. They will vary according to the individual situation as will the interaction patterns, but in general they will be somewhat as follows.

In the elementary school the teacher can assist the nurse to prepare the pupils psychologically for the periodic health appraisal, the medical and dental examinations, immunizations, and other procedures. She is able to give the nurse pertinent supplementary information gained through her observations and close association with the children. She will cooperate with the efforts of the nurses to obtain the child's health history from the parent. If the medical examination is to be conducted by the school physician, it is an advantage for her to be present in order to contribute on the basis of her intimate knowledge of the child, as well as to receive any advice the physician may wish to offer as to the better adjustment of the school routine to the needs of the child.

The teacher is in a position to reinforce the nurse's efforts in follow-up with the child and the parent in the implementation of recommendations and remedial measures. In the case of an exceptional child in her class, the teacher needs to be receptive in regard to ways of dealing with special handicaps and limitations and in working out individual routines. In the event of special testing or immunization programs, the teacher can provide valuable cooperation by supplementing official informative materials with her health teaching. This, in turn, will extend into the home. In the kindergarten and lower elementary grades an informal morning health review permits the teacher to single out those with deviations from the usual. She may arrange temporary isolation until the arrival of the school nurse. Other ways of cooperating with the control of communicable disease have been included in the chapter entitled, Man vs. Disease. All teachers should be familiar with basic emergency care procedures, so that in the absence of the nurse they may carry on in a wise and safe manner. They should be familiar with the policies and procedures prepared for the school district by the chief physician and approved by the Board of Education.

The teacher's personal attitude toward health procedures and toward health personnel is an important factor in reassuring the child, and in encouraging the building of sound mental and emotional attitudes toward health. At all times, the teacher's personal actions should be consistent with the practices and procedures advanced by the school health personnel. She should never allude grudgingly to the time missed by the pupil in meeting dental or health appraisal appointments.

In the junior and senior high schools, the classroom teacher is more remote from contact with the school health service team. At this level, the teacher's own health attitudes are not always quite so convincing to pupils. The home room teacher and the guidance counselor are in key positions for cooperating with remedial measures prescribed for individual pupils, and the tactful and effective management of handicapped pupils. Seeing is believing, and often a visit to the nurse or other school health personnel in the health room will yield more two-way understanding and cooperation than is possible through mere official mimeographed notices.

Teachers should give the nurse in particular full recognition as a member of the school staff. They should welcome her at faculty meetings and case conferences at which times she may be able to provide insight pertaining to the problems of individual pupils and possible clues leading to their solution. Through her daily contacts with the students, an alert nurse often spots significant trends or the first stages of potential group or all-school health problems. Prompt response by teachers to her requests for cooperation could result in an immediate, appropriate preventive program of specific health instruction and action.

All teachers need to realize that an alert health committee or health council in a secondary school greatly facilitates the wise channeling of health problems and allocation of ameliorative measures. Whenever a special sub-committee is assigned to focus upon the possibilities for integration of health education into the content of courses other than specific health classes, teachers should cooperate willingly. Finally, through the sensitive guidance of an understanding teacher in the role of adviser, the student council may actually prove to be a most potent means of securing peer cooperation in the development of desirable health understandings, practices, and attitudes.

The School Health Council

In the individual school, teamwork can be most effectively achieved through a school health council. The structure of such a council will vary somewhat according to the local circumstances. In general, however, an active council would include those persons who have most responsibility for the various parts of the school health program, together with such representative personnel as will permit permeation of the council's influence into all facets of school life.

The scope and functions of a school health council have been admirably expressed as follows in a leaflet prepared for parent information by one of the pioneer school health councils whose record of success during the years has confirmed the soundness of the idea:

> The Health Council, recruited from the various departments of instruction, is a continuously working group carrying on simultaneously many activities pertinent to health matters. At the outset, the following were deemed the legitimate function of such an organization:
>
> 1. to serve as a clearing house for health matters,
> 2. to coordinate health efforts,

3. to evaluate present school health procedures and plan and inaugurate new ones,
4. to provide a healthful school environment,
5. to encourage high standards of personal health,
6. to keep pace with changing ideas in the field of health,
7. to rouse faculty and student bodies to health awareness,
8. to lead to the development of a health program,
9. to use various school resources for health emphasis.[2]

In an elementary school, the health council would include the principal, teacher representatives from all grades, the nurse, the guidance counselor, the custodian, the nutritionist or dietitian, and representatives of the Parent-Teacher Association. The school physician and the school dentist should be invited but usually they are unable to give much time to each school. However, they should be regarded as resource persons, available whenever needed, and should be kept fully informed as to program developments. It is also helpful to include representatives from the public health department and from some of the voluntary health agencies.

In the secondary school, the health council should include the principal, the dean of boys and the dean of girls, the guidance counselor, the nurse, the teachers of health and physical education for boys and for girls, the nutritionist, the custodian, and a representative from the departments of science, social studies, home economics, English—in fact, preferably from all departments so that channels might be set up for having health information carried to all faculty members, home rooms, the Student Council, and the Parents' Association. The chairman of the council should be someone dedicated to health and health education and well qualified in that field. Usually, the principal can function more effectively if he remains ex-officio, for he will need to serve as liaison with the Superintendent of Schools and/or the Board of Education.

Regular meetings should be scheduled and included in the official school calendar. Special meetings may be called when needed. In some schools, monthly meetings have been found adequate. In others, meetings are held bi-weekly.

On both the elementary and the secondary levels it will be found that many of the activities of the school health council will be carried on by means of committees. This permits study groups to focus upon problems of special interest to its members. For example, different committees might focus concurrently on nutrition, safety education, health science instruction, sex education, and on other special areas.

In a large city system in which each school has a functioning health council, it might be desirable to have a city-wide or Central School

[2] Health Council of Senior High School, Reading, Pennsylvania.

Health Council composed of the chairmen or some other representative of each school health council. The chairman of the central group might be the Supervisor of Health Education, the Supervisor of Health, Physical Education and Recreation, the Chief School Physician, or the Supervisor of School Nurses. Such a central council can provide a network of communication among all the schools. In order to extend its influence further, its membership might also include representatives from the local public health department, the Health and Welfare Council, and other official and voluntary agencies concerned with phases of child health. Similarly, it is important to have the Central School Health Council represented on various key community health policy or comprehensive planning committees.

In some cases the term "health committee" has been chosen in preference to the more pretentious "health council." In the case of a large city with an over-all Health and Welfare Council this might avoid confusion. Regardless of its name, basic to the success of any such organization is the whole-hearted, objective cooperation and support of those who comprise the group. A health council is more likely to succeed if at the beginning there is a nucleus of faculty members with a genuine concern for the health of school children, an awareness of existing problems, an urge for action toward improvement, and faith in what a group of dedicated individuals can accomplish by working together in a common cause. Where health councils have failed, it has been observed that usually this precaution has been overlooked or that the approach has been too hurried. In a number of such cases, failure has been due to the fact that the council was imposed upon an unconvinced, lukewarm or indifferent faculty by an ambitious principal or faculty member, in an attempt to keep up with neighboring schools. In still other instances an unsuccessful council was the brainchild of a single well-meaning, enthusiastic teacher who centered activities round herself to such an extent that when she took a position elsewhere the entire structure promptly collapsed.

To illustrate the contrary, the story of the actual steps taken and experienced by one pioneering school in the establishment of a successful school health council may be of interest and value to the reader.

> Clermont Senior High School, with a student body of approximately 3200 and a faculty of 110, was the only public high school serving an industrial city of 100,000. The idea of a Health Council began with three interested staff members; the nurse, the head of the science department and the head of girls' health and physical education.
>
> During casual conversation at lunchtime, it was discovered that one of the home economics teachers and a practical arts teacher had long been concerned about the multiplicity of

student health problems they had observed from day to day. They welcomed the idea of a health council as a possible means of doing something about the situation. With five interested persons as a nucleus, it was felt that the time for action had arrived. Accordingly, it was agreed that two of the group would arrange an appointment with the principal to sound him out on the possibility of a health council for the school.

After thirty minutes of questioning and probing, the principal's enthusiasm matched that of the two delegates. He confessed that he had always been bothered that health occupied top rank in the list of the "Seven Cardinal Principles" and yet so little seemed to be done about it. He proposed that the matter be placed on the agenda for the next regular faculty meeting, and that the five interested persons plan to present it with all five participating in some way. This required careful strategy.

The five finally agreed upon a diagram of the proposed council which they felt would reinforce their presentation if drawn on the blackboard prior to the meeting. To avoid overlapping, it was further decided that each of the five would give a five-minute presentation of the advantages of such a council from the point of view of his particular department, and that one would include an additional five-minute talk about what it could mean to his homeroom pupils.

On the day of the faculty meeting, plans proceeded as outlined. After a brief spirited discussion period, there came from the floor an unsolicited motion for adoption. Several voices seconded it. None of these persons had heard about the proposed plan prior to the presentation. The motion carried unanimously. Thus, the health council began officially with an informed faculty group, each member actively involving himself by his own assenting vote. Furthermore, before adjournment, several members called attention to existing health problems which they felt needed priority of consideration. It was decided that each department would elect its own representative to serve on the council for the current school year.

At its first meeting the newly-formed health council elected as chairman the head of the girls' health and physical education program, and as secretary, the representative of the English department. It was agreed that the student council should be invited to have four members as official representatives to the health council and that the custodian also should be a member.

It was most heartening to the new health council to have its first official action meet with success. Its request to the

Board of Education relayed via the Principal and the Superintendent of Schools, was granted although they knew that the matter had previously been rejected twice when requested by the Principal alone. This time, he had been able to present the matter as coming from the School Health Council which meant that the entire faculty and the entire study body stood behind it.

At first, the focus was upon specific and immediate problems. In a short time, however, the health council found its program growing wider and wider in scope. A number of committees were formed and proved their value. Each centered upon a particular problem or phase of the health program: safety, nutrition and lunch room problems, for example. Membership on committees was not limited to council members but included other staff members interested in the same problems. Usually some students were invited to participate.

It can be truly said that the influence of this health council permeated every phase of school life in this active senior high school. Full use was made of the resources of every department. Its student activities, such as publications and art work and clubs, contributed vitally to every undertaking. Moreover, in its functioning it contributed in untold measure to closer faculty relations and inter-departmental understanding and action.

Presently the Chairman of the Health Council was delegated to serve as a representative to the Community Health and Welfare Council. From that time on, the entire health division of this organization and the Senior High School Health Council collaborated effectively, their joint efforts resulting in many benefits to students and families throughout the entire community.

In-Service Health Education

To enable school personnel to function efficiently in their many-faceted roles as members of the school health team, some in-service education is essential from time to time. New discoveries, procedures, and social changes associated with the new medical and scientific frontiers modify the educational scene. It is important that teachers and health workers be informed in order to teach correct scientific health facts and to emphasize health behavior consistent with current change.

There are different ways in which in-service education can be accomplished. Some school districts utilize the days designated in their states as institute or conference sessions at the opening of the fall term. Opportunities are given the school physician or health specialists to lecture or to demonstrate new procedures. Sessions are also arranged for special groups such as custodians, maintenance workers, cafeteria workers, and others. Sometimes school districts pay all or part of college extension course fees for their teaching staff. In some states, voluntary and official health agencies have made it possible through scholarships or in other ways, to participate in summer health education workshops. In Pennsylvania, Michigan, North Carolina and other states, Inter-Agency Planning Committees composed of representatives from voluntary and official agencies, provide leadership and scholarships in cooperation with colleges and universities in the conduct of School-Community Health Education Workshops.

In certain states the State Departments of Health and of Public Instruction have sent demonstration teams to stage sessions in various locations for the in-service education of physicians, nurses and others in techniques to be used in connection with the implementation of new legislation concerning health examinations, immunizations methods, etc. Various official and voluntary community agencies, at the request of school districts, have cooperated in in-service education through the distribution of literature, exhibits, the use of films and recordings. Public libraries often prove cooperative and valuable in developing lists of professional health publications for local school authorities. An essential point that must not be overlooked is that in-service training programs do not just happen. They require initiative and careful planning and scheduling. This is most appropriately the responsibility of the School Health Coordinator or Director of Health and Physical Education of each school and of the school system in cooperation with representatives of the principals and the Superintendent of Schools.

The Rural Setting

A decade ago, health teamwork in a rural school situation would have been deemed well-nigh impossible. Today, improved means of communication and transportation and the replacement of the one-room school and the small high school by modern consolidated and jointure schools makes this a realizable goal on both the elementary and secondary levels. The office of the County Superintendent of Schools and his supervisory staff is usually conveniently located in the county seat or in one of the centrally located consolidated schools.

In-service health education of teachers in rural schools is also possible, since states require planning sessions or conferences for rural as well as for city teachers.

Sometimes county school health councils function effectively. In Prince George's County, Maryland, for example, there is a health council which has tried unique ways of educating the people. Realizing the difficulties caused by distance in attending meetings, this group instituted the practice of tape recording its meetings. Copies of proceedings, speeches, and the discussion which follows are sent to absent members. Thus, each member is not only kept abreast of developments, but gains deeper insight through the discussion and reactions evoked.

Advisory school health councils, mandatory in some states, have been helpful in bringing together on a working basis, representatives of organizations which share in the responsibility for the health of the school child. These advisory councils have been particularly useful in bringing more health advantages to fourth class districts, particularly in the matter of follow-up of remediable defects among school children.

Where a county health unit has been established, the community profits by increased general health services, facilities, and professionally qualified resource persons. Usually the general health education of the local population improves significantly. Traditionally, the county public health staff works cooperatively with the county voluntary agencies, and the staffs of all serve as resource persons and consultants for school health personnel and teachers. In this manner, rural teamwork sometimes can be of a surprisingly high order.

Where full time county health units have not been established, there may be a part-time health officer who, if non-medical and untrained, is of little use as a consultant, or if a physician, might not readily be available as a consultant or resource person. Moreover, district or regional health units of State Departments of Health in lieu of local health units are too large to permit extensive services by their limited staffs. Nevertheless, even in the face of these discouraging circumstances, an alert county superintendent of schools who feels his responsibilities for leadership, and who has a sound professional background in school health and health education, will find ways of strengthening his present program through the effective utilization of existing agencies. Beyond this, he may play a central role in leading existing cooperative groups in a concerted attempt to secure additional needed county facilities and programs, including a full-time county health unit.

The voluntary health agency has always played an important role in connection with school health. On national, state and local levels their efforts in connection with school health have been consistent throughout the years of their existence. These voluntary agencies have assisted with supplementary literature for the teachers, the pupils, and the parents. Films, slides, and other aids have been made available to teachers for their own development and for use in schools. In rural schools they have been able to make noteworthy contributions because many of them are organized to function on a county-wide basis.

The rural teacher has many of the same child health problems that confront the city teacher. Hers, however, tend to be more complicated because of situational difficulties and lack of resources. The rural teacher needs the same thorough preparation through adequate pre-service courses in school health and health sciences in order that she may meet efficiently the many health situations which call for unusual self-reliance and imagination. Adequate courses in child health, personal and community health, and school health, plus familiarity with health education methods, should comprise a large instruction segment of her pre-professional education.

Summary

An attempt has been made to show how teamwork in school health begins at the top and permeates every level and segment of the school organization. A clear delineation of the responsibilities of each member of the team, and respect for each other's role form the foundation for sound teamwork. In addition, it is essential that each participant appreciate that the total health of the total child in the total school and community setting is the focus of all phases of the school health program. All persons responsible for any phase of the program should share in and understand fully the objectives of the program and be fully aware of their special obligations toward their implementation.

Each member of a troupe of acrobats in a circus must know thoroughly not only his own routine in the act, but also what every member of the team will be doing at every successive moment of the performance. An instant's hesitation or insecurity on the part of any one member can spell failure and even disaster for the entire group. Success of the school health team is built upon this same type of interdependence.

With this brief listing and description of the cast of characters, the members of the health team, upon whom so much of the health and well-being of the school child depends, it is now appropriate to consider in some detail the purpose and content of the three broad program areas with which they are concerned: (*a*) school health services, (*b*) healthful school living, and (*c*) health education.

Questions for Discussion

1. Can you cite some specific examples of accomplishment in the local schools, made possible or enhanced by effective cooperation on the part of the school health team?
2. How may the many professions and agencies concerned with the health of the school child be helped to attain the freedom of communication which is so essential for effective teamwork?
3. What health facilities and agencies are available to the rural school children in your county? To what extent are these resources being utilized? What suggestions can you offer toward the improvement of the situation?
4. Arrange to visit a school health council meeting and to share your observations and experiences with your classmates.

5. Plan a talk which you as a teacher in the elementary school (or a homeroom teacher in junior or senior high school) might give at a Parent-Teachers Association meeting on the topic, "How the School and the Community May Work Together for Better Health for the School Child."
6. Prepare, for possible use at meetings of parent organizations, a list of topics concerned with the activities of the school health team.

Suggested Readings

1. American Association for Health, Physical Education, and Recreation: *Teamwork in School Health: Guidelines for School-Community Cooperation.* A Report of the National Conference on Coordination of the School Health Program, Washington, D.C.: American Association for Health, Physical Education, and Recreation, a Department of the National Education Association, 1962.
2. American Dental Association: *A Preventive Dental Health Program for Schools.* Chicago, the Association, 1970.
3. American Medical Association: *Reports of the National Conferences on Physicians and Schools.* (Annual). Chicago, American Medical Association, 1946-69.
4. American Nurses Association: *Functions and Qualifications of School Nurses.* New York: the Association, 1966.
5. Florentine, Helen G.: *The Preparation and the Role of the Nurse in School Health Programs.* Guidelines for the Use of Administrators, Educators, and Students, New York: National League for Nursing, 1962.
6. Hamburg, Morris and Hamburg, Marian V.: *Health and Social Problems in the School.* Philadelphia, Lea and Febiger, 1968.
7. Joint Committee on Health Problems in Education of the National Education Association and the American Medical Association: *Why Health Education?* Washington, D.C., the National Education Association, and Chicago, American Medical Association, 1966.
8. Mayshark, Cyrus and Others: *Administration of School Health Programs: Its Theory and Practice.* St. Louis, The C. V. Mosby Co., 1967.
9. *New Dimensions in School Nursing Leadership.* Proceedings of the Conference on New Dimensions in School Nursing Leadership, American Association for Health, Physical Education, and Recreation, 1968. Washington, D.C.
10. *Selected Reading Series.* Washington, D.C., National Training Laboratories, National Education Association:
    No. 1 Group Development
    No. 2 Leadership in Action
    No. 3 Human Forces in Teaching and Learning
    No. 4 Forces in Community Development
    No. 5 Issues in Human Relations Training
    No. 6 Conferences for Learning, Planning and Action.
11. U.S. Department of Health, Education, and Welfare: Children's Bureau. *Health of Children of School Age.* Children's Bureau Publication No. 421. Washington, D.C., Government Printing Office, 1964.
12. Van Sickle, Aileen B.: *Bookshelf for the Community Health Nurse Specialist.* Am. J. Pub. Health, *60*:4, April, 1970, p. 618.

Chapter 12

School Health Services

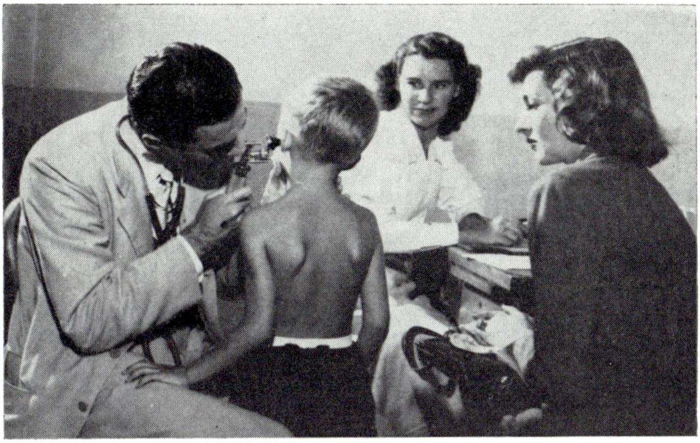

FIG. 56. School health examination.

The Scope of School Health Services

In defining the term School Health Services, as used in all its publications, the Joint Committee on Health Problems in Education of the National Education Association and the American Medical Association, has indicated also the broad scope of the responsibilities carried by this part of the school health program:

> "*School Health Services*: The school procedures carried out by physicians, nurses, dentists, social workers, teachers and others to appraise, protect and promote the health of students and school personnel. Such procedures are designed to (*a*) appraise the health status of pupils and school personnel, (*b*) to counsel pupils, teachers, parents and others for the purpose of helping pupils obtain treatment or for arranging school programs in keeping with their abilities, (*c*) to help prevent and control communicable diseases, (*d*) to provide emergency care for injury or sudden illness, (*e*) to promote optimum sanitary conditions and provide adequate and proper sanitary and safe facilities, and (*f*) to protect and promote the health of school personnel."[1]

[1]*Health Appraisal of School Children.* Joint Committee on Health Problems in Education of the National Education Association and the American Medical Association, 4th ed., Dukelow, D. A., Ed., Washington, D.C., NEA, or Chicago, AMA, 1969. p. 2.

Important guidelines for the practical implementation of these procedures are to be found in the following excerpt from another key publication by the Joint Committee:

> "The ideal school health services program is based on accepted standards and is adapted to a particular community. It is influenced by local customs, the variety of professional personnel and other resources available, and the local awareness of the health needs of children and youth. Health services are designed to protect pupil health and to aid each child to reach and to maintain his best possible state of well-being."[2]

It is consistent with our basic national philosophy that the fundamental responsibility for education lies with citizens on the local level. However, time has demonstrated the wisdom of having the state provide the basic legislative authority as to the type and quality of the health services in schools. The extent and manner in which this is effected varies considerably among the states.

In some instances the State Department of Health carries the responsibility for the establishment and enforcement of standards and regulations concerning health services in schools; in others it is centered in the State Department of Public Instruction. In certain states, the responsibility for the establishment of standards is vested in the Department of Health but the implementation rests with the Department of Public Instruction. In such cases, the two departments usually cooperate in setting up standards and in working out details for their implementation.

Adherence to at least the minimum standards set by the state is mandatory, and usually a heavy penalty is inflicted upon a local school district which fails to meet its state's standards. This has proved to be a wise precaution, for without it the wide disparity in the education and health attitudes of members of school boards coupled with endeavors to "keep the tax rate down" might result in dangerously inadequate standards and procedures, and many children in the state would not be given their rightful health opportunities.

The Administration of School Health Services

School health services are administered in several different ways, depending upon the agency in which authority is placed. In some school districts the health service program is administered wholly by school personnel. The Superintendent of Public Schools is responsible to the Board of Education for the implementation of the entire school health program including school health services, healthful school living, and

[2]*Suggested School Health Policies.* Joint Committee on Health Problems in Education of the National Education Association and the American Medical Association. 4th ed., Washington, D.C., NEA, or Chicago, AMA, 1966. p. 12.

health instruction. The health services constitute a division administered by the Chief School Physician. In a large city system he would be assisted by a staff of part-time school physicians. The nursing division and the dental division would also come under his administration. He would be responsible for the organization and administration of all phases of the service program including the preparation of the budget and the selection and recommendation of qualified personnel. It would be the chief school physician's responsibility to prepare for the approval of the Superintendent and the Board of Education, a detailed written statement of policies and procedures to be followed by the various members of the school staff throughout the district in emergency situations of illnesses and injuries, sanitation, and routine health matters. In all respects, these plans must meet at least the minimal school service standards established by the state, but may be more stringent.

Advocates of this plan point out the advantages of planning the program so that the pupil constitutes the focal point. The ease of communication within the school is another desirable feature. Disadvantages lie in the duplication of staff personnel and the lack of the closest possible relationship with the local Department of Public Health which in the final analysis actually has the responsibility for the health of the child.

A different approach may be observed in some cities where responsibility for the school health services is centered in the Department of Public Health. Obviously this tends toward ease and economy of administration as far as use of personnel is concerned and the centralization and continuity of records. This plan also appears to promote closer interaction among the many official and non-official health agencies concerned with the follow-up program.

Another important advantage of this plan is that it permits closer, more consistent and efficient family contacts rather than to involve a school nurse and perhaps one or two health department or voluntary agency nurses who may be attending other members of the same family. Thus, the same nurse can keep in touch with the child and others in the family in the total family setting over a period of years and give more effective services.

Variations of these two patterns for school health services exist in many places. In some instances the public health department will furnish a requested number of nurses to the school district where they will work under the direction of the school physician. Sometimes nurses from a Visiting Nurse Association or other voluntary health agencies may serve as part-time school nurses. In many rural situations a state-employed nurse will serve in the schools.

Each of these patterns has its adherents, and efficient examples of each can be pointed out. The chief problem seems to be to find the plan best suited to a particular community in view of its goals and objectives, facilities, and finances, and which will permit the closest possible cooperation among all who have something to contribute to the best interests of the child. The rural or fourth class districts usually present the biggest problems, particularly in states with low tax revenues, hence low expenditures for schools.

The Health Appraisal

The health appraisal consists of an evaluation of the pupil's health by means of various procedures conducted by appropriate persons on the school health team with the aim of securing through a composite of all the results an over-all estimate of his health status at a given point in time and over a period of time. The appraisal might include the child's medical history, the medical examination, the dental examination, screening tests of vision, hearing, height, weight, and various other tests.

THE PERIODIC MEDICAL EXAMINATION. The school is responsible for the implementation of the periodic medical examination, for the kind and quality of the procedures used, and for having them conform at least with the minimum state requirements. This includes the selection of suitable quarters in which the examinations are to take place and the provision of appropriate cumulative record forms. Forms vary, but certain items are constant in all. The examination form suggested by the American Medical Association may be considered as a good general example.

Today's emphasis is upon having the child's family physician give the periodic examination using the form required by the school district. The children who do not have a family physician will need to be examined by the school physician. The annual school medical examination has been largely abandoned in favor of fewer but more thorough examinations during the child's school career and with greater emphasis upon follow-up and correction of remediable defects and conditions. Currently accepted standards concerning the medical examination state that

> "During their school years, pupils should have a minimum of four periodic medical examinations: at the time of entrance to school, and at approximately the fourth, seventh, and tenth grades. Additional examinations should be made whenever observations indicate. Local decisions should determine the number of periodic examinations, taking into consideration available medical manpower."[3]

In most instances the school medical examination has been extended to include children enrolled in pre-school activities. In the fall, priority

[3] National Committee on School Health Policies of the NEA and the AMA: *Suggested School Health Policies.* 4th Ed. Washington, D.C.: National Education Association and Chicago, Ill.: American Medical Association, 1966, p. 15.

is given to the examination of pupils planning to participate in athletics or cheer leading. In many states this has been made a requirement. In most situations attempts are made to implement the recommendations of the Committee on Medical Aspects of Sports, of the American Medical Association.

Most states specify the amount of time to be devoted to a pupil's examination and the maximum number of children to be examined per hour. To permit time for counseling, at least 15 minutes per pupil should be allotted. Time schedules need to provide ample time for referral examinations, pre-employment examinations of school personnel, student pre-employment examinations, etc.

The child's medical history is usually secured from the parent by means of a printed form sent to the home. The information is then added or transcribed to the child's cumulative medical record. Included on this form should be the results of screening examinations, referrals, follow-up procedures, health counseling, information concerning school accidents and sudden illnesses. Cumulative records are usually kept in the nurse's office but sometimes they are placed in a separate file in the office of the school administrator. These records are the focal point of teacher-nurse-parent conferences.

A school district should have written policies concerning the handling of medical records: *i.e.*, the recording of information, filing of records, their accessibility, etc. Recorded medical information should be kept confidential and access restricted to the nurse, the principal, the school counselor, the school social worker, the teacher and others concerned with the child's health. Such consideration should be observed in the transfer of the child's cumulative health record if he should change residence and leave the school district.

Screening Tests. Screening tests are usually given prior to the medical examination by the school nurse and trained technicians or, as in some states, by the school nurse assisted by the teacher or aides. Weight, height, vision, and hearing screening tests and an evaluation of the child's physical status, posture, and emotional adjustment are usually included.

Weight. The child's weight record should be regarded along with other significant indications as one general index of the child's fitness. Emphasis should be upon his over-all weight pattern with notation of the changes which occur from month to month. The child's weight should be regarded as an individual matter and not to be compared with scores of other children in the same grade or of the same age. In the northern hemisphere, children of school age usually show gains during the fall months as compared with the springtime records.

It is the responsibility of the person in charge to see that the scale is working properly and that the weighing is done accurately. The weighing should be done under the same circumstances each time with due allowance for clothing. Many schools arrange to have weighing and measuring take place during the physical education period to ensure the same conditions each time. Children should be encouraged to become interested in their own growth and development, and the process should be regarded as an opportunity to teach certain points in hygiene, mathematics, and other subjects.

Height. Height is usually measured by means of a stadiometer or by a sliding rod attached to the weighing scale. However, it can be measured accurately by means of a measure taped to a smooth wall minus a baseboard or moulding. The child stands with his feet flat on the floor, heels pressed against the wall. A wooden box (empty crayon box) held with one surface flat against the wall, is slid down to touch the child's head.

With teacher supervision, junior and senior high school students can maintain their own height and weight records.

Height and weight scores are recorded on the child's cumulative health record; however, a number of excellent individual growth and development record forms are available to schools that prefer to use separate individual cumulative record forms.

The nurse and the teacher should take time to make these weighing and measuring periods meaningful experiences for the children. The important thing is to note whether the child is gaining and developing, not to compare the results with those of other children. Children are naturally interested in their own growth and development. They should be encouraged to retain this interest and their questions should be answered.

Vision. Several tests are used extensively by schools for screening vision: the Snellen Chart Test, the Massachusetts Vision Test, and stereoscopic tests. Usually the vision screening test is given by the school nurse, but certain states permit it to be done by the teacher. The Snellen Test is perhaps the easiest to administer, and actual research has proved it to be just as useful and dependable as the Massachusetts Vision Test.

The Snellen Charts with their horizontal lines of various sizes of letters are familiar to most persons. The chart used in the kindergarten and in lower elementary grades with pupils who have not yet learned to read consists of E's with the arms of the letters extending in different directions.

Several precautions need to be observed when giving the test:

1. The chart should be well lighted.
2. The child should stand at a line marked on the floor 20 feet from the chart. Each eye is tested separately with the other covered by a card.
3. If a wall chart is used, the nurse should have a card large enough to cover the entire line of letters except for an open

space through which a single letter can be seen. In testing, the card is slid back and forth across the letters in the line, thus preventing the child from memorizing the sequence. The chart is obtainable also in roller form with hand control so that the operator can change lines at will.

4. The result is recorded in terms of the smallest letters read successfully. Thus, 20/20 indicates that the child at a distance of 20 feet from the chart can read the line on the chart indicated as 20. A score of 20/100 would indicate that the child at 20 feet can only read what persons with normal vision can read at 100 feet. The numerator represents the distance and the denominator the line score.
5. If the child is wearing glasses, each eye will need to be tested with and without glasses with both sets of results recorded.
6. It is important to understand that this is merely a screening test to discover who needs further help. Referrals should be made where necessary, and the nurse or person notifying the parent should stress the importance of immediate examination by an ophthalmologist.

Most states require an annual vision test in all grades and for pre-school children. However, special tests should be arranged when the teacher feels it is important to the health and educational progress of the child or when a deviation appears to be of significance. The teacher needs to be continuously alert to indications of faulty vision. These might include the child's complaint of blurred vision, frequent rubbing of the eyes, squinting, blinking, red or watery eyes, holding the book or paper too close or very far away or at a peculiar angle, frequent headaches, eye defects, excessive tearing, inflammation of the conjunctiva, poor posture, a disinclination to read or to do close work, poor coordination of eyes and hands, or undue tension.

Hearing. Hearing is tested in various ways but the most accurate school test is an individual pure-tone audiometer sweep check test administered by an audiologist, a trained technician, or by a nurse who has had special instruction. Each ear is tested separately and the score recorded. The child is instructed to indicate with his hand whether the change of tone is higher or lower in pitch. When necessary, this test is followed by the Pure-Tone Threshold Acuity Test.

It is possible to give a group test with the audiometer by means of ear phone attachments. Each child notes in a designated place on a printed chart the number of sounds and the variations. Obviously this is less desirable than the individual test and its use, even with upper elementary or older children, is questionable.

The watch test is still used in places which do not have access to an audiometer. Several lines are marked on the floor at specific intervals.

The child stands beside the line nearest the tester and covers the side of his face toward the tester with a card. The child holds the opposite ear shut. The tester holds the watch beside the child's ear and changes its position without allowing the child to be aware of it. The tester moves it to the various distances measured on the floor and the results are recorded.

The whisper test is also used in some schools. The child closes his eyes and the tester, standing at a designated distance, whispers numbers which the child repeats aloud. The child should be at a right angle to the tester and hold a card against the side of his face toward the tester so he cannot see her lips. This method is obviously very crude and many variables render it inaccurate.

All of these tests are also merely screening tests. The child with apparent defective or questionable hearing must be referred to an otologist for further examination and diagnosis. Most schools require an annual hearing test in all grades. Arrangements should be made for special testing upon recommendation by the principal or the classroom teacher who has observed significant symptoms or deviations. These may include inattention, strained attention, poor coordination or balance, frequent dizziness, poor personal relations with other children, or poor progress in school subjects.

THE DENTAL EXAMINATION. The goals of the school dental health program center upon helping children and parents develop an appreciation and understanding of optimal dental health as a life-long asset and of the need for maintenance of an individual program of correct dental practices under continuing professional advice, with corrective measures when needed. The school dental health program fills a most important place in the school health services program. It is necessary, of course, to meet the requirements set up by the state, but it is important also that the school dentist or director of school dental services consult with his colleagues in the local dental society in the preparation of the program which he submits for approval by the director of the school health services, the superintendent of schools, and the Board of Education.

From a practical point of view, over-all school dental plans must include consideration of the local availability of means of correction: *i.e.*, the number of professional dentists, the number and location of clinics, etc. in relation to the size of the pupil load. If the community does not have a fluoridated public water supply, provision for the topical application of fluoride must be included in the plans. Arrangements need to be made to permit continuing guidance and care by the family dentist and, if necessary, to include permission for such children to be excused during regular school hours.

The American Dental Association states its position as follows:

> "The dental portion of the health appraisal, whenever possible, should be given by the child's own dentist because a thorough dental

examination can be made only in the dentist's office. Less comprehensive inspections and screening procedures, however, can be done within the school setting, often by the dental hygienist.

Frequently, inspections (using mouth mirrors, explorers and adequate illumination) or screenings (using tongue depressors and available illumination) are used or suggested as mass case-finding techniques for dental health programs in schools. Many divided opinions exist regarding the desirability and effectiveness of conducting periodic dental inspections."[4]

The American Dental Association has adopted "a statement on the possible benefits and limitations of school dental inspections" which should be given careful study by all communities planning a dental health education program.[5]

Whichever type of examination is used, the parent should be notified of the results and when necessary, advised to proceed immediately with the corrective program by taking the child to a dentist. The referral should be followed up within a short time by the school dentist, the dental hygienist, or the school nurse. Consistent follow-up is most important. In the case of an indigent family, arrangements should be made for corrective measures at a clinic, a hospital, or a local health center convenient to the child's home.

The results of the dental inspection or examination referrals, corrective measures, etc. must be entered on the child's cumulative health record. Some school districts maintain a separate cumulative dental record for each child. Regardless which method is used, the director of the dental service will find it highly important to plan for continuing evaluation of all segments of the dental program and for keeping accurate statistics and instituting meaningful research projects. The carefully planned research studies in regard to the reduction of caries among school children through the use of fluorides during the past two decades, have established clearly the practical benefit of coordinated research efforts. Today the majority of children in the United States benefit in some degree through some form of fluoridation. In many instances when a community lacks fluoridated water supply, the school program makes the advantage of this valuable preventive measure available to its children in some other approved form.

In some states the dental hygienist under the supervision of the local school dentist, is permitted to conduct the dental inspection for observable defects, the notification of referrals, and the follow-up. Some states also permit the dental hygienist to proceed with the topical application of stannous fluorides. In some school districts, the dental hygienist spends a large part of her time in giving dental prophylaxis and in dental education.

[4] American Dental Association. *A Preventive Dental Health Program for Schools.* Chicago: the Association, 1970. Page 8.

[5] Op. cit. Pages 8, 9.

The dentist, the dental hygienist, and the teacher should work together in the observation of child habits which might have dental implications, and in the prevention of dental accidents. Today the use of a dental mouthpiece in athletics, especially football and hockey, has become a standard practice in most schools and has paid untold dividends in the preservation of teeth of the youth of this generation.

Follow-up Procedures

The evolutionary change of role concept widened by the shift from the term "medical inspection" to school health services, the conquest of the severe ravages of childhood diseases, and the improved mortality and morbidity rates in the school-aged population have made possible more concentration of time and effort upon the findings of the health appraisal. The percentage of children in need of corrective measures remains high, however. As has already been pointed out, the physician and nurse serve as catalysts in instituting appropriate remedial procedures. Suitable notification forms, parent conferences, and home visits are their usual tools.

To the nurse falls the main responsibility for interpreting to the parent the findings of the health appraisal, and for urging of prompt remedial action through the family physician, dentist, or other appropriate health practitioners. When such action has been initiated, the nurse will maintain contact with the progress of the case, making essential notations on the child's cumulative medical record form. When the parent fails to respond, the nurse should try to discover the reasons. This requires patience, tact, understanding, resourcefulness, and skill in parent education. If the difficulty is financial, the physician and the nurse should help the parent avail himself of school-community resources for this type of assistance.

Effective follow-up may entail arrangements for a variety of services and adjustments within the school itself and in the community. The nurse, the physician, the teacher, the guidance counselor, the parent, and the family physician need to plan cooperatively in order to work out successfully the details of the child's daily routine. The policy of having the child remain with his regular class should be adhered to whenever possible and practical. Frequently the nurse acts as the go-between in transmitting to the teacher the necessary information concerning the individual child and in suggesting possible environmental and curricular adjustments.

Health Counseling

Increasing attention is being given to health counseling as one of the most important functions of the health service team. It has long been recognized that psychologically the time of the medical examination or health appraisal is a "teachable moment" for the parent as well as for the child, and that because of the emotions evoked, the counseling or advice is likely to fall upon good ground and bear fruit. It is important that the physician, the nurse, and all members of the school health team utilize such opportunities to the fullest extent. School nursing preparation today includes increased emphasis upon an understanding of family life and family interactions, child psychology, group dynamics, and counseling techniques. The social-psychological aspects are brought into the physician's training too.

If the health appraisal is to be truly effective, the subsequent counseling, referral, and follow-up must be handled tactfully and skillfully. The purpose of referral is to secure correction or, if the defect or condition cannot be corrected, to initiate steps toward the best possible rehabilitation measures or the prevention of deterioration. To do this, the members of the health service team need to be able to communicate satisfactorily with each other to avoid duplication of effort and confusion to parents and children. It is important to be well-informed concerning available facilities and community resources. Usually the results of the appraisal will be routed to the nurse. She should have the vision and the competency to harness appropriate resources to meet any special health needs of the child and to initiate the proper staff and inter-agency action.

The health worker in his counseling role needs to remember that often the slightest comment is significant to the emotionally overwrought parent or child. A tone of voice or even a facial expression can convey unfortunate meanings or nuances. While honesty remains the best foundation for counseling, tact needs to accompany it.

It is important, particularly in a junior or senior high school, that the nurse be available to students during a certain portion of the day for counseling purposes. A nurse's time is always at a premium, but often a job analysis will disclose some duties which can be safely delegated to other persons in order to release time for this vital service.

Prevention and Control of Disease in the School

An earlier chapter has described how the previous prevalence of childhood diseases and the high rate of mortality led to the introduction and evolution of today's health services in schools. It was seen how the nature and scope of school health responsibilities have changed apace with successes and advances in medicine and science. For example, the widespread use of triple DPT antigen (diphtheria, pertussis, tetanus), smallpox vaccination, and now immunization against measles, polio, rubella and mumps during infancy and the pre-school years has changed the task of the school from case discovery, reporting, and quarantine to more follow-up of booster shots at proper intervals and the immunization of those children who through parental or social negligence failed to receive them earlier.

Attention also has been directed to specific ways in which provision may be made for handling cases of chronic disease which are likely to be encountered among school children. Release of staff time due to the diminished amount of communicable disease means more opportunity for effective follow-up of these individual cases of chronic conditions. The importance of cooperation with the local department of public health in disease control and prevention has been stressed. Suffice to say here that there should be constant evaluation of the methods and procedures used in order to maintain such cooperative efforts at a high level of efficiency. At all times, it must be remembered that the local health ordinances and those of the state which govern health matters in schools actually chart the course of the school health service activities. The local medical and dental societies can make valuable contributions in the joint consideration and solution of problems.

Planning for Emergency Care

School procedures concerning emergency care of illness and injuries must be adapted to the total available community facilities and personnel, and to existing local and state regulations. The legal liabilities involved need to be considered carefully, and in many instances interpretations need to be secured through the school solicitor in order to prevent future legal difficulties. These liabilities differ in various states and local communities.

Reference has been made to the importance of a guide or handbook for a school system. Such a document should contain written statements of policies and practices approved by the school physician, the Superintendent, and the Board of Education for use in case of injury or illness to pupils or school personnel. The local department of public health and the local medical and dental societies should be invited to participate in the drafting of such policies and practices. This ensures common understanding and support on the part of all concerned or affected, and promotes the fullest utilization of community resources.

A comprehensive program of emergency planning should include the following provisions:

1. Each school should be equipped with an adequate health room furnished with a cot, blankets, and a properly stocked first aid kit. (A list of supplies and their amounts has been prepared by and is available from the American Medical Association.)
2. Each school should have on file in its office a card for each pupil bearing information which would be needed in case of an emergency. It should list the name, address, telephone number of each

parent, of the family physician or, if he should be unavailable, the name of a substitute physician desired, together with his address and telephone number; also the same data concerning two other adults (relatives or neighbors) to be called in case the parents cannot be reached.

3. In case of accident or illness, the nurse or the principal should be informed immediately by the teacher. One of these, whichever is agreed upon, should get in touch with the parent.
4. It is recommended that in each school building, certain individuals who have qualified in Red Cross first aid should be assigned the responsibility in the absence of the nurse, for handling emergencies. Their identity should be known to the entire staff. Many school districts require that all school personnel, including the bus drivers have some first aid training. Any special limitations as to procedures should be set forth in the handbook.
5. Certain teachers should be assigned the responsibility for transportation of ill pupils, and their cars should be parked in readily accessible locations. The school district should carry adequate insurance on such cars and drivers.
6. Each school should have a special form for the reporting of accidents and illnesses. Teachers and employees should be meticulous in filling them in properly and in filing them immediately with the principal. It is important that such cards provide space for the names of witnesses of accidents.
7. Some schools encourage parents to carry insurance on their school-aged children and often stimulate group insurance plans at low rates.
8. Individual teachers are encouraged to carry personal liability insurance.

School staff members need to differentiate carefully between first aid and treatment, and to be informed as to the grave difficulties which could result from exceeding the limitations of first aid.

Civil defense measures have been worked out with the school authorities everywhere. The implications should be understood by the staff and the children. Civilian defense drills should be carried out faithfully, accurately and with serious objectivity. It is assumed that the school physician will be a member of the local committee charged with the responsibility for providing emergency procedures for schools and school children, in case of disaster of any type.

Exceptional Children

In recent years the attitude of the public toward the disabled and the handicapped has changed perceptibly. Today the term *exceptional* or *special* is applied to these individuals in place of *handicapped* with its negative connotation and stigma. The emphasis upon the remarkable accomplishments in the rehabilitation and re-training of the maimed and disabled veterans of World War II may have helped to stimulate this change of attitude. Parents of exceptional children, formerly reluctant to acknowledge them, have become active in seeking effective help for their children, and their efforts have resulted in the formation of a number of national organizations now promoting research and the establishment of special services on the state and local levels.

State compulsory school attendance laws apply to the handicapped or exceptional children as well as to those who are normal. Those who are residents of state institutions are taught by qualified, specially trained, resident teachers, and the home-bound by visiting teachers or by telephone. In some cases, the state provides funds for children who may require care in special private institutions.

Each state has established standards and provisions according to its particular interpretation of the Social Security Act of 1935 and its subsequent amendments which calls for medical, surgical, corrective and other services and care, and facilities for diagnosis, hospitalization and after-care of children who are crippled, or who are suffering from conditions which lead to crippling. In the various states, channels and procedures have been worked out cooperatively at state level by the various departments concerned.

Included in the group termed exceptional are the blind and partially sighted, the hard of hearing and the deaf, the crippled or disabled, the mentally disturbed and defective, and the many children who have a combination of several of these defects. The term crippled is sometimes interpreted to include victims of cerebral palsy, polio, epilepsy, clubfeet and various other orthopedically disabling conditions. Sometimes the cardiac and the diabetic are included. State institutions are often located some distance from the homes of these children. Moreover, people have come to realize that these children need the affection and support of their families. Thus, the public schools concerned with extending equal opportunity to every child for education to the extent of his capability, have been directing more and more attention to the needs of these children.

The responsibility for the discovery and follow-up of the exceptional child rests heavily upon the division of school health services. Many of these children have been found in the lower socio-economic levels. This means that often their health problems are accompanied by many problems in other related areas. Because of the complexity of these problems, an inter-disciplinary team approach is often needed, involving medical, psychological, sociological, educational, and economic considerations. Some children are permanently handicapped and some may have multiple handicaps. Others may be only temporarily handicapped. Each case requires considerable study by all members of the team involved. Diagnoses and educational placement should be the result of cooperative decision.

Some of the specific responsibilities of a local school program in relation to exceptional children are as follows:

1. early discovery and adequate diagnosis of cases,
2. provision for follow-up and evaluations,
3. the best possible uses of available state and local funds, resources and personnel,
4. the provision of teachers who in addition to their regular qualifications have received special training in working with the exceptional child,
5. provision of the best facilities and equipment for special groups to the extent of the resources,
6. in addition to school health services, the referral for psychiatric, psychological, therapeutic and social services in line with recent standards and as provided by comprehensive health planning,
7. continuous guidance and counseling for the child and the parent,
8. the full use of state funds for vocational training when needed,
9. parent education, and when needed, school staff orientation,
10. provision for continuing evaluation and promotion of research.

Frequently, in a city school system, pupils having the same defect are grouped in classes specially designed for them—the blind, the partially sighted, the deaf, the orthopedically crippled, cardiac cases, the mentally retarded and those with speech problems. In small towns where the number of cases does not make this practical, it is sometimes possible for two or more communities to combine their finances and share the services of a specially trained teacher. Special classes for the exceptional child should be carefully supervised by the physician and the nurse, and every possible help given to the teacher. Children who have been allowed to attend a regular class for all or part of the school day should also be followed up continuously so that every possible environmental and curricular adjustment may be put into effect. In this regard, the classroom teacher, not trained in meeting the needs of the exceptional child, may need special help from the nurse and from a specially trained teacher. The child should be able to participate in the regular classwork without retarding the group progress, and be physically able to take care of himself. The teacher and the school staff must be emotionally ready to accept the child, and encourage the student body to do likewise. Among the handicapped, brain-injured children constitute a large and very special group. These are children who have received an injury to or suffered an infection of the brain before, during, or after birth. Damage of the neuromotor system may or may not be present. Such children may show disturbance in perception, thinking, emotional behavior, or any combination of these characteristics which interfere with or slow the child down as compared with a normal child. Usually the child's mental ability is near average, average, or even above average in general intelligence. Impulsiveness, hyperactivity, emotional instability are common, as are tenseness, talkativeness, awkwardness, and a tendency toward destructiveness and aggression. The school health team should try to cooperate with the treatment recommended by the child's physician. In many cases drug therapy may be used successfully. This requires particularly close cooperation by all concerned with the child's health.

The school representatives on the inter-disciplinary team should bear in mind the importance of orienting the school staff to the problems of exceptional children and allocate this responsibility to definite members of the team. Because of her concern, not only with the physical and emotional health of the handicapped child, but also with his safety in the school environment with normal children, as well as with his ability to learn, the teacher's observations make her a key member of the team. The bus driver will need to give the most intelligent and effective help with due regard for each child's handicap—entering the bus, seating the child, and the use of safety belt. In addition to the driver, another adult should be assigned to a school bus that serves a group of exceptional children. Special class assistants are sometimes needed to aid with toiletting, feeding, and rest arrangements. The selection of the proper building to house a special class would entail consideration of the approach and entrance, ramps or elevators, safe furniture and equipment, floor covering, handrails at strategic spots, and lavatory and lunchroom facilities.

The Mentally Deficient Child. The mentally deficient present a complex problem. Children with an I.Q. between 25 and 50 are regarded as trainable, and in some states are considered the responsibility of the public school. The objectives of their school program are the development of self-care, social adjustment, speech and language facility, work habits and skills, and recreational activities to the greatest extent of their potentialities.

Children with an I.Q. from 50 to 80 are mentally handicapped but educable and are therefore the responsibility of the public school. Their educational goals are centered upon the achievement of personal, social, and economic security and ability to pursue certain work skills without supervision.

On the junior high school level it has been found expedient to form special classes usually grouped according to mental age (mentally 8-11 years but 13-16 years chronologically) and housed in a regular junior high school. The aims at this level are the continuation of skills already learned, and the utilization of opportunities for the greater development of social skills, with emphasis upon jobs and vocational skills. Children permitted to be in one of these classes should be able to adjust to several teachers, to find their way about the building, to use lockers properly, to have socially acceptable sound health habits and practices, and to be able to establish satisfactory social relationships. These pupils may spend most of their time with their special teacher, but assembly attendance and participation in the school's voluntary activities should be encouraged. The special teacher needs to work closely with the child's other teachers in order to be familiar with his learning problems and to help with their solution.

If the special class is housed in a senior high school, the plan would be similar but with more emphasis given to the vocational aspect. It might even include a part-time job experience with follow-up by the school in order to help the pupil with his work adjustment. Each child should be treated as an individual and his program arranged and reviewed accordingly. There is great need for research to determine the most effective methods to use with the mentally deficient.

The Gifted Child. The gifted child is usually included under the heading of exceptional. So much emphasis has been given during recent years to the needs of the gifted that most school districts today are providing challenging opportunities for these children to function at high level and at least during certain periods each week, with their mental peers. Unless there is evidence of undue emotional disturbance or special health problems, these children are not likely to need much attention from the health service division.

Examinations of School Personnel

Most states require that a beginning teacher present a valid medical certificate as to his or her fitness. This usually includes evidence of a smallpox vaccination and a chest x ray for the detection of tuberculosis and other diseases if present. Thereafter, a medical examination and chest x ray should be required each year. In some school districts, the Board of Education permits the school physician to offer this service to the teachers; in others, the teacher is encouraged to go to his private physician. Comparable health regulations should apply to part-time, substitute, and non-professional aides.

In some school districts all school employees are required to have periodic chest x rays. This is strongly recommended both for the protection of the individual and for the protection of the children with whom they have contact. Bus drivers are usually required to have medical examinations every 6 months. Food handlers need to meet additional requirements stipulated by the state or local department of public health.

Other Contributions to the School Health Program

This review of the main responsibilities of the health services division has afforded occasional glimpses of ways in which the interests and activities of the members of the health team extend naturally into the other two divisions of the school health program. The findings of the health appraisal are influenced by the school environment and by the health teaching to which the child has been exposed. Because health problems appear in clusters, a thorough follow-up often finds the roots extending in various directions, sometimes originating in one of the other divisions of the program. There are countless ways in which these roots—causes and effects—are entwined. The following lists have been included that they may suggest other ways in which the members of the health service team can contribute to the strengthening and unifying of the total school health program.

In their visits to schools, the members of the health team by virtue of their training will be able to observe current conditions, and, when necessary to do so, to call to the attention of the person in charge ways of improving sub-standard conditions or of implementing new ideas. Some of the areas of observation might include the following phases of *healthful school living:*

1. The psychological environment of the school as it may affect the child's health
2. Healthful living conditions in buildings and grounds: temperature, lighting, cooperation with building inspector and public health sanitarian
3. The maintenance of sanitation and good housekeeping: cleanliness, habits of workers, *etc.*
4. The types of cafeteria menus, preparation of food, food service
5. The school safety conditions bearing upon accidents and health findings
6. The health and safety aspects of the physical education and recreational programs

These are some ways whereby all members of the team may contribute to *health education:*

1. Strive to make each contact with a pupil a positive, educational experience for the child.
2. Be concerned with the selection of scientifically accurate and appropriate content in health classes.
3. Serve as a resource person to those engaged in curriculum building.
4. Transmit significant health examination findings to the teachers in order to deepen their insight into health problems and to give direction to health teaching.
5. When called upon, evaluate health education materials.
6. Bring to the attention of the staff, new findings in science, medicine and communication media.

7. Prepare the children psychologically for health and dental examinations.
8. Give special health talks to children.
9. Participate actively in the school health council.
10. Seek to effect close school-community relations through health education efforts.
11. Help the teachers to appreciate the importance of relating the health instruction with the school health service experiences whenever possible.

Questions for Discussion

1. In what ways are the school health team and the department of public health in your city (or county) working together toward achieving and maintaining optimal health of the school child in your community? In what ways do you think present procedures and results might be improved?
2. To what extent are the needs of the exceptional child in your community being met? How do the procedures compare with the suggested ways included in this chapter?
3. In your community, how does the number of public school children who receive the periodic medical examination from their family physicians compare with the number examined by the school physician? How do you account for the existing ratio?
4. Assume that you have taken a position as a teacher in the grade of your choice, in an elementary school which has not heretofore emphasized its health program to any extent. The principal has asked you to help with a project which the Board of Education has arranged with the local Tuberculosis and Health Association to offer to the pupils a free tuberculin test and, when necessary, a chest x ray. What procedures would you use in trying to secure understanding cooperation on the part of the pupils, the parents, and the faculty?
5. Outline a sound dental health program for a child from pre-school years through senior high school taking into account the special problems characteristic at particular ages and stages of development.
6. What is the teacher's role in helping the parent understand the purpose and value of the health examination?

Suggested Readings

1. American Medical Association: *Reports of the National Conference on Physicians and Schools.* (Annual) Chicago, American Medical Association, 1946-69.
2. American Red Cross. *First Aid Book.* New York, The Blakiston Division, McGraw-Hill Book Co. Current issue.
3. Cruickshank, William M. and Johnson, G. Orville (Eds.). *Education of Exceptional Children and Youth.* 2nd Ed., Englewood Cliffs, N.J., Prentice-Hall, 1967.
4. Haag, Jessie H.: *School Health Programs.* Revised Ed., New York, Holt, Rinehart, and Winston, 1965.
5. Joint Committee on Health Problems in Education of the National Education Association and the American Medical Association:
Answers to Health Questions in Physical Education, 1970.

Health Appraisal of School Children. 4th Ed., 1969.
Health of School Personnel. 1964.
Mental Health and School Health Services. 1966.
Physical Growth Chart for Boys...
Physical Growth Chart for Girls.
School Health Services. 2nd Ed., 1964.

6. National Committee on School Health Policies of the National Education Association and the American Medical Association. *Suggested Health Policies.* 4th Ed., Washington, D.C. National Education Association, and Chicago, American Medical Association, 1966.
7. National Council of the Chief State School Officers and the Association of State and Territorial Health Officers. *Responsibilities of the State Departments of Education and Health for School Services.* Committee Report. Washington, D.C., the Council, 1951.
8. NEMIR, ALMA: *The School Health Program.* 3rd Ed., Philadelphia, W. B. Saunders Co., 1970.
9. OBERTEUFFER, DELBERT AND BEYRER, MARY K.: *School Health Education.* 4th Ed., New York, Harper and Row, 1966.
10. WHEATLEY, GEORGE M. and Others: *Health Observations of School Children.* 3rd Ed., New York, McGraw-Hill Book Co., 1965.

Chapter 13

Healthful School Living

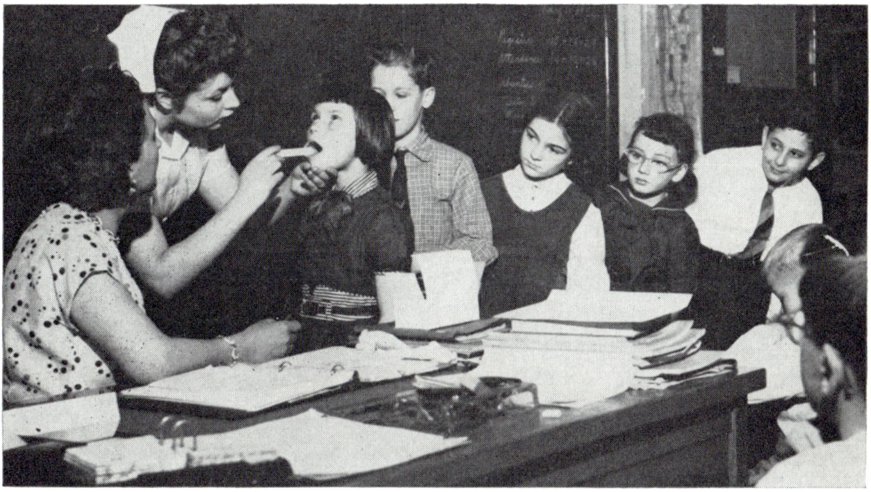

FIG. 57. Classroom screening.

Introduction

Without the effective environmental health programs conducted by the state and local departments of public health, healthful school living would not be possible. A safe, potable water supply in adequate amount, the safeguarding of the milk and food supplies of the community, the sanitary disposal of sewage and waste, and the control of air pollution are basic to the prevention and control of disease and the maintenance of healthful schools and healthy children. Today in most cases these community services are more or less taken for granted. The school cooperates in the routine observance of these and other precautions and preventive measures required by law. When planning a new facility, the school authorities focus intensively upon these basic considerations. On the other hand, safety and accident prevention, food and milk control, rubbish and garbage disposal, insect and rodent control and certain other considerations are daily concerns of school personnel.

Every teacher needs to have a sound understanding of community environmental sanitation as it affects daily living in order that she may teach the basic scientific principles and understandings to children at their particular level of maturity. As future citizens, they need to know basic facts and practices in order to vote wisely, for many of these health precautions concern the quality of family and community living and involve the expenditure of money through taxation. Moreover, to meet the dire need for more trained health personnel at every level, the nation depends in great measure upon the teacher's ability to activate and inspire the youth toward this type of service as a life career. Although the stress upon vocational choice usually occurs during junior and senior high school years, appreciations and understandings can be stimulated in the primary grades by an informed, enthusiastic teacher.

Healthful School Environment

As the stage setting acquaints the audience with the period and the mood of the play and the kinds of characters to expect, so the school environment reveals to the visitor something of the nature of the institution and its program, the attitudes and practices of the staff and the pupils. Conversely, the school environment exerts a very real although subtle or unconscious influence upon the attitudes and the behavior of all within its range.

A healthful school environment has been described as consisting of the physical, social, and emotional factors of the school situation which affect, concern, or relate to the health, welfare, development, and behavior of the individual or the group. In actuality, these factors pertain to the over-all plan and condition of the school plant—the design, construction, sanitation, and maintenance of buildings and grounds—together with procedures and practices which contribute to its efficient and effective utilization, and to the harmonious interactions necessary to the achievement of optimal health and education of the child. So many small details comprise or contribute essentially to the satisfactory functioning of each segment of the school environment that close teamwork involving numerous specialists and resource persons becomes paramount.

The School Plant. Persons or committees confronted with some phase of the responsibility for building a new school plant or renovating an old one, are reminded at the outset that a wealth of material concerning standards and designs is readily available from their State Departments of Public Instruction and Health, the United States Office of Education, the National Education Association, and from professional organizations of the various construction specialists such as architects, illumination engineers, heating, refrigerating, and air conditioning engineers and others. A perusal of such available literature is the first step in the building process. A second step, or perhaps a logical accompaniment of the first, is a series of visits to new structures.

The Board of Education has the over-all responsibility for the selection of the site, the design of the plant to be erected, and the formulation of plans for financing it. Upon the Superintendent of Schools falls the responsibility for presenting to the Board (or to its building committee) a composite picture of the present educational needs and goals and future developmental plans as envisioned by various staff members and other consultants, to serve as a guide in determining detailed plans and features to be included in the new plant. The actual planning of the school should be placed in the hands of a qualified architect, preferably a specialist in school design and construction. He and the Board of Education need to work together constantly to secure the best results.

The planning of schools to meet the enormously increased urban and suburban enrollments entails many unsolved problems. To offset the great annual expense caused by increased vandalism, many urban schools today are being constructed around inner courtyards and present windowless walls to the streets. Soaring real estate values in large cities make prohibitive the acquisition of school sites of sufficient size to include adequate play space and athletic facilities to permit children to develop habits of physical activity, to learn desirable life-time sports skills, and to gain the social and emotional benefits of play. To meet this urgent unsolved problem, Ezersky and Theibert[1] suggest the possibility of the construction of a suitable complex of specialized sports facilities to include gymnasia, swimming pools, etc., so located that each complex may serve a number of area schools, with the pupils being transported by bus according to a daily or weekly schedule. If city youths are to have these important opportunities at appropriate teachable moments of their lives, the idea merits at least an immediate pilot trial. Moreover, such a plan might, through careful scheduling, eliminate the need for the inclusion of cafeterias and food services, and thus further reduce the size and the cost.

In order to provide modern facilities for rural children comparable with urban schools, there is a marked tendency for several small school districts to unite their efforts, to agree upon a common site accessible to all, to plan the equitable sharing of the expense, and to decide upon the design of the plant. Usually a joint school of this type can be located advantageously on the outskirts of a town or village already provided with public water and sewerage systems.

The site of the school plant should be selected with due consideration for

1. the segment of the population to be served, the immediate and future educational needs of the children, and the objectives of the school system,
2. the probable future expansion of the community's population and industry,

[1]Ezersky, Eugene and Theibert, P. Richard: *City Schools Without Gyms.* JOPHER: *41,* No. 4, April, 1970: pp, 26-29.

3. the total building program of the school district,
4. the immediate and future uses of the building, grounds, facilities, and play space, by the school and by the community,
5. the accessibility of the approach with due regard for ease of transportation, proximity to expressways, airports, railroads, and other traffic hazards for children on foot,
6. the proximity of manufacturing plants which may present problems of noise, air pollution, and traffic congestion,
7. the role of the new school in the year-round community recreation program designed to meet the needs of citizens of all ages, and
8. the finances of the school district and the available building funds.

The minimum land requirements for school plants vary according to the number of pupils to be served. The building should be erected on high ground (but not on a hill-top) selected with due regard for exposure and drainage, and the limitation of necessary grading to a minimum. It should be located at a corner of the plot so that a maximum of unbroken space remains for recreational activities, and in order that ready access from the street or highway can make evening community gatherings possible.

The plan of the building, the type of construction, and the materials need to conform with the standards of the State Department of Public Instruction, the state Department of Health, the local municipal building code, as well as with the ideas of the Board of Education, school personnel, and the community. At the same time it should make possible the realization of the objectives and philosophy embodied in the curriculum. All buildings should be as nearly fireproof as possible. Corridors, entrances, stairways, ramps, and fire-towers should receive special consideration as to location and adequacy. The design of the building should permit efficiency in usage, communication, and safe traffic in corridors to and from assembly hall, library, gymnasium, health suite, cafeteria, lavatories, drinking fountains, playgrounds, and storage rooms for audio-visual and resource materials. Planning consideration needs to be given to other features such as the location of service entrances and parking lots in relation to play areas, the various laboratories and shops in terms of use and equipment, the heating plant, the efficient layout of the gymnasium and auxiliaries, and the playfields.

It is important that classrooms be of proper proportions for their intended purposes, allowing 30 to 40 square feet per pupil. Because of essential play equipment and program activities, kindergarten rooms should be about 1½ times the size of the usual classroom. From the standpoint of attractiveness and sight conservation, pastel colored walls and a cream or white ceiling have proved a satisfactory combination. Walls and ceiling should be treated to absorb noise. The moveable classroom partitions featured in many modern buildings, offer the advantages of ready adjustment of space to variations in class size, rich curriculum experiences through greater use of group work, and easier sharing of facilities and equipment.

Heating and Ventilation. In a large city school or a suburban school the control of the heating is likely to be completely in the hands of the custodian. Nevertheless, room conditions play such a basic part in the maintenance of favorable learning situations that the teacher carries a share of the responsibility. Teachers should at least know desirable standards and the proper channels for reporting any failure of operation to meet these standards. If the control of the individual classroom is in the hands of the individual teacher, she should be given adequate instruction as to how to secure the best results.

Classroom temperatures should fall within the range of 68° to 72° F. when taken at a central point about 5 feet above the floor. In a gymnasium, the range should be 60° to 65° F. The thermometer or thermostat should be read at stated intervals throughout the day and the readings recorded on a simple chart. This plan provides objective evidence which has proved helpful in locating heating difficulties. Children enjoy carrying the responsibility and it can prove a practical learning experience.

Steam and hot water systems are most commonly used, probably more of the latter. Radiant heating beneath the floor is also used quite extensively. In some heating systems, mechanical fan ventilation is attached; in others open window ventilation suffices. In the latter case, a window glass or board, designed to slant backward toward the room, functions satisfactorily in order to direct the current of air upward and out through a duct near the ceiling on the opposite wall. If there is no duct system, the window may be lowered from the top thus permitting the warm air which rises, to flow out.

The comfort of the children depends not only upon the temperature and the air circulation, but also upon the relative humidity. High humidity of the atmosphere prevents the human body from ridding itself of heat through perspiration, and the individual feels uncomfortable. Low humidity has the opposite effect. When the body loses too much heat, the nose and throat feel dry and the mucous membranes can no longer serve their function as the first line of defense against respiratory infections. Restlessness, inattention, listlessness, and sleepiness on the part of the children are indications that room conditions need attention.

Air Conditioning. During the past decade this nation has given practically unanimous recognition to the advantages of air-conditioning. Research studies have confirmed enthusiastic reports from business and industry as to improvements in efficiency and production as well as the health of the workers. Certainly these benefits would be highly desirable in schools, too; but the expense of installation has probably prevented its inclusion in many new schools. Its introduction in some sections of the country has made year-round use of school buildings possible. Where included, central air-conditioning is the plan most often used. Some schools have provided for room type of installation in cafeterias, health suites, and offices, and special situations.

Lighting. The marked progress in illumination engineering is substantiated by the generally attractive and satisfactory lighting observable in most of the recently constructed school plants. Whether a new building or the renovation of an old one is involved, the planning of this most important feature of a school plant requires a specialist in lighting. Preliminary calculations give due consideration to the purposes for which a particular room or area is to be used at various hours of the day, the degrees of reflected light from the surfaces of walls, ceiling, furniture, the kinds and quality of the glass areas, etc. Informative publications on school lighting are available for use by building committees. Space permits the inclusion here of a few facts essential for the classroom teacher to bear in mind.

Classrooms should be so designed that daylight enters from but one side. Windows should be unobstructed by partitions which cast heavy shadows, and should extend as near the ceiling as possible. Provision should be made for the regulation of outdoor light by means of Venetian blinds or translucent shades. Two roller-type shades placed at the middle of the window and rolling in opposite directions permit the best control of light.

Fluorescent lighting fixtures today are planned to provide diffused light with practically all shadows on desks eliminated. Standards of lighting call for 50 to 70 foot-candles in the classroom for close work. A gymnasium too needs good light for accuracy and safety in athletics; 50 foot-candles should be sufficient. A light meter should be available to test the light at various times during the day. Whatever lighting plan is devised, it should be possible for the classroom teacher to make adjustments to changing conditions.

Attractively colored chalkboards are commonly used today, but it is important that they be placed with due regard to light reflection and to the height of the pupils, and that dustless crayons of sharply contrasting color be used. It must be remembered that glass in a picture frame, in the doors of the room or in bookcases, can cause annoying glare. When individual small tables are arranged for various groupings, the teacher needs to watch that all children are protected from facing the windows and from glare. Ordinarily, the children should be seated with the light from the windows falling over their left shoulders, and with chairs slightly turned so that they are facing toward the front right-hand corner of the room. The teacher needs to be careful while teaching to avoid standing with her back to the windows thereby forcing the pupils to face the glare as they look at her.

Lavatories. Lavatories should be ample for the enrollment. It is desirable to have wash stands in the ratio of 1 per 40 pupils, at proper height to accommodate the children to be served. Hot water, soap, paper towels or electric hand dryer should be available. A ratio of 1 toilet per 60 boys and 1 urinal per 30 boys, and 1 toilet per 30 girls is considered standard for elementary schools. Secondary school standards call for 1 toilet per 90 boys and 1 urinal per 30 boys, and 1 toilet per 45 girls. Toilet paper should be supplied and sanitary napkin dispensers should be available for girls. Boys' lavatories are usually at opposite ends of the building from the girls'. Kindergartens and first grades are often provided with lavatories adjoining the classroom so that they may be readily supervised. Terrazzo floors, walls of glazed tiles, and fixtures of vitreous material impervious to the retention of odors permit a high standard of sanitary maintenance. Provision for careful supervision must be arranged by the principal.

Drinking Fountains. For safety reasons, drinking fountains should be recessed in the walls. They should be of standard sanitary design, providing a jet spray which does not permit contamination at the nozzle. Fountains should be placed at appropriate heights for the users, about 25 inches from the floor in the lower grades, 29 inches in the upper elementary grades, and 32 to 35 inches in the high school. Drinking fountains, in the ratio of about 1 to 75 pupils, should be readily accessible with at least one on each floor.

Physical Education Facilities

In planning for physical education facilities basic considerations include the philosophy, goals and objectives of the curriculum, the varied activities which are to make these realizable, the numbers, age level, and sex of the pupils to be served. Whether facilities are to be used exclusively by the pupils or shared by other groups during vacation, or whether the facilities are to be used jointly throughout the year by the community population of all ages under the aegis of the recreation department of the community, constitute decisions which should antedate the actual planning process. Certainly the Board of Education, the school administrator, the director of the physical education program, and the director of the recreation program need to confer with the school architect and the city planner to ensure a common understanding of the entire situation as a basis for the wise selection of the site with due regard to the necessary space for desirable activities at all seasons of the year, and with attention to possible problems involved in proper grading, drainage and safety.

All plans should include provision for outdoor and indoor activities. If the school is a lower elementary school housing kindergarten and the first three grades, the playfield should be ample in proportion to the enrollment. Space should be reserved for pre-school and kindergarten activities, preferably near the building. Play apparatus for the grade school children is usually located in a corner of the playfield where its use can be readily supervised and thus leave the maximum amount of space unobstructed for active group games. The playing surface should be as dustless as possible and of a substance least likely to cause injury when children fall. Many synthetic types are now available. Some turf is desirable for quiet activities.

Indoor facilities should include one large gymnasium or playroom, an adjoining office for the instructor, and ample storage closets for equipment. If adapted or individual exercise is to be offered, an additional, smaller, adjoining room would be desirable. If the children merely change from street shoes to sneakers for their play periods, it is not necessary to provide locker rooms. In some schools a multipurpose room is expected to serve both as assembly hall and gymnasium. This is undesirable from several viewpoints, however, and should be avoided.

The middle school (Grades 4, 5, and 6) should be equipped with separate locker rooms and shower rooms for girls and boys.

In the secondary school, if pupils are to have an opportunity to develop and carry over into adulthood the physical and social skills and values which accrue from satisfying experiences in sports and activities, outdoor and indoor facilities must be provided in sufficient quantity and of official dimensions to accommodate the daily class load, the intra-mural program, and the inter-school athletics as well. Often a stadium for inter-school athletics is included in the over-all plans. All courts, track and field plans need to meet the required dimensions and the official specified playing surfaces. School plants are usually so planned that locker rooms and storage facilities may serve for both outdoor sports and indoor needs to eliminate the additional expense of a field house. Playing courts and swimming pools are sometimes made suitable for year-round use by the inclusion of retractable roofs or plastic domes.

Pupil enrollments and official measurements of playing courts are equally important considerations in planning the indoor gymnasiums. Separate gymnasium facilities for girls and for boys at this level are highly desirable. With moveable partitions it is possible to divide a large gymnasium into two or more areas. In addition to the main gymnasium, there should be a smaller auxiliary gymnasium for adapted or individual exercise. Offices for the staff should adjoin the gymnasium and preferably afford a view of the entire gymnasium.

The gymnasium floor should be of an approved, resilient material. All markings should be plainly visible and clearly indicated by the use of colored paints. The walls should be free from protruding obstructions. Safety glass should be used in windows and door panels, and further protected by gratings or other safety devices to prevent accidents. Drinking fountains should be recessed and located away from playing areas. Doors should not open directly upon playing areas. Storage closets should be ample and there should be provision for the sanitary care and storage of mats. Today mats are available in a variety of materials. Usually plastic covers make them easy to care for and sanitary for use.

Adequate, even lighting at all hours of the day and evening is essential to safety. Shadows, glare, and reflected light can be hazardous to players. All lights need to be protected by metal guards.

Separate locker rooms readily accessible to their respective gymnasiums should be provided for boys and for girls. Locker rooms should be of ample size to permit efficiency of movement of the largest scheduled class. Locker rooms should be well-lighted and ventilated. Stationary benches should be provided.

Various types of lockers may be used. The basket type has the advantage of compact storage space and of permitting the clothing to dry readily. Full-length lockers for the storage of street clothes need to be provided in sufficient number to accommodate the largest class. In other instances, a half-length locker is provided for each pupil and so assigned as to afford convenient space for each pupil in a class. Lavatories should adjoin the locker rooms. Girls appreciate plenty of mirrors and hair-dryers in addition to the usual automatic hand dryers, and sanitary napkin dispensers.

The shower rooms should adjoin the locker rooms. The gang shower is used in many schools while others have booths clustered in fours or in pairs round a shower. Nearly all schools include at least a few individual showers for handicapped pupils and others who prefer them. Shower rooms should be tiled to a height of about 7 to 8 feet, be well-drained, and have central control to regulate the flow and temperature. It is desirable to have the shower room open directly into a drying room, which in turn communicates with the locker room. Soap and towels are usually provided by the school. A system of automatic soap dispensers is convenient. In some instances a nominal towel fee is charged to cover the cost of laundering. The same locker room can serve both the gymnasium and the swimming pool.

The swimming pool should be of regulation size to permit its use for inter-school competition and community events. The walls of the room should be of tile at least a third of the way up. The pool itself should be completely tiled, equipped with adequate scum gutters, and properly installed under-water lights. If there is but one pool for all purposes, the floor should be sloped at one end to permit a diving zone. The decks round the pool should be of terrazzo or non-skid tile. The diving board should be of regulation type and properly mounted. State and local health agencies have regulations which apply to swimming pools and their care. There should be an approved type of chlorinator and other provisions for sanitizing the water as may be prescribed. The pool should be flooded each morning before the first class for surface drainage.

Daily testing of the water and the addition of chlorine and other chemicals need to meet prescribed regulations. Life buoys, and rescue poles should be placed at the poolside and a resuscitator should be available nearby. In addition, every precaution should be taken in regard to safety including instruction to pupils, and constant enforcement of sanitary regulations in regard to individual health standards, possible dangers and ways of avoiding them, the hazards involved in non-observance of safety regulations pertaining to deep water, diving, horse-play, etc., and methods of meeting emergencies.

The aim has been to include here sufficient general information regarding what is obviously a specialized field, to give the non-specialist a glimpse of some of the main problems involved in planning for a healthful environment as it concerns the physical education program. Actually, the ramifications are so numerous and there is such variation in the types of programs in effect, that the American Association for Health, Physical Education, and Recreation for many years has sought to improve the programs and their results in terms of health and skills by cooperation in the preparation and publication of a handbook setting forth the best standards based upon research and the judgment of physical education teachers and specialists representing all parts of the United States.[2] This guide is revised from time to time to keep it up to date. It can be regarded as the most valuable resource in determining the dimensions of various facilities, the number appropriate for various enrollments, and questions pertaining to materials, choice of equipment, designs and the like calculated to give the best results. The reader is advised to examine this manual in order to appreciate something of the magnitude and complexity of the entire problem.

The Health Unit

Every school should have a well-equipped health unit planned to meet the needs of the pupil enrollment. The unit should consist of a waiting room or reception room, several conference rooms which can also serve as examining rooms, and, in an elementary school, a rest room, and lavatories for boys and for girls. In a secondary school, separate rest rooms should be provided for girls and boys. The health unit should be so located as to be readily accessible to pupils, to the school office, and in case of need for transportation by wheel chair or stretcher, to an exit which would permit ease in transferring the patient to a vehicle.

Equipment should include adequate supply closets, files, cabinets, office equipment, and in the examining rooms foot-operated washstands,

[2] National Facilities Conference. *Planning Areas and Facilities for Health, Physical Education and Recreation.* Revised edition. Chicago and Washington, D.C.: Athletic Institute and the American Association for Health, Physical Education, and Recreation, a department of the National Education Association, 1965.

scales, necessary medical equipment and supplies. The enrollment should determine the number of cots per rest room and therefore the size of the rooms. In secondary schools more cots will be needed for girls than for boys.

The reception room offers an excellent opportunity for health education by means of exhibits, displays, books, and materials. Plans should include provision for bulletin boards and display cases.

The Role of the Custodian

A large share of the responsibility for the daily health, comfort, and safety of the school population rests with the custodian. The scope and seriousness of his duties demand that he be an alert, intelligent individual with at least average education and highly skilled, possibly with technical training in one or two areas. He needs to have a thorough understanding of the heating, ventilation, lighting, plumbing, and drainage systems of the school plant, and the health and safety standards and operating procedures required by law for their day to day maintenance. The custodian cooperates in the management of the fire-drills, civilian defense drills and activities, the parking of cars and bicycles, and the maintenance of the playfields and grounds. He is responsible for the daily care, cleanliness, and sanitation of the building, therefore he must possess knowledge of basic health practices. Certainly, the health objectives and practices of the occupants are of concern to him. Hence, it is most important that he serve as a member of the school health council.

To ensure the maintenance of the best standards, it is essential that the custodian be allowed an adequate staff. A job analysis would lead to efficient planning and an equitable division of labor and time among the members of the janitorial staff. The custodian is directly responsible to the principal of the school and to his supervisor who is usually the school district superintendent of buildings and grounds. To prevent confusion and misunderstandings, channels for handling necessary requests from teachers should be clearly defined and adhered to. The teachers in charge of swimming pool, gymnasia, shops, and laboratories should inform the custodian about their special problems and projects so that he may provide proper and safe handling of their equipment during the daily cleaning, and maintain periodic inspection, upkeep, and repairs. Because of their close contacts with the children, all members of the janitorial staff should be required to have periodic health examinations including chest x-rays.

From time to time in-service education should be provided for the custodian and his staff so that they may learn new procedures and methods of maintenance of buildings and grounds; and from members of the school health service team, pertinent health facts. Instructive pamphlets setting forth the duties and procedures of the maintenance workers are available from the NEA and other sources.

The Teacher and the School Environment

While it is within the province of the school to provide facilities and conditions to meet the approved standards, all the occupants of the school share the responsibility for their maintenance and proper usage. Because of her constant contact with the children, the greatest share rests with the classroom teacher. In the secondary school, the teachers of health, science, physical education and home economics should be especially alert to utilize opportunities within the scope of their subject courses for the integration of such understandings, with emphasis upon desirable health practices in daily school living. A common understanding of proper classroom temperature, ventilation, and lighting is necessary so that all expend their efforts in the same direction and toward the same ends. In the upper elementary grades and high schools, a study of lighting problems and eye care could incorporate pupil surveys of classrooms and activity rooms as to intensity of light and glare. Seating problems relate readily to the teaching of posture and activity habits. Certainly a part of every child's introduction to kindergarten and first grade will include instruction in the proper use of drinking fountains and the dangers of teasing and tricks, particularly the hazards to teeth.

A feeling of responsibility for the cleanliness and proper usage of lavatory facilities needs to be developed. Group pride in care and maintenance can be encouraged along with emphasis upon sound habits of handwashing before eating and after visiting the toilet. These should be stressed at all levels if needed, and in a manner best suited to the group.

The opportunities of the health and physical education teacher for emphasis upon the relation between personal health and environmental health are ever present. Such situations as the following involve all the pupils and offer meaningful opportunities for firsthand application of teaching:

1. Proper use of locker and shower facilities
2. Sanitary care of towel and gymnasium costume
3. Avoidance of special hazards from accidents due to thoughtlessness or horseplay
4. Cooperation in the observance of pool regulations such as refraining from spitting in the pool, running, and other dangerous acts
5. Individual use of toilet articles
6. Inspection of play equipment before using to ensure safety
7. Assistance to performing pupils when safety precautions are needed

8. Use of mats and other protective devices when needed
9. Care of street clothes during physical education class
10. Personal grooming before going to classroom after activity
11. Prompt reporting of accident or sudden illness

At a time when the young adolescent may not be interested in careful grooming, an appeal to his sense of social responsibility will often prove effective. The wise teacher will utilize accidents or other critical incidents as opportunities for incidental health teaching.

The School Luncheon

The school luncheon presents many health problems but at the same time it is replete with opportunities for teaching and learning. In some schools, the lunchroom may be merely a room equipped with tables and chairs to accommodate the children who bring their packed lunches from home. In some situations an active parents' organization has been known to provide one hot dish—a bowl of soup or a cup of cocoa—to supplement the children's packed lunches, with the mothers taking turns in preparing and serving. In large secondary schools, suburban and urban, the cafeteria becomes a highly organized affair, sometimes accommodating several thousands of students in relays during several successive periods of 30 to 50 minutes' duration. Despite these contrasts, it is possible to offer some basic principles and practices as they may involve school and teacher responsibility, and which are conducive to the best results in terms of the child's health, educational experience, and social satisfaction. Each individual school situation would need to make its own adaptations according to its needs, personnel, and finances.

The Role of the School. The following considerations are definitely responsibilities of the school:

1. The cafeteria or lunchroom should be well-lighted, well-ventilated, cheerful and attractive, and located above ground.
2. The lunchroom should be large enough to meet the needs of the student body and so designed and located as to permit efficient and safe movement of traffic.
3. As nearly as possible, the walls and ceiling should be soundproofed, the floor covering unwaxed, sound absorbent, and readily cleanable, and the chairs equipped with silent tips.
4. The kitchen and serving room should be separate from the cafeteria.
5. The equipment should be durable and sanitary and meet the requirements of the local and State Departments of Public Health as to type, materials, installation, and use.

6. Counters and steam tables should be ample to accommodate the numbers to be served within the allotted time and so designed as to protect the food from lines of passers by.
7. The counters should be so arranged that the desserts and sweets are the last foods to be encountered by the passing lines.
8. Ample provision should be made for seating in order to prevent pushing and crowding.
9. Time spent in line for service should not prevent the child from eating an unhurried lunch.
10. Cafeteria workers should be trained in sanitary handling of food. State or local Departments of Public Health make this type of training available.
11. Employees need to conform to local health department and school requirements as to health examinations and requirements.
12. Lavatories and locker accommodations should be provided for workers, and handwashing after the toilet and before food handling should be required. Hair nets should be required.
13. The cafeteria should be under the supervision of a trained dietitian employed by the school district rather than an outside concession.
14. Volunteers should not be permitted to serve food to school children unless they have undergone health examinations and unless proper sanitary equipment has been installed: safe cooking facilities, proper refrigeration, sanitary methods of dishwashing and waste disposal.
15. The implementation of current federal school food programs should provide maximum benefit to all needy, eligible children.

The Role of the Dietitian. A well-run cafeteria in the charge of a trained dietitian, can make a unique contribution to the total school health program. In order to realize its fullest possibilities, the cafeteria should be operated entirely under the Board of Education rather than controlled by an outside concession. The dietitian is usually directly responsible to the administrator. In a large city system with lunchrooms in all junior and senior high schools, special schools, and perhaps in elementary schools, there is usually a supervisor of food services to whom the dietitians in the individual schools are responsible.

The dietitian should meet the qualifications established by appropriate professional groups. This implies the usual training in home economics, with additional preparation in institutional cookery and management, marketing and buying, and other related areas. Considerable business and executive ability and skill in management of personnel are also required. In some instances a portion of her time is reserved for special nutrition education in the elementary schools.

These are some of the ways in which the trained dietitian functions in a typical school lunchroom situation:

1. Seeks to establish an attractive, inviting atmosphere in the cafeteria
2. Observes carefully such room conditions as temperature, humidity, air circulation, and cleanliness
3. Supervises the personal appearance, health habits, and service skills of the workers
4. Maintains the best standards of food handling and kitchen sanitation
5. Operates food service on a non-profit basis with meals served at lowest possible cost to pupils as may be permitted by the plan adopted by the Board of Education and the meeting of requirements for a balanced food service budget
6. Utilizes government food subsidies and surplus foods wisely
7. Gives due consideration to local, cultural and religious food habits and nutritional needs
8. Provides a place in the lunchroom for students who bring packed lunches from home
9. Offers individual nutrition instruction to students referred by the nurse or guidance counselor
10. Provides supplementary feedings for referred cases
11. Encourages the formation of a nutrition committee as part of the school health council and works with it willingly
12. Cooperates with special school events involving the cafeteria service, such as open house for parents, teas, and other functions
13. Cooperates with the student council in special projects
14. Works closely with the home economics department in surveys and special projects, and with all student groups in visits to the kitchen and other parts of the lunchroom organization
15. Makes full use of school publications, morning bulletins and the art department for nutrition publicity
16. Provides pertinent exhibits and bulletin board information for the lunchroom area
17. Prevents monotony and maintains student interest and cooperation by the observance of holidays, the introduction of new recipes, and occasional surprises
18. Initiates research and plans periodic and continuing evaluations
19. Represents the school in community affairs concerned with nutrition and related community problems
20. Strives to implement current federal school food programs to benefit all eligible, needy children.

The Teacher's Role. The teacher's responsibilities will vary according to the situation. The school lunch offers a wide variety of opportunities for the implementation of health and science concepts and social experiences at all levels. In an elementary school in which there is no food service, the teacher can make the lunch period and the mid-morning snack time valuable social events during which teacher and children eat together and converse in a natural friendly atmosphere. Children need to experience mealtime as a pleasant occasion providing opportunity for satisfying conversation. The teacher's social attitudes and table manners should present a fine example to the children. At the same time, she is able to observe the health and social needs of the group and of individuals in it. These needs will vary from time to time, but they may serve as the subjects for informal discussion periods and related experiences when they can be brought in naturally. Included at some time or other might be such topics as food needs for growth and nutrition, food likes and dislikes, balanced meals, and such experiences as the introduction of new foods through "tasting parties," food shopping expeditions, the selection of foods for a picnic or special occasion, and entertaining others such as the children's parents or the grade next door.

In the junior and senior high schools, teachers frequently have a separate lunchroom so that they too may benefit by relaxation in a calm, quiet, social atmosphere. Students at this level should be expected to assume the major responsibility for their own conduct and for having a smoothly run luncheon period with a minimum of supervision. Appropriate classes in health, science, home economics, and the home room programs might offer opportunities for the students to learn more about wise choices from lunchroom menus and the value of the government-subsidized lunches in terms of nutritional gain and budgeting their allowances. Student nutrition problems at this level center mainly upon the failure to eat breakfast, or an inadequate one, experimentation with exotic diets, the omission of lunch in order to save money for social or other purposes, and the snack habit in place of regular meals. Convincing experiences might include practice in working out balanced meals possible from the cafeteria menus to discover how to get the most for one's money. The tendency among girls to diet to maintain a slim figure might be offset effectually by stress upon the need for the high school girl to build optimum health through adequate nutrition to assure safer motherhood and stronger children. A tie-in with the physical fitness program often proves effective, particularly with boys.

At this level it is important to examine advertising in all communications media in order to help students realize the need for accurate specific knowledge, establish the habit of appraisal of new products, and to learn the proper sources for obtaining reliable information. The students need to realize also, the extent to which advertising is aimed directly at teenagers and young adults, and at the uninformed. Visits to food processing plants open new worlds as will surveys of food transportation, consideration of the food habits and problems of other nations, experimentation and research to discover new and untried ways of storing surpluses, and conversion of various substances into nutritious foods for human consumption. The wide range of health careers connected with nutrition and foods should be called to the attention of students whenever possible. Included would be professional careers in biochemistry, home economics, nutrition, public health, agriculture, science, pathology, and non-professional careers such as food inspection, preparation and service.

Teachers and guidance personnel need to bear in mind that individual nutritional problems often stem from an emotional base, particularly during adolescence. The approach to solution requires consideration from every angle. As the student nears the beginning of his vocational career, nutritional problems may assume vital importance. Close cooperation with the school health service is highly important.

Home economics classes might cooperate with the guidance department, the school health council, and with the cafeteria management in the conduct of various types of surveys of food habits. In some of the smaller schools the lunchroom is under the supervision of a teacher of home economics. In this type of situation, it is often possible to afford the pupils opportunities for actual practice in food preparation and food service. The Student Council might appoint a cafeteria committee with a faculty sponsor. This committee would seek means of cooperation between the students and the cafeteria management. Students like to feel that they have a voice in affairs and frequently they point out existing needs of which adults have not even been aware. Their suggestions for improvement are usually practical and satisfying. In some schools the ten or fifteen minutes of the period which remain after the majority of students have finished lunch, constitute a problem. To obviate possible disciplinary problems, student councils sometimes set up a number of quiet activities in various locations, such as listening to recordings, social dancing, table games, and study rooms. However, care must be taken that these should not become an inducement for students to omit lunch.

Pupils permitted to go home for luncheon should be required to have a valid reason and written permission from parents. This rule should be strictly adhered to at all times in the interest of school liability for the pupil at this hour. All other pupils should be required to remain in school and not patronize outside restaurants or stores. Students who bring their lunches from home should always be made to feel comfortable and welcome to eat them in the cafeteria. In the case of indigent pupils needing financial help, it is important to handle the distribution of luncheon tokens or funds discreetly and inconspicuously so that the student does not feel embarrassed before his peers.

School Safety

Safety in the school is everyone's responsibility and should be given prime consideration at all times. It should be recognized that accidents are the leading cause of death among children of elementary and high school age. The Board of Education and the Superintendent of Schools carry the over-all responsibility for safety and accident prevention. It is essential that the handbook on policies for the district include written policies covering safety and accident prevention and that these be reviewed frequently and kept up-to-date. In a city, the responsibility for a planned program should be delegated to a qualified director or coordinator of safety who serves as a member of the Superintendent's staff. In every school the responsibility should be assigned to an individual, to a safety committee, or to a school safety council. Written regulations and policies should be drawn to fit the particular school situation and be approved by the principal and the faculty.

The school safety committee might well be a part of the school health council. At least, the members should study their task in the setting of the total school situation. The range of responsibilities is enormous and impossible to describe here. The list which follows contains some of the duties which commonly fall within the scope of the school safety committee:

1. The planning and implementation of adequate fire drills
2. Provision for periodic surveys of fire and safety hazards within the entire school plant
3. The planning for safe school parking of bicycles and motor vehicles of faculty, students, and visitors, and of delivery trucks and buses
4. The alerting and indoctrination of all staff members at the beginning of the year concerning their special responsibilities for instructing their classes about the possible dangers and hazards related to their course experiences, the precautions and safety measures to be followed, and the need for continual follow-up and eternal vigilance on the part of each teacher
5. The responsibility for the formation of a functioning school safety patrol in each elementary school, with appropriate leadership and instruction
6. The planning of safe traffic regulations for school corridors, lavatories, cafeteria, locker rooms, stairways, assembly hall, and other similar locations
7. Cooperation with the public safety department in the periodic inspection of the school and the prompt compliance with recommendations which they might offer
8. Cooperation with the police department protection at the opening and closing of school and on special occasions, traffic and crossing protection
9. Cooperation with special security guards assigned to daily permanent or temporary emergency duty within the school plant

10. The alerting of those responsible for the selection and purchase of equipment and supplies to the need for consideration of safety factors and accident hazards
11. Cooperation with the health service program in the planning of emergency procedures and in evaluation and research pertaining to various phases of the safety program
12. Cooperation with community agencies and civic organizations which have an interest in or bearing upon school safety and accident prevention
13. Cooperation with comprehensive community planning for the pooling of means and resources to meet unpredictable disasters or post-disaster conditions: (such as power failure, tornados, riots, etc.)
14. The planning for in-service safety education of faculty, maintenance staff, and parents as well as pupils (such as hazards attached to new products, chemicals, environmental hazards, etc.) making full use of available resources such as consultant services, qualified speakers from agencies on national, state, and local levels, audio-visual aids, etc.
15. Cooperation with school library and audio-visual departments in keeping safety and accident prevention materials up-to-date

The Safety Patrol. The Safety Patrol movement has proved its effectiveness and has gained wide respect and support of school personnel and the public. The responsibility for its organization and functioning should be assigned to an interested teacher who can give it the requisite amount of time and attention. The sponsor needs to keep up-to-date as to legislation which may relate to its activities, and work cooperatively with police authorities and civic safety groups. Excellent materials are available for guidance from the National Safety Council and other sources.

Safety in Secondary Schools. In the senior high school, the person who carries the responsibility for driver education should be a member of the safety committee and coordinate his teaching with their efforts in every way possible. At this level pupil representatives from the Student Council should be included on the safety committee.

In the area of safety much can be accomplished at all levels through the joint efforts of pupils and faculty. On the secondary school level, it is particularly satisfying to students to feel that they are working on adult problems, as adults, with adults. Moreover, students can often suggest effective ways of coping with student attitudes toward safety problems (such as experimentations with fire alarms, drug abuse, daredevil stunts with motor vehicles, etc.). Accident figures among youth at this age level point to this as an area of major concern. Moreover, outdoor education, sports participation, aquatic activities, and camping are on the increase. This means the need for more safety education with stress upon new types of problems as they may relate to scuba and skin diving, winter sports, boating and canoeing, camp cookery and other recreational activities.

Liability

Wherever large groups assemble, there are likely to be some unavoidable accidents. However, it is of utmost importance that teachers and other personnel do everything possible to prevent accident or injury to pupils. Many of the accidents at school occur in connection with physical activity, sports or recreational activities, or in the shops and laboratories, or on stairways. They can, of course, happen anywhere and at any time. State laws and regulations concerning liability of school boards and teachers vary greatly, but in some states teachers as individuals and even school boards can be held liable for injuries suffered by pupils on school property.

Careful planning will reduce the possibility of accidents. Usually such planning is the teacher's direct responsibility. Inspection of playfields, swimming pools, gymnasiums, apparatus, and equipment should be systematic and frequent to ensure freedom from defects. Bleachers and grandstands need to be included. Charging admission often increases the liability. The prompt reporting in writing of a defect or needed repair is most important, and the teacher should, for his own protection, keep a duplicate dated copy of the report. The teacher needs to observe care (*a*) in the use of mats and protective devices; (*b*) in the choice of activity appropriate to the age and developmental level of the children; (*c*) in the teaching of proper skills and precautions before permitting participation, and in careful supervision of the activity or apparatus; (*d*) in the safe location of an activity in relation to dangers from other groups or objects; and (*e*) in the prompt administration of first aid with recourse to a physician as soon as possible. Obviously, play apparatus of a dangerous character should not be chosen for a playground which is to be unsupervised during part of the time. School districts or departments of physical education should agree upon policies and procedures and include them in the handbook not only to the teachers of physical education, but to all preschool and elementary school teachers as well, for they too are usually responsible for the conduct of physical activities. Under ordinary circumstances, if the teacher has observed "due care and reasonable precaution" and negligence cannot be proved, there is little basis for liability. Many teachers, however, carry liability insurance. In any case, prompt and adequate reporting of accidents and injuries, and a complete and accurate description of the circumstances by the teacher constitute an important part of the protection of the legal interests of the teacher. Whenever possible, such written statements should be countersigned by witnesses, and the names and addresses obtained for subsequent reference if needed. An excellent sample form for the reporting of accidents is available from the National Safety Council.

The Recreation Program

The shorter work day, the increased amount of leisure, and the disappearance of land for recreational purposes from many localities, point to the increasing need for education to focus upon greater emphasis upon the development of leisure time skills, interests, and values. Such emphasis must be a part of school experience beginning with kindergarten and extending through all grades. Happily the old stereotyped playground equipment is rapidly being superseded by attractive, innovative types which stimulate the imaginations of youngsters and lure them into participation in activities which are satisfying and developmental. If such experiences are really to become part of the warp and woof of everyday living, participation must bring genuine satisfaction to the child at each succeeding maturity level. Moreover, the experiences must cover a range sufficiently broad to include the development of skills and interests which will be usable and which will stimulate active participation at all stages of life.

The schools and the community should share the responsibility for making such a program an actuality. This can be done by cooperative study, planning, and financing, and through the joint use of facilities, equipment, and leadership. Therefore, the present and future recreational needs of the community and the school need to be considered together when designing the lay-out of the school grounds and recreational areas or rooms in the building. Equipment and space should be adequate in amount, not only for the present needs, but also for the estimated future needs of the school and the community population. The quality of leadership and the objectives of the program should be continuous throughout the year. Often persons with training and interest in recreation can be recruited from the teaching staff or from a nearby college or university to carry on late afternoon, evening and summer programs. The program itself should be flexible in meeting the needs of groups, stimulate creativity and imagination on the part of the participants, and have high standards of excellence in leadership. Such pooling of effort represents the best economy for the community, the peak use of facilities, and, it is hoped, the best character results.

Organization of the School Day

Aside from the environmental factors which have already been discussed in this chapter, there are certain other factors which have such significant effects upon the health, comfort, and performance of the child as to merit inclusion here. These largely concern administrative or classroom arrangements and procedures pertaining to the educational experience, but all carry emotional and social implications relating to the child's progress and development.

Correlation between the organization of the child's school day and his educational progress is needed at all levels. Effective organization of the child's day is the product of over-all coordinated planning on the part of those concerned. The over-all pattern should provide ample proportionate time allotments for the various subjects and experiences in the curriculum. In the elementary grades, it is important that the child's best teaching-learning hours be allocated in turn to each subject. Thus, the over-all plan should provide for wise alternation or rotation of subjects and periods on different days. In the primary grades, a block plan permits this desirable flexibility and places the responsibility in the hands of the classroom teacher for the inclusion of the required work at the most favorable time, with part of a large project needing great blocks of time on certain days and perhaps tapering off proportionately at another time. A skillful teacher can save a great deal of teaching-learning time through effective integration and correlation of subject matter at propitious moments.

The length of the school day should be such as to prevent undue fatigue on the part of the child. Work and rest periods can be alternated to advantage. Frequently, a mere change of task provides a rest. Periods of big-muscle activity and vigorous free play should be introduced when they will be most beneficial to the child. The teacher needs to be constantly alert for fatigue symptoms. The day's schedule should permit a calm, unhurried lunch period for both teacher and pupils. Supplemental feedings and mid-session snacks should be scheduled in relation to the entire day's program as well as the lunch period.

On the secondary school level, the time schedule is more complex and consequently more rigid. Class periods vary from 45 to 60 minutes in length according to the philosophy of the school. In some schools, the last period of the day is reserved for special activities and conferences; in other schools these take place before or after the regular school hours. Time between classes should be sufficient to permit the brief relaxation and socialization which is so necessary to relieve tension after a class period. Lunch periods should be kept free from activities, rehearsals, teacher conferences and other appointments. Homeroom teachers, nurses, and guidance counselors need to be on the lookout for the "chronic joiner"—the student who loads himself too heavily with extracurricular activities. A time budget kept for a week will often help this student see his own problem more objectively and help him become more willing to make intelligent adjustments.

Schools utilizing the module in their scheduling, report more flexibility in scheduling, better use of special facilities and audio-visual equipment. The Philadelphia experiment with the "high school without walls" has attracted interest as a promising innovation which provides maximum flexibility and independent study. For success it demands mature, qualified, imaginative teachers, and cooperation from many community agencies.

Teaching-Learning Procedures. Classroom procedures should stem from concepts of child development, the dynamics of psychology, and total health. Today's concept of sound discipline implies on the part of the child the development of inner controls based upon understanding and emotional satisfaction derived from work and play experiences, and accomplishments. Basic to all class procedures are the following considerations:

1. The need for clearly understood, common goals to be established cooperatively by pupils and teacher
2. At all times, respect for the individual
3. The recognition of and provision for individual differences in rates of speed in learning, the need to provide challenge for all pupils, and for each child to receive a proportionate share of the teacher's time and attention
4. The inculcation on the part of each pupil of a feeling of responsibility for his own unique role in the class and in the school as a whole
5. The development on the part of each pupil of the ability to relate happily to others, and to work successfully as a member of a group
6. The need for each child to grow and progress both "*vertically*" and "*horizontally*," *i.e.*, in sequential learning and in personality development
7. The recognition of evaluation as a continuing process to be participated in by teacher, pupils, and others.

In actual classroom practice there should be a pervading sense of orderliness, cleanliness and good use of time, economy in routine procedures, everyday courtesy, and increasing tendency to consider the comfort of the group ahead of individual whims or desires.

The Testing Program. If the child is to develop a healthy attitude toward the testing program of the school, and, in a larger sense, toward life in a competitive world, such attitude must be demonstrated to him by the administrator and the faculty. The school assumes responsibility for determining the type and the amount of testing, the selection of the best available standardized tests for the purpose, and the decisions as to when they are to be used, and who is to administer them. If properly used, such tests can help to measure the educational progress of the child and to some extent his capabilities. Some children enjoy the self-tests provided by certain teaching machines. While all tests must be considered as possibly contributing to the total picture of the child, they should by no means be regarded as a final or complete means of categorizing him. A common complaint is the failure of tests to indicate the unusually talented or gifted child.

The teacher-made test is used frequently for diagnostic purposes, to discover what the child or group already knows and what remains to be taught about a certain topic. Tests when used for teaching-learning purposes and followed as soon as possible by discussion and interpretation by the teacher, can be very helpful to the class. The test which really educates is not a mere memory test, but elicits critical thinking on the part of the child by requiring the selection and actual application of principles or concepts he has learned. Frequent and varied tests of this kind help the child to retain concepts. Children tend to prefer frequent tests to merely one final test given at the end of a term.

Grades and Marks. The methods of arriving at grades and marks have much to do with the emotional health of the child. The child needs to be helped to a realization of his own powers and to make the most of them. At the same time, he must learn to face his own shortcomings objectively and to understand the reasons for them, and what, if anything, he can do to improve matters and to seek the kind of help he needs.

The teacher needs to adopt a wholesome, objective attitude toward grades and marks, and to use them along with an analytical conference with the child. Children respect justice and readily recognize it. Discussion of test grades and marks should follow a test as soon as possible to minimize possible negative mental health effects, such as needless tension and anxiety. Finally, the teacher's philosophy and that of the school should possess a certain consistency which the child will eventually recognize for himself.

Progress reports to parents should be objective. At the same time, it is important that they be handled without emotional harm to the child. Many schools have substituted a descriptive report or letter for the time-honored report card with its list of impersonal numerical or letter grades. A home visit or a pre-arranged visit by the parent to the school is often an essential supplement to grading and marking. It is highly important that parent, child, and teacher feel a sort of partnership in connection with the child's educational progress and realize that evaluation is a useful and continuous process.

Administrator-Teacher-Pupil Relationships

The social and emotional atmosphere of the school reflects the existing administrator-teacher-pupil relationships. Within the school, the principal, by his own personality, attitudes, and actions, sets the keynote for these relationships. Its tone, however, might be modified consciously or unconsciously by his own relationships with his superiors and the pressures which he feels, not only from that angle, but from various community angles as well.

The teacher, in turn, sets the keynote in her classroom. Her relations with her pupils reflect her attitudes and practices as they in turn, may be affected by her interactions with the principal, her colleagues, her supervisors, and the various pressures and demands inherent in any profession which entails responsibilities, judgments, and decisions. It is the accumulation of unreleased tensions which so often results in the feeling of hopeless inadequacy and frustration that leads to a breakdown on the part of the person who has not learned to cope with them successfully, as they arise.

The administrator can alleviate his pressures by learning to share his burdens with his staff, by discussing his problems with staff members, and by delegating some of his responsibilities to others. Many feel that this is inconsistent with the role of the administrator, not realizing that such old-fashioned concepts of the need for isolated dignity and aloofness prevent release from tensions and the realization of sound mental health. The person who possesses genuine respect for the individual will not hesitate to risk his self-importance by sharing his problems. Thus, it is possible not only to minimize one's inner tensions, but to avoid the dissipation of energy through worry and to allow more complete concentration upon the task at hand.

This applies to the teacher, too. Insecurity, frustration, inability to attain one's aspirations, or a lack of sense of humor can cause tensions which children are quick to detect. Outbursts of temper or irritation also have traumatic effects upon children and colleagues. Hence, by her constant proximity to the pupils, the teacher can exert a negative influence upon their mental health.

The preliminary selection of students for teacher education should include careful screening as to personality and mental health. From time to time during their years of preparation, and throughout their student teaching experiences, they should be observed carefully. They should be given therapeutic help if necessary, or, at times, guided into a different type of profession rather than be allowed to carry a negative attitude into the classroom.

Opportunities for Health Teaching

The school environment abounds in opportunities for functional health teaching. At all levels, the focal point is a problem which is meaningful to the child, one which concerns him as an individual, affects his comfort, or presents a group problem in which he shares. The alert teacher will utilize such practical opportunities to the fullest extent, involving the child in problem solving which might include various activities such as investigations, research, surveys, or special studies at his own maturity level. From this, it is not too difficult to widen the scope to a community viewpoint. The following list is merely suggestive of some topics which might be adapted to all levels. The possibilities, however, are practically endless.

Water: safe water; uses of water; relation of water to bodily health; water-borne diseases: conservation
Sanitation: waste disposal and health; insect and rodent control
Heating and ventilation: temperature, humidity and the human body; air pollution; body defenses against respiratory diseases
Lighting: principles of illumination; eye health; school lighting survey; home lighting; study conditions
Safety and accident prevention: bicycle safety, traffic safety, hiking safety; recreation hazards; first aid
Health Room: purpose; the school health program; school health services; duties of the members of the health team; disease control; health careers
Recreation: uses of play space; values of recreational skills; family recreation; balanced living; vacation health; life-time sports; physical fitness; care and beauty of school grounds.

Questions for Discussion

1. Compare the regulations and standards governing school buildings in your state with those of a neighboring state.
2. As a newly appointed teacher in an elementary school, how would you proceed in seeking to influence favorably any existing undesirable principal-teacher-pupil relationships?
3. What are the school-community recreation plans for the next decade in your community? How adequate are they in terms of the needs of persons of all ages?
4. Let us suppose that an elementary school is troubled by poor lavatory conditions. The lavatories are not being kept clean by the pupils and the problem has been brought to the attention of the school health council. What means of approach might be employed toward remedying the situation?
5. What are some of the effects upon the pupils of the marking and grading plans in use today at various grade levels in schools?

Suggested Readings

1. American Association for Health, Physical Education, and Recreation in cooperation with the Athletic Institute. *Planning Areas and Facilities for Health, Physical Education, and Recreation.* Washington, D.C.: the Association and Chicago, Ill.: the Athletic Institute, 1965.
2. American Association of School Administrators: *Schools for America.* Washington, D. C.: the Association, a department of the National Education Association, 1967.
3. Anderson, Carl L.: *Heating and Lighting.* NEA Journal, *51,* No. 7, October, 1962: 23-29.
4. Bogert, L. Jean, Briggs, George M., and Calloway, Doris H.: *Nutrition and Physical Fitness.* 8th Ed. Philadelphia, W. B. Saunders Co., 1966.

5. Educational Facilities Laboratories. *The Cost of a School House.* New York, the Laboratories, 1960.
6 Joint Committee on Health Problems in Education of the National Education Association and the American Medical Association. *Health Aspects of the School Lunch Program.* Washington, D.C.: the National Education Association and Chicago, Ill.: the American Medical Association, 1962.
7. Joint Committee on Health Problems in Education of the National Education Association and the American Medical Association and other contributors. Eds.: C. C. Wilson, M.D. and Elizabeth A. Wilson, Ph.D.: *Healthful School Environment.* Washington, D.C.: the National Education Association and Chicago, Ill.: the American Medical Association, 1969.
8. Leu, Donald J.: *Planning Educational Facilities.* New York, Center for Applied Research in Education, 1965.
9. Mittelstaedt, Arthur H. Jr.: *Planning School Grounds.* J. Health, Phys. Educ. and Recr., *40,* No. 5, May, 1969: 37-40.
10. National Commission on Safety Education: *National Conference on School Transportation.* Rev. ed. Washington, D.C.: the National Commission on Safety Education, National Education Association, 1965.
11. National Commission on Safety Education: *The Expanding Role of the School Safety Patrol.* Washington, D.C.: the Commission, of the National Education Association, 1953.
12. National Commission on Safety Education, of the National Education Association: *Who is Liable for Pupil Injuries?* Washington, D.C.: the National Education Association, 1963.
13. National Safety Council: *Accident Facts.* Chicago, Ill.: the Council. Published annually.
14. Seaton, Don Cash, Stack, Herbert J. and Loft, Bernard I.: *Administration and Supervision of Safety Education.* New York, The Macmillan Co., 1968.
15. Stack, Herbert J. and Elkow, J. Duke: *Education for Safe Living.* 4th ed. Englewood Cliffs, N.J., Prentice-Hall, 1966.
16. Turner, Clair E., Randall, Harriet R., and Smith, Sara L.: *School Health and Health Education* 6th Ed. St. Louis, The C. V. Mosby Co., 1970.

Chapter 14

School Health Education

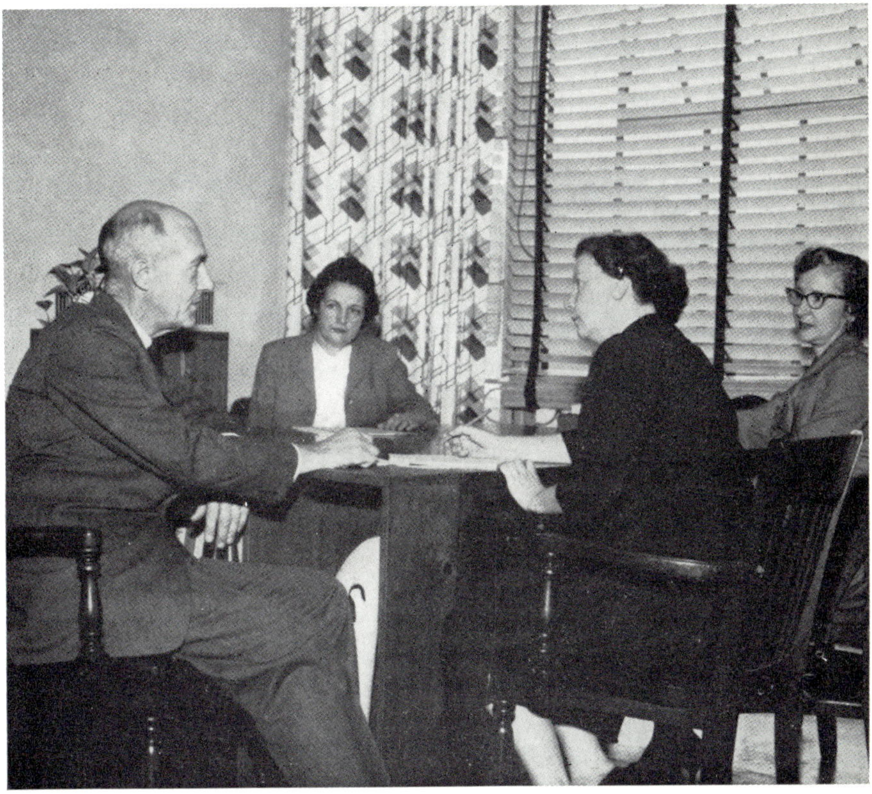

FIG. 58. Health Education Requires Planning.

The Meaning of Health Education

Health education, according to one accepted definition, is "the process of providing learning experiences for the purpose of influencing knowledges, attitudes, and conduct relating to individual and group health."[1] Learning experiences can take place anywhere that an appropriate combination of learning conditions exists; and understandings, attitudes, and conduct in the form of practices, skills, or habits are associated with every learning process. Thus, health learning experiences are not merely

[1] Report of the Committee on Terminology in School Health Education. J. Health, Phys. Educ. and Recr., 22:7, September, 1951, p. 14.

those which occur in relation to or as the result of planned health instruction in school or community. They can occur in all three of the major divisions of the school health program—health services, healthful school living, health instruction—or in any segment of the curriculum. In other words, health education can occur at any time or in any place; it is not synonomous with or limited to planned health instruction. Hence, health education becomes the responsibility of everyone with whom the child comes in contact during his school experience. It is of utmost importance therefore, that his school health educational experience be consistent throughout. It is equally desirable that this consistency should extend also to his health education experiences in the home and in the community.

Although the exact scope and dimensions of health elude concise definition, they extend deeply into "the four domains of knowledge within which are implied quite clearly the objectives of education and the kinds of learning that schools are concerned with. These dominions are by recent tradition, physical science, biological science, social science, and humanistic studies."[2] Health in itself can hardly be regarded as a separate science. It is concerned mainly with the functioning of man in relationship to and in conformity with the observed and accepted laws and processes included within the range of all of the root sciences; that is, with the application of science. While science itself is regarded as abstract and free from the various cultural beliefs and attitudes of man, social sciences and humanistic studies have great bearing upon man's functioning, and therefore upon the ways and means whereby the application of science can be made effective in everyday living. Thus, to be really effective, health education must be functional in character.

Health Education as a Learning Process

Health education is concerned with the building up of useful and desirable understandings, attitudes, and practices in regard to health. Scientific facts constitute the bedrock of health concepts or understandings, but accurate comprehension and interpretation of these facts must precede their wise utilization and practical application in daily living. An understanding of health facts can serve as impetus to intelligent health behavior. For example, understanding what possible dangers may be lurking in a clear roadside spring will cause the informed person to refrain from drinking even though he may be desperately thirsty. To another passer-by who lacks this knowledge, such restraint appears senseless. Thus, sound knowledge may lead to wise health conduct.

Knowledge of facts alone, however, will not ensure desirable health practices and attitudes in an individual. For example, the mere possession of sound information about tuberculosis and the means of protection

[2] Thelen, Herbert A. *Education and the Human Quest.* New York, Harper & Brothers, 1960. p. 35.

will not ensure conduct leading to prevention of infection by bacilli of the disease. During his health class the robust high school athlete may absorb many important facts pertaining to the disease; but if he fails to see any relationship to himself or to his daily activities or his goals, the facts may not influence his conduct in any way whatever. The student is likely to react positively to just those facts which appear important to him in his own private world composed of his inner self, as he perceives and accepts himself, his interests, his friends and peers, his life goals and value system. His private world includes his physical and socio-cultural environment with its human relations and interactions, pressures, and prejudices. Moreover, it embraces not merely the present, but also the experiences and resultant attitudes of his previous years. However, an undesirable health practice may persist in spite of exposure to correct scientific knowledge, particularly if the practice was begun early in the person's life and pursued for a long time without observation or knowledge of any other practice. Actually, primacy may be a factor in its persistence long after exposure to the correct knowledge.

In similar fashion, practices if reinforced by sound, scientific knowledge can build up definite appreciations or attitudes toward health. These may be favorable or unfavorable, negative or positive. A two-year-old child, for example, gradually forms the habit of brushing his teeth because his mother, day after day, patiently teaches and supervises his performance. As the reasons for the practice grow increasingly clear to him, the habit, through its daily repetition, is likely to become strengthened if the emotions accompanying the practice are positive and satisfying; that is, if his mother praises his efforts, the dentifrice is pleasant, the clean feeling is emphasized, and his appreciation of the attractiveness of clean, white teeth is developed. If the emotions aroused should be negative—involve constant nagging, scolding, or even punishment for a lapse or failure, and an unpleasant, gritty dentifrice—when he finally assumes full responsibility for his own health decisions, the practice is likely to be irregularly and carelessly performed. Sound practices reinforced by sound knowledge can lead to the building up of favorable attitudes and appreciations toward health. In turn, these favorable attitudes inspire sound practices and the acquisition of more health facts. Thus, in cyclical fashion, knowledge, practices, and attitudes are linked together inseparably and one cannot identify the exact points or zones in which one merges into another. As health knowledge increases, and practices and habit patterns are intensified, attitudes are strengthened. Whether the health experience occurs in the home, the school, or the community, these considerations are basic to an understanding of the learning process in health education. However, the great gap which exists between health knowledge and health practices has long baffled teachers, physicians, health educators, and others concerned with changing health conduct. The bridging of this gap constitutes one of the great unsolved problems confronting health education in school and community. Recent research into the learning process—the motivational, psychological, and sociological facets—has shed some light upon it, but it still remains unsolved.

The home, the school, and the community share in the common task of helping each child to realize optimal health, and apace with his increasing maturity, gradually to assume more and more responsibility for his own health. In a school situation, it is not possible to provide opportunities for actual practice or experience in all areas of health. Obviously, the home, the school, and the community need to plan and work together so that the health education to which the child is exposed is scientifically sound, unified, and consistent, and that the efforts of one supplement and reinforce the others effectively.

Motivation in Health Education

To the individual or group with a cause to promote, a product to sell, or a fact to teach, the problem of motivation is of major concern. In recent years intensive study and research have centered upon motivation as it pertains to business, industry, politics, and education, and many of the findings have common application. Because of the need for health education to function in daily living, the processes preceding and involved in changing health behavior have been subjected to special scrutiny by the behavioral scientists. This concern extends to motivation in health education as it applies to the individual, to the group or class in school, to the neighborhood, and to the community.

Motivation has to do with the inner movement or response of the individual as regulated by his biological drives and by the effects of his own past experiences, toward that which holds meaning for him—that which is associated with his values, goals, desires and needs. The results of research studies are in general agreement that the well-spring to action arises *within* the individual. Movement toward action may result from, be modified or directed by organic changes, environmental pressures, the individual's own values or aspirations, or by all or any possible combination of these.

It is indeed difficult to fathom the precise motive which underlies an individual's health behavior. The teacher or leader or any extrinsic force may contribute to or set the situation with the aim of encouragement or stimulation to desirable action. Various devices calculated to incite a glow, or fan a faint flicker of interest already there may be used. But unless the glow or the flicker is fanned to the point of actual flame, the result is likely to be complete failure, or at most, short-lived, feeble and non-productive. On the part of the teacher, therefore, there is need for sensitivity in discovering pupil needs, interests, goals, and values *as the pupil himself sees them.*

It is essential too, that the teacher remember that many of these goals will change at various ages and stages of the child's development and growth toward maturity. They are prone to be tenuous and fleeting, changing without warning, from month to month, week to week, and even to some extent, daily and hourly. The range of these goals varies not only with their importance to the child, but in relation to his development. The young child thinks in terms of short range or more immediate goals; the older one, if maturing according to the usual pattern, will have long-range goals for which, if they are of sufficient significance, he will sacrifice immediate satisfactions. Therefore, at the outset, in addition to discovering what knowledge the pupil already has concerning a particular health topic or area, the teacher will find it advantageous to determine what value and significance the pupil attaches to it and any misconceptions he may have in regard to it. She must then decide what new essential learnings are needed and how they can best be approached. To arouse and maintain the interest of all members of a class or group in a specific health topic the teacher will need imagination and skill in using various approaches and motivational devices.

The teacher needs to be aware of the effects of motivational forces upon group behavior and to become skilled in the application of group methods in the teaching-learning situation. To a school-child the mores of his group are all-important. To the adolescent, status with his peers ranks above almost everything. The alert teacher makes a point of finding out about these small social groups and their relative importance to the various pupil members. Some exist outside the school but the teacher will hear of them through discussion periods, casual conversation or by means of planned devices. The beliefs and standards which these peer groups uphold can often serve as powerful influences, favorable or unfavorable to desirable health conduct. The teacher, aware of the potentialities of group motivation, can sometimes introduce health experiences which will utilize these forces in guiding the health conduct in the desired direction. She can set the stage or use devices, but these will not bring the desired responses unless the group as a whole and each member of the group, is involved in the activity—doing, thinking and feeling. She should strive to utilize the group's motivational forces in pursuance of *their* worthwhile, long-range goals. With younger children, her focus will be upon helping them discover answers to their questions and grow in maturity, and upon gradually leading them to set long-range goals for themselves.

Concepts in Health Education

A basic core of essential health knowledge consists of clusters of related facts and understandings generally accepted as effective in helping the student meet his present needs as an individual and his future needs as a citizen and possible head of a family. Included also are skills and experiences and a stock of resources which might serve as tools adapted to the discovery of solutions to future problems of living in the swiftly paced latter part of the twentieth century about whose nature we can, at this point, merely speculate. To become functional, this core of essentials would need to be undergirded and reinforced at all points by principles, concepts, and attitudes sufficiently crystallized as to constitute a flexible, resilient base or springboard for effective health behavior.

However, functional health knowledge is not acquired through the mere acquisition of accumulated, discrete facts. Facts need to be related and built into generalizations or concepts. These are built up gradually by the student himself from a variety of sequential experiences much as a picture puzzle takes form with piece added to piece, each contributing toward the completed picture. Just as the player in working the puzzle sometimes needs to try a fragment in numerous locations before the exact fit is found, the student will need to examine many facts and experiences to which he has been exposed during the teaching-learning process and evaluate each in the light of his own life values or goals, in terms of its worth to him. After due reflection, he accepts or retains only those which are meaningful to him and which seem related to his goals or ends. During this period of reflection the student tests, judges, or appraises, and finally decides what is acceptable and useful to him. Some of these experiences should involve the student in activity for these are the most likely to be retained as meaningful and, because of the self-involvement, will make him want to know more. He will not discard his present pattern unless the new one seems to him, more desirable. But he will not arrive at this point of change by reading or hearing about it. Precisely what inner motivational forces actually move the student, nobody can know. The teacher can merely observe and try to judge by his behavior.

A new concept is not established quickly. The process involves repetition and in the traditional school this meant *drill.* Today's concept of education recognizes the need for repetition but stresses the importance of adding a new feature or making a new application in a different setting each time. This provides a challenge to the pupil to test out the new understanding or skill and to further his grasp of it. During this stage the teacher serves as guide and points out his successes. Tests, commendations, and self-evaluations are indispensable means of helping him chart his own progress. Thus, the conceptual approach to teaching-learning leads the student to establish for himself fundamental understandings resulting from a variety of experiences, and which after due reflection on his part, assume definiteness or are built into him, so that they are sufficiently meaningful to him as to influence his health conduct now and in the future. If the student has received sound and skillful teacher guidance during the teaching-learning process, the resultant concept would be consistent with sound health facts and future desirable health conduct.

An Illustration

To see this in action, let us look briefly at a tenth grade class whose intense interest has been roused by a dramatic news headline concerning the plight of a popular movie star who has taken an overdose of sleeping pills. The class teems with questions about sleeping pills—their content, how much is an "overdose," and myriads of other questions. Taking advantage of this intense interest and emotional involvement, the teacher after pursuing the topic to the point of their present satisfaction, gradually widens the focus and leads the class to see that there are other health practices under individual control which can be just as dangerous: neglecting a wound, staying in a game after injury, taking medicine prescribed for another member of the family, and other examples. In leading the group to examine a wider range of health behaviors, the teacher is assisting the pupils to gain a broader view which will presently make generalization possible. Thus, the class will be led to build up a significant concept: "Self-medication is undesirable and may prove dangerous to life."

The mere reading of such a statement in a textbook is not likely to involve the student sufficiently to apply this concept to himself or to his future health decisions. A varied sequence of experiences with each designed to contribute in some ways to the building of the desired concept is needed. These experiences may involve trying to find examples in newspapers and magazines, discussions of examples gleaned from reading, interviews with local health authorities or prominent adults, and the process of analyzing underlying causes and meanings. A generalization is deduced after the student has examined all the evidence gleaned from situations meaningful to him or which involve him emotionally as well as intellectually.

From time to time there needs to be a pause to permit an appraising look backward at the route which has been traveled, and then a look ahead. Has our search uncovered facts and facets which we had not anticipated? Are we still moving toward the goal we set? Are the goals precisely the same when viewed from various angles? A self-evaluation by the teacher and the students should measure the stockpiling of facts, growth in skill and practices, decision-making skills, and attitudes, and help the teacher discover to what extent the desired concept is beginning to crystallize in the mind of the student. A joint teacher-student evaluation shows also the degree of communication which has occurred and the level of maturity. Out of such evaluation should come new agreement as to necessary directions and next steps. Through this process, the teacher is leading the children to think. The subject matter covered may not have followed precisely the original systematic plan, but the student will have made it his own as the learning progressed. In this type of procedure he is constantly sharpening his powers and abilities to meet new conditions and situations. The teacher needs to uphold high standards within the reasonable grasp of the pupil and constantly help him set high standards for himself so that eventually he will find satisfaction in no other kind.

The Curriculum

The philosophy of the school or institution determines the curriculum which should assume such nature and form as to permit the most complete realization of the aims and objectives inherent in the philosophy. The two are inseparable. The philosophy and curriculum determine the choice of content and learning experiences, predict the outcome of each course or subject area to a great extent, and provide for and inspire the best development and self-realization of the individual child. Together they design the "image" of the school and the behavior patterns of the administrators, the faculty, the staff, and the pupils.

Curriculum has been defined in various ways. Here it is considered in its broadest sense as including all teaching-learning experiences and activities offered to the pupil in the over-all education pattern of the school. Curriculum patterns vary according to such conditions as the pupil enrollment; the size, type and quality of the teaching and administrative staff; the needs of the pupils; the facilities and resources available; the financial budget; the state requirements; and the attitude of the community toward education. A form of curriculum which appears to work well in one community may not be effective in another.

Responsibility for the Curriculum

Most states bear the responsibility for the minimal standards as to the quality and extent of education within their boundaries. The state is responsible for the certification of qualified teachers, the length of the school term, for standards and facilities, and for determining what is to be taught. The curriculum is defined in a general way with minimal standards indicated and recommendations and suggestions as to their implementation. Courses of study in most fields and subjects are provided, but again, these are broad and general in tone and usually intended to be suggestive rather than mandatory. The local community is responsible for the implementation of the minimal requirements, but it may extend the content as far beyond as it chooses.

The preparation of a course of study or guide in a special field such as health education, is usually a cooperative affair authorized by the state superintendent of education and initiated by the specialist in the department of education who is designated as the person responsible for its construction. The next step is the appointment of a central committee composed of several teachers from various sections of the state representing the level for which the course is intended, a curriculum specialist, persons from official or voluntary agencies whose interest impinges upon health education, a university or teacher education specialist, if possible, and additional resource persons when needed. The committee will collect and examine the best available courses of study, in terms of the needs of the state. The committee then prepares the guiding philosophy, objectives, and scope of the proposed curriculum guide, and sets up a work plan. The preparation of the proposed units or section is usually divided among the various committee members, each of whom will probably head a sub-committee. Each sub-committee is composed of special teachers of health education, a school physician, a school nurse, a parent or two, and some representatives of official and voluntary health agencies whose work is related to the health of school children. Special consultants and experts might be called upon as resource persons. The completed units are tested in actual health class situations by designated teachers, who then return the units to the sub-committee for revision in the light of their evaluations. The final drafts of the completed units are sent to the central curriculum committee for further testing, editing, and publication.

This method of curriculum making may require more time to produce results but it has many advantages. A number of persons have been involved in its construction and will therefore be more keenly interested in its implementation. The fact that all parts of the state have been represented means that the completed instrument will more nearly fit the area needs. But in spite of careful democratic procedures, the state guide must be regarded as minimal and suggestive in spirit. The final adaptation of its contents to meet the particular needs of a class or group must be made by the classroom or subject teacher herself. Pertinent local problems or special situations, available teaching materials or facilities, the general curriculum pattern of the school, and the time allotment must all be taken into account. A really sound course of study or guide will provide generous latitude and suggestions for all types. When curriculum building is undertaken by a local group, as in a large city system, the procedure just described may be utilized with some adaptations in the selection of appropriate personnel. The initiative and responsibility would devolve upon the supervisor of health education. But the final product would need to incorporate at least the minimum state requirements.

Curriculum Patterns

The most typical curriculum pattern encountered in our schools today, particularly at the secondary and college levels, is the categorical approach of a simple series of *independent subjects.* A separate course of study for each subject, one of which may be health education, is worked out independently by individual departments or teachers. The integration of health concepts in other subjects is far more effective if the planning is done cooperatively by the health teacher and the subject teacher. If selected health units are carried in related subjects, they should be planned in relation to the content of the regular health education courses to avoid undue overlapping and duplication.

Even better is the curriculum pattern in some schools which takes the form of what is commonly designated as *broad fields.* Under this plan, related subjects are fused into one field; for example, social studies encompasses history, civics, and geography. In this pattern, principles and concepts are stressed and the content is arranged accordingly. In a school using this plan, health education is very likely not found as a separate course. The content might be included in social science or in general science, or divided between the two. It is important that teachers designated to teach these courses have definite interest in health education and training, and skill in health teaching methods. Experience has shown that frequently under these circumstances, health fails to be presented as functional in daily living.

A *core curriculum* is in effect in some schools. The core area is usually centered upon some broad topic such as Personal and Social Living, or Problems of the Community. In this type of curriculum, emphasis is upon the process of exploration and problem solving rather than upon the mere acquisition of facts. The core teacher is usually with the same class during a large portion of the day, and therefore is able to integrate and correlate material to a great extent. Obviously, a functional type of health teaching could receive a central place in many core areas and excellent results might be attained.

In some places, there exists a *child-centered* or *laissez-faire type* of curriculum plan. With the child as the focus, teaching-learning is based upon his immediate needs and then proceeds in ever-widening circles as determined by its significance to the child. Facts and general concepts follow in sequence as determined by the child's immediate needs, so this plan is not conducive to orderly organization and developmental sequence from grade to grade. Unless there is constant evaluation, its use could result in undue repetition and in many gaps in the child's educational background and progress.

Current Trends in Planning

Current thinking appears to favor a curriculum plan determined or shaped by the philosophy of the school, with consideration of individual differences among the children. It provides vertically for consistent educational progression throughout the child's school years, and horizontally for a pattern of teaching-learning experiences which will contribute to the social and personal development of the child. Emphasis needs to be given to the encouragement of a spirit of inquiry on the part of the child, and opportunity to discover, to think, and to reflect. This type of curriculum calls for teachers able to function effectively in this kind of situation and with a mastery of skills calculated to bring a high quality of results. Obviously, there is need for research and experimentation to determine the best and most productive pre-service and in-service programs to help teachers meet this need.

Sequential Progression

In planning the health curriculum, consideration must be given to a sequential program extending from semester to semester and from grade to grade. Apathy from undue repetition should be avoided. Because there are continuing problems extending throughout the child's growing period, certain topics will need to be included during successive years. But the approach and the angle of emphasis should be different each year and slanted toward the particular problem of the group. In the sixth grade, for example, bicycle safety may need to be stressed; in the seventh grade, safety in sports. In their attempt to avoid repetition, some secondary schools have found it practical to introduce a cycle plan whereby the same health units are taught to all the pupils in a given year and rotating so that at the end of a period of three years, each pupil will have had the same health material.

Provision should be made for the articulation of elementary school health instruction with that of the junior high school, and of the junior high school with the senior high school. This should apply not only to content but to experiences, audio-visual aids, and resources too. Certainly, careful cooperative planning is basic to vital health instruction.

Health Education Curriculum Publications With a Conceptual Approach

Against this background of principles of curriculum making and their possible application to health education, special reference should be made to several current innovative curriculum publications based upon the conceptual approach and which might well be regarded as milestones in the upgrading of health instruction throughout the nation.

I. In 1967, the Curriculum Commission of the Health Division of the American Association for Health, Physical Education, and Recreation, after considerable study, discussion, and research, completed and published a guide in curriculum development, entitled, *Health Concepts: Guides for Instruction.*[3] This guide has stimulated much thinking and

[3] American Association for Health, Physical Education and Recreation. *Health Concepts: Guides for Health Instruction,* The Association, Washington, D.C., 1967.

discussion in the education profession and has proved of sound, practical use to curriculum makers.

II. The School Health Education Study was a comprehensive, well-organized study approached as an integrated whole, financed by the Samuel Bronfman Foundation of New York City, under the excellent, continuing leadership of Dr. Elena M. Sliepcevich aided by an eminent Advisory Committee, and with the cooperation of the American Association for Health, Physical Education, and Recreation. The study began in 1961 with a survey to determine the practices in regard to health instruction in a random sample of public school districts in the United States and to explore the status of students' health knowledge and behavior in grades 6, 9, and 12. The resulting *Summary Report of a Nationwide Study of Health Instruction in the Public Schools,*[4] published in 1963, aroused keen interest and corroborated many findings long suspected by professional educators. The results pointed up specific weaknesses, unmet needs, untouched areas, and misconceptions, and clearly indicated the need for a further study.

III. The School Health Education Study (known as SHES) then focused upon the preparation of a research monograph encompassing completed research related to health education. This was accomplished with the cooperation of the officers of the Health Division of the American Association for Health, Physical Education and Recreation, and other health educators. Certain individuals well known for their interest, experience and research were invited to contribute to the development of a manuscript and comprehensive bibliography. In 1963 the compilation entitled, *Synthesis of Research in Selected Areas of Health Education*[5] was published. It has proved to be a valuable resource to health educators in general, and highly useful to the Study itself.

IV. The Director of the School Health Education Study and Advisory Committee then began careful over-all planning for curriculum development which culminated in the publication, in 1967, of *Health Education: A Conceptual Approach to Curriculum Design.*[6] Persons involved in any phase of curriculum development would find it especially profitable to read Appendix B, School Health Education Study Chronology of Procedures, in order to fully appreciate the infinite care and thought given to each procedure, the provision for experts in special areas such as evaluation, and the pre-involvement of teachers and supervisors in four school

[4] School Health Education Study. *Summary Report of a Nationwide Study of Health Instruction in the Public Schools.* Elena M. Sliepcevich, Director of the Study, 1961-63. Sponsored by the Samuel Bronfman Foundation of New York City.

[5] School Health Education Study. *Synthesis of Research in Selected Areas of Health Instruction.* School Health Education Research Monograph, edited by C. Harold Veenker, Purdue University. Publication of the School Health Education Study sponsored by the Samuel Bronfman Foundation of New York City, 1963.

[6] School Health Education Study. *Health Education: A Conceptual Approach to Curriculum Design.* Grades Kindergarten through Twelve. Curriculum Development Project 1967. Published by The 3M Education Press, St. Paul, Minnesota, 1967.

systems selected as trial centers, etc. A small group of dedicated, creative professionals concentrated upon the actual writing and the preparation of the two completed units which appeared at the same time.

The design is based upon three key concepts which extend vertically from kindergarten through Grade 12: (1) *Growing and Developing,* (2) *Interactions,* and (3) *Decision Making.* The Study recognizes content as part of process; *i.e.,* the latter provides reason for the content. Ten organized concepts are used with thirty-one sub-concepts or substantive points. Instructional materials are arranged for four levels: elementary, upper elementary, junior high, and senior high. Goals are stated in terms of *cognitive domain, affective domain,* and *action domain.* Throughout, inter-relatedness of all phases of health is stressed and there is always opportunity for critical thinking, student involvement and discovery, concern for value development, and conceptual thinking, with increasing complexity as the grade level advances. Through its Visual Products Division, The 3M Company, St. Paul, Minnesota, (which has taken over the financing of the Study) is involved in the production of excellent aids to accompany each unit as it is developed.

This Study, with its sound approach based upon research, commands the respect of educators generally. It is proving instrumental in arousing states, communities, and school personnel to envision a better program in health education. The curriculum is not planned for use as a nationwide course, for any curriculum to be truly successful must be adapted to the local needs. It was designed as a guide to curriculum makers in health education everywhere in their attempts at revision and in the inclusion of new health information as it appears. Its wise usage holds great promise for the future quality of health instruction in the nation's schools.

V. Two other publications in the late sixties which have proved of value to classroom teachers, health educators, and curriulum makers are the product of Study Committees of the American School Health Association. *Mental Health in the Classroom,* Revised Edition, 1968,[7] prepared by the Committee on Mental Health in the Classroom, is designed for the convenience of the teacher with its content arranged in three parallel columns under the headings: *Concepts, Learning Experiences,* and *Materials.* Lists of references for pupils and for teachers accompany each grade level. The report's practicality is further enhanced by brief over-views of the emotional characteristics and problems common to children of a particular grade level.

Health Instruction: Suggestions for Teachers, Revised Edition, 1969,[8]

[7] *Mental Health in the Classroom.* Revised Edition No. 3. 1968. Report of the Committee on Mental Health in the Classroom of the American School Health Association, 515 East Main Street, Kent, Ohio 44240.

[8] *Health Instruction: Suggestions for Teachers.* Revised Edition, 1969. Report of the Study Committees on Pre-school, Elementary School, and Secondary School Health Education of the American School Health Association, 107 S. Depeyster, P.O. Box 416, Kent, Ohio 44240.

follows a three-column form with these headings: *Concepts, Suggested Learning Experiences or Activities,* and *Evaluation.* The sections on secondary level with their explorations of problems of special concern to students, should prove particularly helpful to teachers.

Both publications reflect the well-rounded view characteristic of the ASHA study committees composed of representatives from various health professions and agencies.

Time Allotment

No matter which type of curriculum plan prevails, an adequate portion of the total time needs to be reserved for health education. The report, "Suggested School Health Policies," contains the following widely accepted statement concerning standards:

> "The time allotment for health instruction in a quality program should equal the time devoted to other instructional areas in the curriculum. Health teaching at the primary level is largely concerned with health and safety practices. At the upper elementary level less time is spent in health practice sessions, and more time is allotted to considering the reasons for desirable health attitudes and practices.
>
> At the junior high school level, health teaching should be in keeping with that scheduled for other academic areas. Recommended time allotment for the health education or health science course is one semester at the seventh grade and one semester at the ninth grade, or a year course at the eighth grade, or an equivalent plan. Many schools are trying marked changes in time schedules. Health education should have an important role in the new plans.
>
> Time allotment for health instruction at the senior high school level also should be equal to that of other academic areas. A recommended plan is providing a semester course at the tenth grade with content primarily concerned with individual and family health, and a semester course at the eleventh or twelfth grade focused on family health and community health problems. An equivalent schedule should be adopted for schools using an 8-4-4 plan."[9]

The Selection of Content

What basic learning—facts, content, subject matter—does the pupil need to help him toward optimum realization of a "state of complete

[9] National Committee on School Health Policies of the NEA and the AMA. *Suggested School Health Policies,* Fourth Edition. Published by The Joint Committee on Health Problems in Education of the National Education Association: Washington, D.C. and the American Medical Association, Chicago, Ill., 1966. p. 9.

well-being" that he may live happily now and in the years ahead, and realize his life goals to the greatest extent possible? What learning experiences will induce sound thinking and exercise of judgment which will lead the pupil to wise health decisions now and in the future? These questions are separated merely for clarity. Any attempt to find answers would show that actually the two are inextricably entwined. These questions have been explored fully in several well-known textbooks; such exploration here would not be consistent with the purpose of this chapter.

Attention has already been called to certain related considerations such as the personal, family, and community health needs of the children; their age, grade, and maturity; the health content of the preceding courses and what is to be included in the following years; the time allotment in the curriculum; available resources; special local community problems; and the future health needs in so far as these are known. The following list of questions may serve as general guidelines to the selection of content:

1. Are the problems or topics and experiences appropriate to the maturity level of the children?
2. Are the learning experiences consistent with or correlated with the interests and goals of the children?
3. Are the health questions and needs of the children given due consideration?
4. Are the concepts and methods keyed to the children's daily living experiences or related to them?
5. Are the materials scientifically accurate?
6. Are the individual differences of children given consideration?
7. Are the resource materials appropriate for their intended application?
8. Are the teaching-learning methods and procedures consistent with recognized educational principles?
9. Do the references and activities encourage independent study, discovery, and further explorations by the pupil?
10. Has consideration been given to the children's previous health courses and those scheduled to follow?

Kindergarten and Primary Grades

In the kindergarten and the primary grades the objectives of health education are centered upon changes which improve the child's health and the establishment of sound health practices and attitudes. Health experiences and practices should be accompanied by emotional satisfaction which will result in favorable attitudes toward health. At times, in response to questions for example, reasons for health practices might be offered in terms appropriate to the child's maturity level; however, how the children "feel about health" is more important at this level. Health experiences would center round the child's daily living and be drawn from such areas as the following:

Sleep, rest	Health protection:
Food	Communicable disease control
Activity and play	Clothing
Safety	Cleanliness
Family life education	Medical examination, immunizations
Teeth, eyes, ears	Mental health
	Growth and development

Teachers in kindergarten and the primary grades can integrate and correlate their health teaching effectively with such areas as social science, language arts, fine arts and others. This means careful planning in order that important health topics be given due emphasis as planned in the over-all curriculum. Many supplementary aids are available and almost endless possibilities exist for variety and creativity. Whenever possible, the health teaching should tie in with the activities of the school health service and the maintenance of a healthful school environment as suggested in preceding chapters. Incidental health teaching is likely to occur frequently and the alert teacher will utilize these opportunities when they appear to be timely. The teacher's best means of evaluation of health changes in her pupils would be her own observations, interviews with parents, group discussions, children's drawings and play activities.

Upper Elementary Grades

At this level the emphasis upon health practices and attitudes will continue but with increasing stress upon facts and knowledge. Children are interested in their own growth and development, in understanding the workings of their own bodies, in their common illnesses, and in activities. During these years, it is important to rouse interest in and appreciation of community health problems such as water and food supply, cleanliness in relation to prevention of illness, and some understanding of the organization needed to maintain community health. The children need to realize that assumption of some responsibility for daily health practices indicates progress toward adulthood. Field trips, investigations, problem solving, and projects offer a variety of opportunities for genuine learning experiences and for growth toward citizenship. Special stress would be upon problems common to this age group pertaining to such areas as:

Growth, height, and weight
Cleanliness and self-care
Exercise, rest, relaxation
Teeth and dental program
Structure and mechanism of the human body
Accident prevention and simple first aid
Mental health and social relationships
Community health-school health
Outdoor play and fitness
Common diseases: communicable and non-communicable

Junior High School

In the junior high school more emphasis is given to health knowledge than in the previous grades. For many pupils, ninth grade is the terminal point of their schooling, and this fact should be given consideration in planning the health courses. The junior high school years are considered as time for exploration when pupils are given opportunity to try many skills and to learn about occupations and careers. The main emphasis in health education is usually given to personal health and self-realization. Pupils are interested in their own development as adolescents, physical and emotional particularly. This is a period of rapid physical growth involving special health problems of puberty, and anxieties, conflicts, and disturbing emotional problems. Postural difficulties, dental needs, and food excesses are frequent, and accidents are a leading cause of death at this age level. These problems merit curriculum inclusion if the course is to be functional. The main interests of the boys center upon physical prowess and sports, but the girls are absorbed in problems of personal appearance and social skills. The health teacher is in an excellent position to give effective individual health guidance which is so often needed. Although it is recommended that health should be a separate course, in some schools the bulk of the content is carried in the general science course. Regardless of where or in whom the responsibility is centered, the course should be functional and the opportunity for personal guidance should be a factor in planning. In some schools boys and girls are taught in separate health classes; in others, the classes are coeducational. The content of the health course usually includes some of the following areas:

Personal Health: appearance; making the most of one's self; good grooming; neatness; cleanliness
Growth and Development: body mechanics and posture patterns; developmental exercises and fitness; values of activities; changes of adolescence; individual differences
Mental Health: getting along with others—family, peers, authorities; mental health a part of total health; handling emotions
Family Life Education: social skills; friendships with both sexes; boy-girl relations; pubertal changes, menstruation, seminal emissions; heredity and environment; reproduction
Food and Nutrition: adequate diet for daily activity; food selection; eating habits; foods and health
Stimulants and Depressants: alcohol and tobacco; coffee, tea, and cola drinks; drug abuse and related problems

Common Diseases: communicable and non-communicable diseases with emphasis upon respiratory diseases, certain skin diseases such as acne and athlete's foot; venereal diseases

Safety and Accident Prevention: school safety; safety in sports and outdoor activities; vacation safety precautions; assuming responsibility for safety of self and others

Health Maintenance: dental care; medical care; dangers of self-medication; care of senses; activity-rest-fatigue; immunizations

Community Health: school health services; water; food and milk control; local health department activities; health careers

Senior High School

In the senior high school, the objectives of the health courses will center upon the pupil's life goals—career, citizenship, adulthood, and family life—with emphasis upon health knowledge and the development of favorable health attitudes. At this level the student should assume more and more responsibility for his own health, for keeping health appointments, and for the observance of sound health practices. While it is desirable to avoid undue repetition of content, teachers realize that differences in maturation and cultural experiences often make it necessary to include some personal health teaching at this level. The main emphasis is upon health problems of the consumer, problems pertaining to family life, and to the community in its broadest sense including global health. Since this is the last formal health course many of the students will have, it is important that ample opportunity be provided for individual health conferences. Each student should be encouraged to think in terms of his own personal goals and to work toward their achievement. Opportunities for evaluation of progress should be frequent, but the student needs to realize that not all goals can be attained, and that progress in the right direction deserves commendation too. Cooperative planning is required on the part of all teachers concerned if the health units are scattered in various courses such as social science, home economics, and science courses instead of being centered in a separate health course. At this level, if the health teaching fails to be functional in daily living, the loss to most pupils is quite irreparable. Usually the range of topics and areas of emphasis includes the following:

Mental Health: emotional maturity; adulthood; mental disease; addictive diseases

Family Life Education: family living; choosing a mate; marriage; responsible parenthood; child care

Safety and Accident Prevention: traffic safety; safe driving; first aid; home nursing; community safety; safety in sports

Health Maintenance: balanced living; physical fitness; recreational values; disease problems of adulthood; occupational health; environmental health

Consumer Health: evaluation of health products—foods, drugs, and cosmetics; resources for evaluation; hospitalization plans; health insurance

Community Health: voluntary and official health agencies—local, state, and federal; global health; health careers

Health Units in Other Courses

Practically every course in the junior and senior high school curriculums offers some opportunity for health education either by means of a special unit or through natural association of content. If the school has a health council, the matter of cooperative planning is readily arranged; if not, the health teacher should take the initiative and meet with all teachers involved. The possibilities for correlation with science, home economics, and physical education courses are quite obvious. Mathematics and certain business education courses can extend the students' understanding of insurance plans, hospitalization costs, health statistics, and public expenditures for health. Courses of study in social science might appropriately include housing with its health implications, the care of the aged, and community health problems and the responsibilities of the individual citizen in regard to them. Courses in literature present opportunities for insight in human behavior and personality development; history can show how disease and environmental health problems have affected political, social, and cultural developments and population movements. Art courses can assist in accentuating the functional character of health in daily living. These are mere suggestions; the possibilities are endless. This type of emphasis by correlation supplements the regular courses, strengthens the total results, and enriches the student's experience by helping him to integrate his health knowledge.

Methods in Health Education

The very breadth and variety of areas and topics included in health education suggest the need for a number of methods to meet the individual differences among the pupils. The following sections will include brief descriptions of some of the most commonly used methods and techniques which every teacher needs to master as part of his professional equipment.

Unit Planning. A unit is the teacher's plan for arranging the aims and objectives or desired outcomes, content or subject matter, related activities, and teaching materials, in order to ensure adequate coverage of a topic, area or problem so that a maximum of learning may take place. Sometimes various subject areas contribute to the unit; again, the unit may center upon a single, definite problem. The types of unit in most common use in schools and colleges are the resource units and the teaching-learning unit, the latter sometimes designated as an experience unit or a subject matter unit.

A resource unit consists of an organized assemblage of facts, materials, references and other resources focused upon a particular area but gleaned from all related subjects. In actual use, the teacher draws from the assembled mass those particular facts and materials which appear to fit the needs of her particular class. A resource unit to be really useful and a genuine time-saver for the busy teacher, needs to be kept up-to-date with new material added and old deleted.

A teaching-learning unit, although somewhat similar in structure, is designed for a particular class. Its content may be drawn from a resource unit and adapted to the class needs, as in the case of the much used subject matter unit. However, the teaching-learning unit is often developed by the teacher and the class cooperatively, including the questions or problems to be answered during its progress, and their evaluations. An experience unit is developed around a particular topic and is used to a great extent in the elementary grades. A subject unit is one which is prepared in advance on a particular topic, the usual kind found in a state guide or course of study. The teacher needs to make necessary adaptations to fit the needs of her particular class and teaching situation.

Various unit patterns have been found useful in health teaching and the health teacher is advised to examine many sources.

Some of the advantages of the unit plan in teaching are:

1. The unit plan assures more complete coverage of the topic or area.
2. The teaching is more likely to move in sequential progression.
3. The teacher and the pupil plan together, evaluate, and agree upon conclusions.
4. The unit offers ample opportunity for original work and individual enterprise as well as group work.
5. The unit introduces a variety of pupil experiences and provides for individual differences.
6. The teacher is readily able to discover a pupil's difficulties.
7. Undue gaps in the pupil's health knowledge are less likely to occur.
8. Units are a great convenience to the teacher: the materials are at hand and may be readily revised to fit the needs of specific groups.

Problem-Solving. Health education abounds with problems to challenge the pupil's interest or arouse his curiosity. Frequently the problem is the student's own personal problem and he is deeply intent upon solving it. Sometimes it concerns one or more members of his family, or it may be a school or community problem.

The problem-solving method is characterized by certain specific steps or stages:

1. *The Statement of the Problem.* The problem must be clearly defined and understood by the individual or the class. Sometimes a casual

question may be sufficient to challenge the attention; at times, the teacher, through skillful questions, may be able to increase the interest by making the student aware of additional ramifications. In other words, the teacher helps the class to gain insight into the extent and nature of the problem and intensifies the desire to find the solution. The selection of the problem and the setting up of possible approaches to solution are important parts of defining the problem. It is the teacher's responsibility to see that the problem is appropriate to the educational maturity of the group, is of such stature as to justify class attention and time, and that it will offer the learning opportunities which the class should have. While the pupil may see and phrase the problem according to his point of view and vocabulary, the teacher must possess sufficient imagination to see possibilities and ways of preserving his interest, and at the same time, guide his statements into a clear definition of the problem.

2. *Working Toward a Solution.* There is a need for gathering information on many phases of the problem. The class will need to determine the areas in which information is desired and the sources likely to yield this information. As the pupils proceed, additional sources will be discovered. This step is sometimes called the collection of data. The data need to be scrutinized and evaluated as to their contribution toward the task of solution. The class will have to decide what must be retained and arranged in logical order. The task will probably be divided among committees, so the teacher's role at this point is to help the pupils form a functioning working organization. She may help them discover appropriate sources and thus prevent the discouragement of undue frustration. The results of the committees will need to be grouped and integrated into wholes.

3. *Summarization and Drawing Conclusions.* The class now concentrates upon the important task of determining possible solutions and deciding upon the best one. Obviously not every health problem can be solved. Some can be ameliorated or eliminated by focusing upon contributory situational conditions; others have a number of possible solutions and each possibility needs to be evaluated against the background of the problem itself to determine the best or most acceptable one.

Frequently during the problem-solving process other impinging problems are uncovered. Sometimes these need to be explored and solved before the major one can be approached, or, the group may agree to table them as special problems for future exploration. Problem solving permits the utilization of the full resources of the school and the community, and in the process, the children often realize the interrelationships which, when discussed, seem quite nebulous. At the same time, the problem-solving method offers opportunity for originality and creativity on the part of the children. To see how a well-drawn map or a logically constructed graph made by one of his peers can contribute to the solution of the problem, is a truly broadening experience. Then too, one problem can touch off another or inspire the entire semester's work. The children experience genuine satisfaction in their accomplishment and this incites them to go on to further achievement. With modifications commensurate with the age and maturity of the group, this method can prove effective at all levels.

Discussion. Whether used to resolve international differences or to arrive at one's simple day to day personal decisions, discussion is recognized as a most valuable method. The give-and-take of discussion offers excellent practice in verbal expression and quick thinking. In the process, one idea grows out of another. The ability and readiness to discuss grows with the pupil's maturity, and should be encouraged throughout school life. Group discussion provides opportunities for the individual to practice self-control, self-expression without undue timidity, fairness of judgment, and to experience the satisfaction of group participation. Discussion is a basic tool in education. It can be used alone as a means of solving a health problem but certainly at every stage of problem-solving it is a prime essential. Today's emphasis upon teamwork in health involves constant use of discussion.

It is impossible in a large class or group to give everyone a chance to air his views. Committee work, buzz sessions, symposia, and forums provide discussion opportunities. The use of a variety of methods proves stimulating. Usually the more secure students will be the most vocal, but, by breaking the large group into a number of small ones, each student is afforded an opportunity to express his views and feel that he is an active participant. The wise teacher or leader usually makes a point of providing this type of discussion situation the first day of class to start everyone in the habit of participation. Sooner or later, everyone needs to be given a chance to try his wings as leader, beginning first with a small group.

Many health topics become controversial because so often emotions are involved, or family or cultural traditions or customs are challenged. When helped to approach the topic objectively in a discussion group, the student often becomes aware of his misconceptions or errors. At least, he will learn about all sides of the question. At the same time, the teacher is enabled to discern misconceptions on the part of the student, gaps in his health knowledge, or to discover the existence of deeply rooted health needs and problems. Actually, from pre-kindergarten through college, it is a most useful method. In fact, in the kindergarten and lower grades informal discussion is one of the principal tools of learning.

The teacher needs to develop her own skills as discussion leader and, at the same time, know how to help the pupils develop their skills. At times a teacher-led discussion is a stimulating affair particularly if it centers upon a controversial question which the student could not be expected to handle because of insufficient background and poise. The teacher needs to provide the pupils with an example of calmness and justice, exemplifying ways of bringing out all aspects of a problem and also involving all members of a class or group. After such discussion, it is important for the class to engage in an objective review of the discussion techniques used, the reasons why the discussion sometimes strayed, and what the leader did about it in each case.

Demonstration. As applied in health education this method could be used in many forms. It could involve a simple scientific experiment performed for the class by the teacher or by a visiting specialist. One class might demonstrate for another, for example, a fitness test, or a particular health skill such as an exercise, or it might be a long-range demonstration such as a nutrition demonstration. The teacher needs to decide whether this is the most appropriate method to use, whether it is practical in her situation, and whether the appropriate materials are available. Careful planning must precede every demonstration, and ample time allowed for adequate discussion, interpretation, and conclusions. This method is often used in conjunction with other methods.

Role Playing. In the hands of a skillful teacher, role playing can contribute effectively to health education. One of its main uses is to promote understanding of the feelings and emotions which underlie an individual's behavior. For example, two children may play the roles of a mother and daughter, discussing bedtime hour, with the daughter pleading for a later hour than the mother wishes. The child in the role of mother is likely to understand something of the feelings the mother has about the situation. In a committee meeting called to discuss whether or not to appeal to the health department to institute fluoridation of drinking water, the person known to be opposed would be asked to play the role of one in favor of it. This method has proved especially successful in helping people develop insight and understanding about controversial questions or situations. However, its success depends upon the thorough understanding of its uses and its limitations, and upon the skill of the leader in drafting the situation and in securing whole-hearted unself-conscious cooperation of the individuals in their respective roles. The wise teacher would involve the entire class by having special "listening groups" concentrate upon particular players and their feelings. The discussion which follows role-playing demands analytical skill on the part of the teacher and sound preparation in psychology, and practice in role playing as well as in leading it. However, she needs to be warned never to become involved in deeper feelings or emotions, or to allow the class to get beyond its depths.

Lecture. Quite obviously, the lecture method is inappropriate as a teaching method in the elementary school. With secondary school pupils, occasional short talks by the teacher or a resource person can be stimulating and are sometimes necessary for the presentation of new materials within the limits of the teaching period. Such talks should be followed by class discussion or activities which provide opportunity for the application of the ideas gained from the talk. If accompanied by illustrative materials, the usefulness of the lecture is likely to be intensified.

Experimentation. In a scientific age it is logical that experimentation should be stressed. Its use in health science teaching is particularly useful and effective. Children possess boundless curiosity, and even in the intermediate grades they are eager to work with a magnifying glass or a microscope and perform simple and safe investigations under teacher supervision. They learn to be objective in approach, thorough, and painstaking, and to build deep appreciations of the meaning of science and truth. The vital challenge to the teacher is to keep alive this spirit of inquiry. Much can be accomplished by a perceptive teacher with a sound background in science and health education, even with a small amount of equipment. Frequently in an elementary or junior high school, careful scheduling permits classes and departments to share equipment and supplies.

The various teaching methods which have been mentioned in this chapter are often used in combination with one another or with audio-visual aids, trips, and visits. Considered thus, the imaginative teacher has at her command, an almost endless variety of methods. When variety is introduced, the pupils approach the health class with interest and lively anticipation and the results are usually rewarding to pupils and teachers alike.

Team Teaching

A number of schools use team teaching in health science classes in the upper elementary grades and in junior and senior high school. Certainly, careful pre-planning is essential to the smooth functioning of any team. At a planning session the entire teaching team is familiarized with the objectives of the unit or lesson, the concepts to be emphasized, and the procedures to be utilized by the master-teacher; and the experiences and the activities to be used by the other team members in their respective small group sessions are agreed upon. An evaluation session following the class enables the team to chart progress and accomplishments and to decide upon the next steps. In situations in which each member of the team serves in turn as the master teacher, one individual is designated as the team leader who assumes the responsibility for continuity and sequence. This arrangement permits a particular unit to be assigned to the teacher best equipped to teach it.

The following precautions are vital to the success of team teaching:

1. The team needs to maintain a steady focus upon meeting the health needs of the children and to avoid over-attention to mere excellence of subject-matter presentation.

2. Sufficient roster time must be allotted for planning and evaluation.
3. Since lessons and units vary in time requirement, the schedule needs to have considerable flexibility to ensure the best results.
4. If audio-visual aids are used during the master-teaching, it is often desirable that they be available for repeated use by the small groups.

Teaching Resources

Health instruction can be enriched by the imaginative use of a wide variety of supplementary materials and aids. The flood of available materials, constantly increasing in numbers, types, and attractiveness, makes the matter of selection a truly difficult and sizeable task. In some school systems, special committees of teachers and other professional school personnel are appointed to evaluate textbooks, supplementary library books, and other types of health reference materials for use at the various grade levels. Most school districts find it advisable to establish policies regulating classroom use of commercial advertising materials.

Health textbooks have grown increasingly functional in content and interesting as to format, and most teachers and pupils rate them as practically indispensable. Certainly their use adds to the stability of the health course not only because of the range in reading comprehension among the pupils, but because all children need time to re-read and reflect. It is a broadening experience for a class to have access to several texts and thus enrich their understandings by different approaches and emphases, and comparisons of viewpoints. Extensive opportunities for readings in health-related biography, fiction, essays, science, social science, and foreign languages add new dimensions to health understandings and appreciations. Happily, inexpensive paperbacks make such enrichment possible at every grade level. Magazine articles and newspapers provide orientation to the range of current health problems, local to global, and help the pupils realize that *health is daily living*. Workbooks at practically all levels are available but should not be used as "busy work." Constructing one's own cumulative health workbook can be a valuable experience for a child.

Today's classrooms are so designed that the teacher may utilize modern audio-visual and other materials readily. This refers to moveable furniture, space, electric outlets properly placed, ample closet space prepared for the storage of all types of materials and specimens. Often the school will provide a so-called resource room just for health education materials, or a common resource room to be shared by all departments (to house viewing machines, micro-film card readers, etc.). In the latter case, a portion might be set aside for the supplementary materials required for health instruction.

Learning experiences can be intensified through the wise use of many aids and devices. The following list suggests the richness of the resources available to-day:

Speakers and resource persons
Field trips, visits, participation in a community health event
Dramatizations: plays, skits, pageants, pantomime, puppets, role playing, sociodrama, spontaneous dramatics, dramatic games, unfinished problem plays for discussion
Printed materials: textbooks, supplementary books, pamphlets, magazines, newspapers, leaflets, guides, teachers' manuals, reading lists, catalogues
Student publications: newspapers, newsletters, leaflets (utilization of health facts, articles, experiments, surveys concerning the school)
Drawings, maps, cartoons, graphs, pin-maps, silhouettes, diagrams
Posters, exhibits, bulletin boards, flip-charts, charts with text overlays, etc.
Models, objects, peep-shows, diorama, school health museum, specimens
Flannel board, chalkboard, opaque projector
Pictures, slides, photographs, films, filmstrips, motion pictures, stereoscopic pictures, kineoscope, combinations with recordings
Radio, tape recordings, recordings, television, videotapes

The teacher needs to bear in mind that these are *aids* to teaching and that the real success of the lesson depends upon the teacher's methods of using these materials. Some of the aids—films, filmstrips, recordings and others—are frequently accompanied by a special guide for the teacher. Careful step-by-step preparation precedes each lesson. In the case of a film, a recording, and other audio-visual aids, necessary steps include a preview, a study of the guide, and familiarization with sequence and details. The showing is followed by discussion and evaluation. Always, the teacher, familiar with the backgrounds of the children, has to make necessary adaptations to meet the needs of her group. Many times the most meaningful supplementary aids are those which grow out of a project and are made by the pupil himself or by his group.

Useful guides to the selection of audio-visual materials are obtainable. They contain annotated descriptions, suggestions as to wise uses, precautions to be observed, evaluative criteria, and grade or group listings. Lists are available from local and state health departments, and the Public Health Service, as well as from many of the voluntary health agencies on national, state and local levels.

Television

One of the most striking changes in the cultural habits of the people of the United States is the tremendous importance which radio and television have come to occupy in their lives. Children, conditioned to the speed, spread, and the strength of conviction conveyed through visual, oral, and auditory sensual impressions, have gained much factual knowledge ranging over world-wide focus along with many partially assimilated, fragmented impressions. At the same time, they are building up learning habits, aptitudes, and skills as required by the technical characteristics of these popular media. It would seem then, that these media would hold enormous potentials for the enrichment of teaching-learning processes if utilized properly and adapted to appropriate situations.

Many states and areas have made television programs available in schools. In some instances closed circuit television has been arranged. Much excellent experimental work has been done in the preparation of educational films, videotapes, etc. but much more is needed to determine the most effective approaches and methods in health education. In spite of the high cost, many schools throughout the nation to-day have made these audio-visual opportunities constantly available for the pupils through the purchase of excellent equipment. In some cases the teacher may have access to a video camera or to monitoring devices and can start, stop, and re-play portions according to the needs of the class.

Video-tape has the advantage of uniform presentation of facts, viewpoints, and concepts. One advantage, of course, is that a single presentation can reach a large group. But no matter which medium is used in health education, best results depend upon the wise selection, planning, and follow-through by the teacher supplementing the audio-visual experience with other classroom techniques as may be needed for reinforcement, in rounding out the cognitive and the affective concepts. Thus, the viewing by a large group might be followed by small group discussions, the handling and examination of specimens already viewed on the screen, and further exploration by committees of pupils or by independent study by individuals. Panel discussions, dialogues, and teach-ins with or without audience participation, are techniques already familiar to pupils through their viewing experiences at home. Students sometimes enjoy taping class discussions for comparison. All can benefit by re-play and examination of their own skills in participation or other details which might have contributed to the success of the lesson. Slides taken with an ordinary camera can be made meaningful through skillful usage by the teacher in providing necessary reinforcement, rounding out experiences, building up concepts, etc. However, assignments, explanations of debatable points, and reviews under teacher leadership establish good rapport. At all grade levels, pupil experience in verbal and written responses, inter-actions with their peers and with the teacher, constitute integral elements in effective teaching-learning situations. Thus the teacher will always be essential to the situation and is not in any sense to be displaced by television or any other machine.

Teaching Machines

Programmed instruction has been used with marked success by some teachers. Many of the interesting and useful teaching machines available today utilize principles formerly applied through simple teacher-made devices such as matching games, flash cards, and others. The child is enabled to use these with the aid of the machine and thereby the teacher's time is released for other purposes. Teachers need to be open-minded and adventurous in exploring the new and the different, and to make full use of whatever may be of value. At the same time, it is important that teachers evaluate continually, objectively, and critically, the actual contribution of such machines to the child's educational progress.

Lesson Plans

The lesson plan should fit the subject and the purpose of the lesson and be comprehensive, flexible, and meaningful to the teacher, her supervisor and others concerned. Lesson plans may assume a variety of forms and should suit the convenience of the teacher while fulfilling their purpose of securing logical progression and thorough coverage of material. They usually center upon material drawn from the unit and are prepared prior to the class period by the teacher. Sometimes they are planned cooperatively by the teacher and the pupils at the beginning of the class period or at the initiation of a unit. The children's questions concerning the topic are listed on the chalkboard. When grouped and perhaps re-arranged in logical sequence they comprise a framework for the development of the lession. Usually a lesson plan contains the following elements, but the variations may be manifold:

- The topic or specific problems
- The relation of the lesson to the entire unit
- General aim of the unit
- Specific objectives of the lesson (purposes; goals)
- Materials needed
- Introduction or approach to the lesson
- Development of the lesson (body):
  - Content (concepts)
  - Methods and procedures
  - Conclusion or summary
- Evaluation
- References: pupil, teacher
- Assignment

The assignment is an important part of the lesson, linking one period's accomplishments with the next. It is not necessarily made at the end of the lesson, but in unhurried fashion whenever it fits in naturally with the flow of the lesson.

Evaluation

An effective design for evaluation is part and parcel of every health education program and should be planned at the outset. Evaluation is an attempt to appraise the program or some part of it, not merely as to extent, but also in terms of value or quality. Evaluation is directly related to the objectives of the program or activity concerned, and the more clearly and specifically these are stated, the more useful the appraisal results. But foremost in everything is the *learner* and what is happening to him through this program or activity.

The usual purposes of evaluation as applied to the school health program, to each of its major divisions, or any of its component parts are:

1. To determine the extent to which the objectives have been realized
2. To measure accomplishments in terms of quality, value, or extent
3. To determine strengths or weaknesses
4. To point out unmet needs
5. To measure progress and improvements
6. To point out places in need of teaching emphasis
7. To compare records or accomplishments with standards
8. To use as a basis for re-direction of program or activities
9. To determine trends and new directions

All persons responsible for or affected by any feature or activity included in the program or for the program as a whole, may participate in evaluation. Appraisal procedures must be appropriate for the particular feature to be evaluated and in each case the instrument used must be suitable for the purpose. A baseline must be established. It may be a pre-test, a dateline, a survey, or take some other form. Evaluation is a continuing process. For comparative purposes it may be done at periodic or stated intervals, at the completion of a lesson or project, or at the beginning and the end of a designated term or year. The tests must be administered as efficiently and objectively as possible, and the test results interpreted so that they may be clearly and properly understood by all who use them.

Some evaluative instruments in common use in school health programs are listed here:

Survey	Observation
Check list	Inventory
Questionnaire	Interview
Opinionnaire	Conference
Rating scale	Self-appraisal chart
Record	Test (standardized; teacher-made)
Parents' opinions	Photographs
Graph	Examples of pupils' work

A periodic evaluation of the entire school health program proves most valuable from every point of view. It might take the form of a self-evaluation in which all persons involved might participate. During the process a great deal of insight is gained by the school personnel about their immediate problems, a realization of the roles of the various members of the health team, and improved relationships. The self-evaluation is often followed by an evaluation by a team of experts. Because of the self-survey, the members of the team are usually ready to implement the recommendations of the survey team or at least to determine priority of implementation.

In the previous section, evaluation was indicated in numerous places as a part of the teaching-learning process involving teacher and pupils. The school health service division finds it invaluable to establish constant comparison of records from year to year, to discover trends, shifts in health needs, illnesses, successful referrals, the study of accidents, and other problems. Appraisal of healthful school living usually involves the services of trained sanitarians, firemen, safety experts, nutritionists, and others. The school and the community might join in such evaluative projects as the follow-up of effectiveness of health teaching, the carry-over power of instruction into the health practices of adulthood as shown in attitudes and practices of young mothers, the application of safety procedures in households, in traffic accidents, and other situations. Facilities and resources for evaluation studies can be shared by the community and the school to mutual advantage.

The Role of the Teacher

In health education, the teacher as catalyst, plays many roles. At various times she is leader, guide, consultant, observer, and at all times, an example to her pupils.

In the last-mentioned role, she has no choice. If the teacher is accepted, loved, and respected, her own example—her health practices, attitudes, and conduct—may prove a powerful influence leading to conscious or unconscious imitation on the part of the pupil. Since the teacher's health behavior reflects her own attitude toward health, her example may prove more powerful than her words. The majority of teachers in the United States derive from the middle-class component of our social, economic and educational structure. These are the cultural patterns which she is likely to impress upon her pupils by example whether or not these patterns are practical or consistent with their own cultural backgrounds or experiences. If the pattern happens to coincide with those of her pupils or the middle class pattern satisfies an ambition and, in the eyes of the child, seems worthy of adoption, a desirable change in health behavior may ensue. If not, the resultant frustrations and confusions may negate the child's acceptance of the new, and possibly block future changes of conduct. If a new idea should appear to flout the social structure upon which rests the individual pupil's value system, the perceptive teacher will seek to discover the foci of resistance in the group, and to estimate the various strengths of the attached values. The teacher needs to chart her approach carefully and to utilize opportunities to point out new angles and cast side-lights upon the prevailing values, and gradually make it possible for the pupil to see his own attitudes in a different light. Thus, the child begins to realize that various cultural patterns exist and that one can learn to live with them comfortably.

The concept of *leader* has largely replaced the traditional image of the teacher. Today the teacher and the children plan and work together cooperatively to reach certain goals. By means of skillful questioning and other devices the teacher leads by calling upon and drawing forth their capabilities. She knows that domination and step-by-step, over-detailed directions stunt the child's initiative and creativity and crush him into a sadly dependent, apathetic person. The teacher seeks to establish through the sound application of leadership principles, a learning atmosphere which will encourage the full development of each child's potentialities.

Throughout this over-view of the school health program, it has been pointed out that the teacher, in her attempts to understand the total child, is almost constantly observing him. The teaching process witnesses the utilization of these observations as guidelines in the selection of subject matter, experiences, and materials suited to the child in particular situations. Throughout the entire teaching process the teacher never deserts her role as observer.

However, during the process of observing the children and involving them in activities, the teacher often slips into the roles of consultant and guide. To make an experience truly educational, she permits the pupils to adventure in collecting, analyzing, categorizing, and coming to decisions. When difficulties arise, she serves as consultant and advises, but the pupil makes the decision. Again, the teacher may unobtrusively guide the child toward experiences within his developmental range and in the direction of accomplishment. Here a searching question, a phrase or indication of source materials may suffice. Thus, the art of teaching is inherent in the teacher's ability as a catalyst, to perceive the precise role behavior likely to be effective in a particular situation, and to slip into it easily and naturally.

The observant teacher often recognizes the beginnings of health faults or problems and can offset them by timely action before they assume serious proportions. When a particularly disturbing or frustrating community health problem or condition emerges suddenly or assumes an alarming slant, emotionally aroused legislators, community groups, parents, or individuals may rightly recognize the need for protective education for the young and clamor insistently for speedy action. Thus, the school sometimes finds itself faced with an overwhelming demand (or even a mandate) for some immediate special health education of its pupils. Usually this results in exposing the pupils to a series of lectures, speeches, films, exhibits, etc., crammed into an absurdly brief period of time. The teacher needs to be aware that a crash program of this sort seldom brings lasting results in terms of changed health attitudes and practices. The problem, if really important, needs to be considered in the context of the entire health education curriculum and integrated through a conceptual approach at appropriate grade levels. A wise teacher can often bring this about tactfully and, at the same time, educate the advocates of the crash program as to more desirable procedures in a similar future situation.

Sometimes the public health educator is inclined to regard with envy the potentialities for health education which confront the teacher with her captive group of children day after day. But it must be remembered that the parents of these children are part and parcel of the community and that the health practices and attitudes which these children have developed during their pre-school days are likely to be a perpetuation of those of the parents, and, therefore, subject to the same obstacles which block the way to new community health patterns. At times the resistances which reappear in the children may be somewhat attenuated. Again, they may be even more formidable. The teacher's main advantage lies in the opportunities for prolonged observation and study of the children and the multiplicity of chances to draw upon a broad spectrum of possible means and materials for finding the vulnerable points at which to try to trigger changes toward the improvement of health conduct. Because of his understanding of community attitudes, facilities, and resources, the public health educator can be of inestimable help to the teacher in suggesting and providing supplementary materials for classroom use and for reaching into the home. On the other hand, the community can serve the teacher as a vital health laboratory. Obviously, the teacher and the public health educator need to work in partnership for school and community health.

Parent Education

In seeking to help the child attain the best possible health and education, it is logical that the school, as a part of the total process, should assume some responsibility for the health education of the parent.

The enthusiastic classroom teacher soon becomes aware of the very real possibilities of extending the school's positive health influence into the home by way of the children. A teacher who has succeeded in establishing warm, friendly relations with the parents has actually created a climate conducive to influencing favorably the health behavior of the entire family. The teacher's opinion and advice are likely to be sought on some of the most pressing family health matters. Her day will often begin with questions: "Mother says to ask you . . ." "Mother says, what do you think we should do about . . ?" In responding, the teacher familiar with community health resources, is often able to draw into the picture the official or voluntary agency which can best help the family toward a solution to their problem.

A great deal of individual health education is accomplished by the nurse, the physician and other members of the health team in connection with the medical examination and the follow-up or referral procedures, particularly if the parent is present during the examination. Home visits in this connection also prove fruitful.

Parent-teacher organizations provide many opportunities for group education concerning the common health problems of school children. If the organization includes a health committee, the school nurse or the health teacher should prove a most valuable member and thus be able to promote effective coordination of effort in meeting problems and in extending education. The program suggestions which follow have proved successful with various parent-teacher groups:

- Talks by the health teacher or school health service personnel
- Organization of study groups on special health problems, child development, psychology, family life education
- Panel discussions with school health personnel representatives
- Interpretation of children's health records
- Talks by professional persons: child growth and development; mental health; drug abuse
- Nutrition programs and demonstrations
- New health measures initiated by the school (immunizations)
- New developments in health sciences; health careers
- Community health resources; comprehensive health planning
- School-community health problems (*e.g.* addictive diseases, venereal diseases)
- Health films and discussions

All talks and programs should include discussion periods so that parents' specific questions may be answered.

Some ways in which the school might take the initiative and invite the parents to participate are listed here:

- Visit the school health council at an open meeting
- Hold a visitors' day with a health theme, demonstrations, exhibits
- Invite the parent-teacher organization to stage a health exhibit in cooperation with local community health agencies

If there is no organized parent-teacher group, the teacher may wish to seek the cooperation of room mothers as a helping group. Often a group or individual parents will be pleased to be called upon for help with some health project, particularly if their own children are involved.

The inclusion of the children in the program provides an added attraction at all school events.

The real crux of the problem of parent education is not the parent active in the home-school organization, but the one who cannot be reached or will not respond to requests for interviews or conferences. Working mothers will often keep an appointment for an evening visit if one can be arranged. The problem of establishing communication is sometimes a truly difficult one, but its very importance makes experimentation necessary. The goal is to try to have all parents working along with school personnel to find ways of meeting the health problems of the children.

Teacher Education

The most effective preparation of the prospective teacher of health education and of the classroom teacher for his responsibilities in all phases of the school health program, has been a major concern of colleges and universities charged with this important task. Today's trend is toward having all prospective teachers include in their undergraduate work at least one course in school and community health in addition to the usually required undergraduate course in health. The reason is to enable the student to gain greater insight into and to appreciate the responsibility every teacher has for the health and safety of all pupils with whom he or she comes in contact, to acquire some skill in the health observation of children and in the recognition of deviations from the usual, and to understand the functions of the school health program, the inter-actions among its three segments, and the role of the teacher in relation to each. It is important that health teaching and experiences in other phases of the health program be included in the student teaching experience.

In 1969 the Joint Committee on Health Problems in Education in its resolutions expressed as follows the urgency of the need and some desirable guidelines concerning the special certification of teachers of health:

> "*Whereas,* a number of states have recently adapted their regulations on teacher certification to include separate certification of health, and
> *Whereas,* as is true for other curricular areas, such certification involves the requirement of a major or minor (including both health content and professional education course) in health education for eligibility to teach health, and
> *Whereas,* in states where such certification regulations have been instituted, significant improvement in the quality of health education programs has occurred, therefore be it

Resolved, that states not having separate certification of teachers of health institute such regulations at the earliest possible time, and be it further

Resolved, that certification provisions for teachers of health include the requirement of at least a minor and wherever possible a major in health"[10]

States which seek to implement these certification regulations, should include in their plans date lines which would permit present teachers to meet the new requirements.

In-service Education

The broad implications of health and the rapid change in concept due to new discoveries in science and medicine, imply the need for continuing in-service education for teachers and others with responsibilities for the school health program. Ways in which school districts utilize the school health service staff and the supervisor for direct in-service education concerning an immediate acute health problem have been mentioned in previous chapters. Most states have arranged their teacher certification procedures so that all teachers are required to have some graduate work. Unless specified otherwise, some of these additional college credits might well be in the field of health. A full-time teacher of health in a secondary school should have at least one degree in health education. Teachers of science in the secondary school who may be responsible also for the health teaching, should be expected to take additional courses in health curriculum and methods.

Some school districts that offer total or partial subsidization of courses for teachers at a nearby college or university or arrange for a local extension course, might plan certain years for this to be in the field of health. In a number of states, where there are summer school-community health education workshops administered cooperatively by a college or university, official and voluntary agencies, scholarships have been provided for teachers, administrators, and health service personnel as well as public health workers. Some of the health agencies provide fellowships for the regular college year which teachers may use during a sabbatical leave. Occasionally grants from foundations are available for research by teachers, and often in the process of carrying a study or experiment through to completion, the teacher's gain may equal or excel the benefit derived from a college course. Information concerning fellowships, stipends, and research grants should be centered in the office of the superintendent or in some designated person.

Parent-teacher organizations and teachers' professional organizations

[10] Adopted by the Joint Committee on Health Problems in Education of the National Education Association and the American Medical Association, Washington, D.C., February 9-11, 1969. *School Health Review:* September, 1969, Page 23.

sometimes sponsor educational lecture series which might occasionally be health oriented.

A school district should work closely with the local library to ensure the provision of current well-selected periodicals, textbooks, and other literature pertaining to health. The school health council might include a library committee whose function would be the review and recommendation of library acquisitions and the fostering of discussion groups on subjects relating to health.

Questions for Discussion

1. What are the certification requirements for teachers of health in the elementary schools of your state? In the secondary schools? How do they compare with the requirements in neighboring states? With the requirements in California?
2. What is the plan of the health education program in the local public junior high school as it relates to time allotment, teacher assignment, grade level, and the basis of grouping pupils in sections or classes? In the local public senior high school?
3. How can a course of study or curriculum in health education be kept vital and up-to-date?
4. How would you justify the inclusion of courses in health in the crowded secondary school curriculum?
5. Assume that you are a teacher in an elementary school (or a junior or senior high school, according to your choice). Explain how you might utilize the school health council or committee in seeking to make more effective the teaching of a particular health topic.
6. What are some of the practical ways whereby the senior high school and the college might endeavor to articulate their health education programs?
7. Considerable concern has been voiced by some educators as to the dichotomy between science and the humanities. Secondary school instruction in health involves both areas. What can the teacher of health do to prevent this dichotomy from being perpetuated by her students?
8. Cite important advances which have been made in medicine or science during the past several years which, in your opinion, might modify the content or merit inclusion in the school health courses at specific levels.
9. In what ways may the health education programs of the school and the community be coordinated and mutually supportive? To what extent are these practiced in your community?

Suggested Readings

1. American Association for Health, Physical Education, and Recreation: Curriculum Commission of the Health Division: *Health Concepts: Guides for Health Instruction.* Washington, D.C.: the Association, 1967.
2. ANDERSON, CARL L.: *Health Principles and Practice.* 6th Ed. St. Louis, The C. V. Mosby Co., 1970.
3. BEYRER, MARY K., NOLTE, ANN E., AND SOLLEDER, MARIAN K.: *A Directory of Selected References and Resources for Health Instruction.* 2nd ed., Minneapolis, Burgess Publishing Co., 1970.
4. BYLER, RUTH V., LEWIS, GERTRUDE M., AND TOTMAN, RUTH J.: *Teach Us What We Want To Know.* Mental Health Materials Center, 419 Park Avenue South, New York, N.Y. 10016.

5. Bloom, Benjamin S. (ed.) *Taxonomy of Educational Objectives.* Handbook I: *Cognitive Domain.* New York, David McKay Co., 1956.
6. Bruner, Jerome S. *The Process of Education.* Cambridge, Harvard University Press, 1963.
7. Center for the Study of Instruction, National Education Association. *Rational Planning in Curriculum and Instruction.* Washington, D.C.: the National Education Association, 1967.
8. Conner, Forrest E., and Elena, William J. (Eds): *Curriculum Handbook for School Administrators.* Washington, D.C.: American Association of School Administrators, 1967.
9. Cornacchia, Harold J., Staton, Wesley M., Irwin, Leslie W.: *Health in Elementary Schools.* 3rd. Ed., St. Louis, The C. V. Mosby Co., 1970.
10. Fodor, John and Dalis, Gus T.: *Health Instruction—Theory and Application.* Philadelphia, Lea & Febiger, 1966.
11. Goodlad, John, von Stoephasius, Renata, and Klein, M. Frances: *The Changing School Curriculum.* New York, The Fund for the Advancement of Education, 1966.
12. Grout, Ruth E.: *Health Teaching in Schools.* 8th Ed., Philadelphia, W. B. Saunders Co., 1968.
13. *Health Instruction*: Suggestions for Teachers. (Rev. ed.) Report of the Study Committee on Pre-School, Elementary School, and Secondary School Health Education of the American School Health Association: 107 S. Depeyster Street, P.O. Box 416, Kent, Ohio 44240.
14. Hein, Fred V., Farnsworth, Dana L., and Richardson, Charles F.: *Living.* 5th ed., Oakland, N.J.: Scott, Foresman, College Division, 1970.
15. Humphrey, James, Johnson, Warren R., and Moore, Virginia P.: *Elementary School Health Education.* New York, Harper & Row, 1962.
16. Johns, Edward B., Sutton, Wilfred C., and Webster, Lloyd E.: *Health for Effective Living.* 5th Ed., New York, McGraw-Hill Book Co., 1970.
17. Joint Committee on Health Problems in Education of the National Education Association and the American Medical Association; *Health Education.* 5th Ed., Bernice R. Moss, Warren Southworth, and John Lester Reichert, M.D., eds. Washington, D.C.: the National Education Association of the United States, 1961.
18. Kilander, Holger F.: *School Health Education: A study of the Objectives, Content, Methods, and Materials.* 2nd Ed. New York, The Macmillan Company, 1968.
19. Krathwohl, David R., Bloom, Benjamin S., and Masia, Bertram: *A Taxonomy of Educational Objectives,* Handbook II: *The Affective Domain.* New York, David McKay Co., 1966.
20. Roberts, Beryl J., Grossman, Jerome, Griffiths, William: *The Public Health Education Bookshelf.* Amer. J. Public Health, 53:4, April, 1963: 531.
21. Rogers, Carl R.: "The Interpersonal Relationship in the Facilitation of Learning," P. 2: *Humanizing Education: The Person in Process,* ed. by Robert R. Leeper. Washington, D.C.: Association for Supervision and Curriculum Development, 1967.
22. School Health Education Study: *Health Education: A Conceptual Approach to Curriculum Design.* St. Paul, Minn., 3M Education Press, 1967.
23. School Health Education Study (sponsored by the Samuel Bronfman Foundation of New York City). *Synthesis of Research in Selected Areas of Health Instruction,* C. Harold Veenker, Purdue University, ed., Washington, D.C.: Publication-Sales, National Education Association, 1963.
24. SIECUS (Sex Information and Education Council of the United States). *Study Guides.* SIECUS Publications Office, 419 Park Avenue South, New York, N.Y., 10016.
25. Sliepcevich, Elena M., Director, School Health Education Study: *Summary Report of the School Health Education Study.* Washington, D.C.: SHES, 1965.
26. Turner, Clair E., Randall, Harriet R. and Smith, Sara L.: *School Health and Health Education.* 6th Ed., St. Louis, The C. V. Mosby Co., 1970.

27. Tyler, Ralph W.: *Basic Principles of Curriculum and Instruction.* Chicago, University of Chicago Press, 1950.
28. Tyler, Ralph W.: "Implications of Behavioral Studies for Health Education." J. School Health, 33:1, January, 1963.
29. Willgoose, Carl E.: *Health Education in the Elementary School.* Philadelphia, W. B. Saunders Co., 1969.
30. Wittich, Walter A. and Schuller, Charles F.: *Audiovisual Materials: Their Nature and Use.* 4th Ed., New York, Harper & Row, 1967.
31. Woodruff, Asahel D.: *Basic Concepts of Teaching.* San Francisco, Chandler Publishing Co., 1961.

Chapter 15

Health Careers

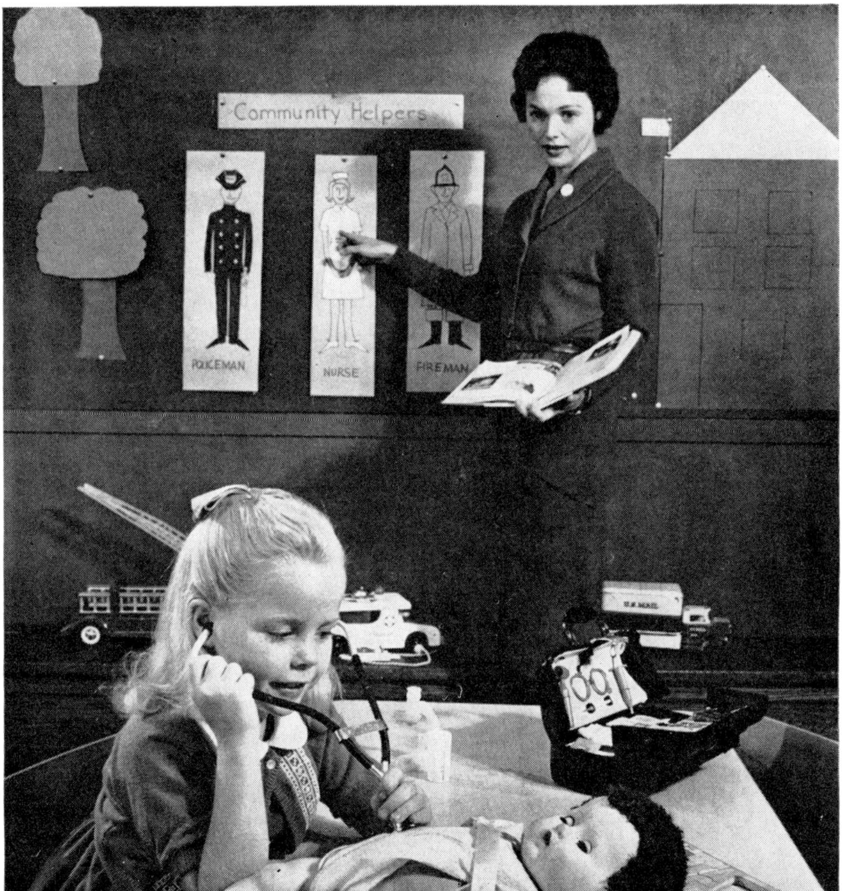

FIG. 59. In Good Hands.

"Health Needs People"[1]

This plea, the repeated cover-motif of a challenging brochure issued in 1957 by the National Health Council, voices the crucial need for workers in all types of positions. To maintain the present high level of health in the nation, to promote research along the many frontiers of health-related sciences, and to explore the possibilities for improvement in procedures and relationships demands a huge task force. Paced by a fast-growing population with its additional quota of health needs, an ever-increasing task force is required to provide personnel for new situations, present under-staffed agencies, and the annual percentage of replacements.

The present high national level of health has been attained gradually with the greatest gain occurring during the past fifty years. The amazing developments since the achievement of atomic fission have resulted in new scientific tools which speed the accomplishment of research—new machines for fractioning and computing, the utilization of isotopes and light rays, for example. Moreover, the trend toward national and international cooperation and creative application of scientific effort bespeaks great future advances. At the same time, there is a marked increase in the population at both ends of the curve, infants and the aged, the two groups which need the greatest amount of personal health care. New discoveries, new devices, and new problems require appropriately trained workers.

The Present Situation

From official and voluntary health agencies and professional groups come reports of serious shortages in the availability of new personnel, and great alarm is expressed concerning possible future curtailment of services because of personnel shortages. At the present time about 3,400,000 people are employed in professional and related health service occupations. Table 21 shows the numbers of men and women in certain of them. It should be noted, however, that shortages exist in many of the categories shown. Thus, the nation now needs 48,000 more physicians, 17,800 more dentists, 150,000 more nurses, and many thousands of other health workers. Obviously, the great population increase is accentuating the problem all the time.

The shortage of physicians is due largely to an inadequate number of medical schools, high costs of education, limited class sizes, and length of curriculum rather than to a dearth of applicants. It is estimated that merely to maintain the present ratio of physicians to population in the United States will require the establishment of one new additional medi-

[1]*Some Perspectives on the Path Ahead in Health Careers.* Prepared for the Commission on Health Careers by the National Health Council, 1790 Broadway, New York 19, New York, 1957.

Table 21. Health Manpower, U.S. Present Supply, Needs and Shortages

		Supply	*Need*	*Estimated shortage*
PHYSICIANS	Now	325,000	373,000	48,000
	1980	412,000	438,000	26,000
DENTISTS	Now	102,200	120,000	17,800
	1980	119,400	176,000	56,600
NURSES	Now	700,000	850,000	150,000
	1980	890,000	1,100,000	210,000
ALLIED HEALTH	Now	925,000	1,191,000	266,000
MANPOWER (Total)	1980	1,344,000	1,776,000	432,000
At Least Baccalaureate	Now	210,000	271,000	61,000
Medical Allied	1980	320,000	413,000	93,000
Environmental Health	Now	64,000	124,000	60,000
	1980	90,000	155,000	65,000
Less Than Baccalaureate	Now	325,000	396,000	71,000
Medical Allied	1980	475,000	580,000	105,000
Dental Allied	Now	138,000	167,000	29,000
	1980	151,000	246,000	95,000
Environmental Health	Now	188,000	233,000	45,000
	1980	308,000	382,000	74,000

Source: Amer. Med. News, Aug. 3, 1970.

cal school each year for some years to come. Then as each appears, a problem of staffing arises. The shortage in nursing and other professions whose personnel consists almost entirely of women, is due in significant degree to the annual loss through marriage. On the other hand, the role of the public health educator is not well understood by most people; the same is true of the health teacher and the health coordinator in the school, the sanitarian, the medical technician, and many other important workers whose exact roles have not been dramatized for the public.

The need for intensive recruitment is urgent. The approach to the problem needs to be aimed at two main groups as manpower reservoirs: the youth now in secondary school and college who are about to choose a life career, and those mature persons who wish to re-direct their careers either because of a desire for advancement or for more personal satisfaction. So general is the need for recruitment, that since 1955, the more than fifty member organizations that comprise the National Health Council have pooled their efforts in a cooperative appeal through printed materials widely distributed, and through the appointment of a special Commission on Health Careers which has sponsored conferences and stimulated nation-wide efforts in recruitment.

The National Health Council in 1955, with the support of the Equitable

Life Assurance Society of the United States, published "Health Careers Guidebook,"[2] a most useful book which listed approximately 150 different health careers together with details concerning the duties and responsibilities inherent in each, the expected salary range, and the personal qualifications and educational preparation needed by the prospective worker. The book and the condensed version were designed for the junior or senior high school student himself, and the Council arranged for their distribution to every junior and senior high school in the country. This valuable reference has since been updated and expanded by the U.S. Department of Labor.[3] The responsibility for recruitment falls mainly on the guidance counselors in these schools, but since all members of the school health team and every home room and subject teacher contribute to the total guidance plan of the school, everyone needs to be fully informed about the potentialities of health careers in order that the information to the students be consistent and up-to-date.

A truly functioning worker in the field of health is a dedicated person vitally interested in certain phases of health and motivated by a sincere desire to be of service to his fellow-man. This desire can come about only through an understanding of some of the major forces in the health situation and a feeling of personal involvement. A well-administered school health program should abound in situations stimulating recruitment: the school-child's contacts with the health services, for example, a clean, attractive building, and especially relevant health education classes rich in arousing this quality of interest. The satisfaction from actual participation in some form of community health activity can be most convincing in helping a teen-ager to discover his future area of service. Wise counseling will enable him to obtain an over-view of the wide range of possible health careers, and then to focus upon those compatible with his aptitudes, abilities, interests, and finances (the short-range goals and long-range career possibilities), financial help available, and finally, his immediate need to choose as a first step toward his own goal, school subjects prerequisite to his future field.

Under the leadership of the Commission on Health Careers of the National Health Council, organized recruitment efforts have been initiated on a nation-wide scale. Many states now have a state committee on health careers and many of these committees have in turn stimulated the formation of local or area committees composed of representatives of key professions and health agencies. These committees are largely advisory in character, but members often serve as speakers and panel members, and are active in the preparation and distribution of pertinent literature, and in the utilization of mass media for education and recruit-

[2] *Health Careers Guidebook*, published by the National Health Council and Supported in the public interest by The Equitable Life Assurance Society of the U.S., 1955, New York 1, N.Y.

[3] *Health Careers Guidebook*, Washington, D.C., U.S. Dept. of Labor, 1965.

ment. The Commission on Health Careers has emphasized that recruitment efforts must span all types of careers. For those requiring college background and additional graduate training, it is important for the student to plan in ninth grade or senior high school in order to include the science prerequisites. However, many health careers require training other than scientific, such as the mental health attendant, the medical secretary, and numerous other auxiliary but most necessary occupations. The Commission seeks to stimulate research into various unanswered problems involved in recruitment—for example, why a person chooses a particular career, and what methods of recruitment prove most effective and why.

Professional organizations also encourage their members to ply their own recruitment methods. The nursing profession faced this problem early and over a period of years has tried many methods and has met with a high degree of success. In addition to the dissemination of attractive brochures, their efforts have included future-nurse clubs in schools, participation in career days in secondary schools, special

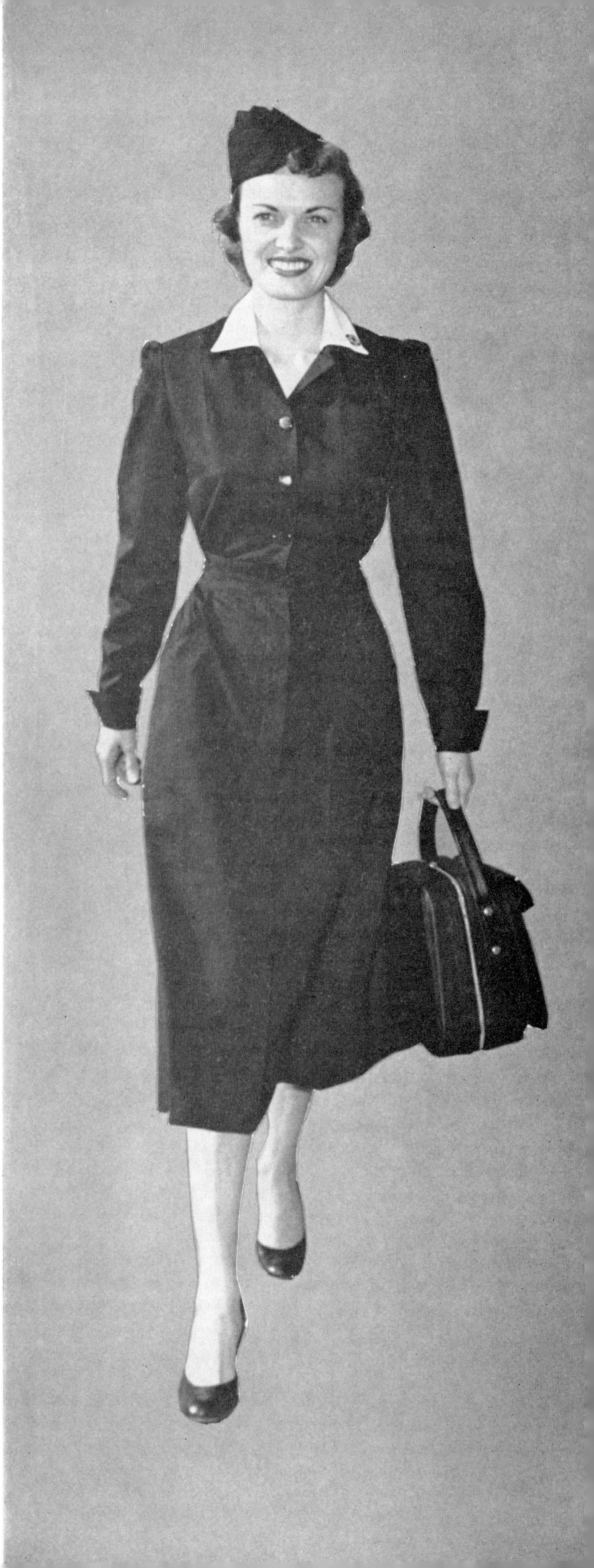

FIG. 60. A Health Worker in Action.

nurse career days at hospitals, tours of hospitals, and cooperation with the American Hospital Association in the arrangement for volunteer teen-age services in hospitals after school and during the summer vacation periods. In many communities, considerable prestige has become attached to the wearing of the "candy-striped" uniform and this community recognition has been satisfying to the students. In some communities, summer volunteer hospital service now includes boys who have given excellent services of many kinds. One hospital reported that it had expanded its annual hospital career day to include medicine, medical technology, occupational therapy, x-ray technology and dietetics.[4] Some of the colleges have had success with the plan of sending students as speakers at high school career days. Libraries, scout meetings, and recreation centers should not be overlooked as possible places for health career education.

Efforts must also be made to overcome the unwise and rigid barriers to entrance into the various professions and occupations. Each of us in our respective professions should take the initiative to seek out and encourage others to participate in the great movement for improved health, education and social service. Currently, much attention is being given to the employment of groups such as discharged military corpsmen, and to the training and trial of a wide variety of auxiliary non-professional aides to take some of the burden off the more highly and expensively trained professional. This has the virtue of providing much needed services to many who otherwise would go without. It also has the added value of providing initial career opportunities for many, especially the young and disadvantaged who otherwise might have little to look forward to in the form of a rewarding life.

Parent education should be stressed, for unless they are acquainted with the details of a proposed career, parents can neither share their children's enthusiasm nor inspire it. Parent-Teacher Associations, Women's Clubs, civic clubs, unions, church and other community groups include many parents who might wish to extend their knowledge of the situation if they were aware that speakers or a panel would be available to them. Radio and television programs and panel discussions by members of local Health Careers Committees have brought forth numerous inquiries in most places. A planned sequence of news stories scattered through the entire year has proved effective. Student publications should not be overlooked, for they are read not merely by the students but by their parents too.

Many college students are uninformed about the possibilities of a career in health work. More emphasis might well be placed upon acquainting students interested in the biological sciences, the physical sciences, and the behavioral sciences with the existing opportunities.

[4] Einstein Medical Center, Philadelphia, Pennsylvania. Oral report to the Philadelphia Health Careers Committee by Mrs. Nancy Goldsmith, June 22, 1962.

They should be given a wide view of the field with particular emphasis upon careers for which the prerequisite is a bachelor's degree (such as dental hygienist, radiological technician, etc.) and those requiring post-graduate work such as psychiatric social worker, therapeutic dietitian, pharmacist, sanitarian, etc. The English major needs to know about the possibilities of becoming a science writer or a medical librarian, while the person possessing an interest in art as well as science, should become familiar with the work of the medical illustrator.

Teacher education too frequently overlooks its responsibility for informing students about the position of health teaching and the possibilities of adding health courses to supplement a major in science. Physical education and health education have long been associated, but they differ widely in their appeal to pupils and often to the teachers responsible for instructing in both fields. There is a growing, nation-wide movement toward the special certification of teachers of health education, however, which calls for special guidance in planning. A recent national Conference on Teacher Preparation in Health Education, held under the sponsorship of the American Association for Health, Physical Education and Recreation for the purpose of "appraising existing undergraduate and fifth year programs in health education reaffirmed that a health education major is recommended for all teachers of health in secondary schools."[5] The Conference focused upon recruitment as a major problem and agreed that efforts should be directed toward all groups that are sources of prospective health education professional students. These would include secondary school students and selected groups of college students. The Conference Report includes excellent specific suggestions for making health careers "more visible" by means of campus activities, printed materials, visual aids, and through the development and utilization of placement services on all levels.

To meet the current manpower needs, there is considerable emphasis upon recruitment and training for the paramedical type of position, such as inhalation therapist, radiological technician, physician's office assistant (*i.e.*, receptionist, secretary, bookkeeper, etc.) for which the usual prerequisite is graduation from an approved standard high school. Training courses for positions in this category are sometimes provided by medical schools or by hospitals; but many community and junior colleges are now prepared to offer them. It has been stated that "Among programs now being offered by community and junior colleges are those in nursing, dental assistance, dental hygiene, hospital ward management, x-ray technology, operating room technology, medical secretarial work, medical librarianship, radiology, medical laboratory technology, inhalation ther-

[5] Recommended Standards and Guidelines. *Teacher Preparation in Health Education.* Reprinted from the Journal of Health, Physical Education and Recreation, February, 1969, by the American Association for Health, Physical Education, and Recreation, 1201-16th Street N.W., Washington, D.C., 20036.

apy, environmental health technology, child care, and prosthetic technology (making and planning artificial limbs)."[6]

Interested students need to be advised to include in junior and senior high school subjects related to their future career training, such as biology, chemistry, English, commercial subjects, etc.

The more mature person who wishes to advance or re-direct his career, is likely to scan the professional journals and recruitment literature, so the task is to make these available. The United States Office of Vocational Rehabilitation has offered many stipends which permit the individual to work and to go to school at the same time. The United States Public Health Service and many state and local health departments have made educational stipends available to physicians, nurses, and many other professional people in order that they might advance into administrative, public service, professional education or research positions. Scholarships and fellowships are sometimes available from voluntary health agencies and foundations. Often mature workers widen their experiences upon completion of a fellowship by a tour of duty in a foreign land, thus adding to their professional equipment.

In a number of instances experienced military medical corpsmen returned from active duty, have been recruited, given further training, and are being utilized as assistants to work with and under a physician's supervision.

Over the years well-trained and devoted health workers have been discouraged by their many failures to secure permanently improved health or health conditions among the underprivileged. Interesting new methods are being tried in various places through the utilization of persons recruited from the area involved. An intelligent housewife, for example, may be trained in simple relevant health procedures which she may then share with her neighbors whom she has known for some time. Usually such efforts are received with confidence and are most likely to be adopted quite promptly by previously recalcitrant or indifferent persons. Successful projects such as rat control, have been carried out in similar fashion by recruitment of indigenous manpower.

In Pennsylvania "a new training program which will provide both career opportunities for underprivileged persons and a team of trained technicians to assist the State's environmental protection program was recently initiated by the Department of Health. The program . . . represents a one-year course for Technical Aides aimed at preparing participants for a career in the environmental health field. Following completion of their training, the aides are eligible to take the Civil Service examination for Environmental Health Technician. As they advance in class they can choose a specialty in either air pollution, water pollution,

[6] News Notes for Health Educators. School Health Review, September, 1969, Page 44. American Association for Health, Physical Education and Recreation, 1201-16th Street, N.W., Washington, D.C. 20036.

radiological control, environmental medicine or housing and environmental control."[7]

It is interesting to note that the average age of the participants is 24, ranging in age from 19 to 36 and that their average educational level is 11th grade. The Department is making use of its own professional resources as instructors in the program. During their training program, the aides are regular salaried employees. "The Pennsylvania Health Department is the first agency to adopt this concept of career training which was developed through the Governor's office."[8]

These illustrations merely suggest the enormous amount of imagination and innovation which characterize the developments in the health field today. The freedom and willingness to experiment indicate a genuine awareness of the acuity of the nation's needs and the existence of the will to meet new challenges with open mindedness and new methods.

Schools of Public Health

Specific training in public health is now available at the 18 accredited graduate Schools of Public Health located at University of California at Berkeley, University of California at Los Angeles, Columbia University, Harvard University, University of Hawaii, Johns Hopkins University, Loma Linda University, University of Michigan, University of Minnesota, University of Montreal, University of North Carolina, University of Oklahoma, University of Pittsburgh, University of Puerto Rico, University of Texas at Houston, University of Toronto, Tulane University and Yale University. Ordinarily, an academic year at the school plus about three months of field training is required for the Master of Public Health degree. Several of the schools also award the more advanced Doctorate in Public Health, which follows a previous doctorate in another field and ordinarily requires two additional years of more advanced study and/or research.

In line with the increasing recognition of the inter-relatedness of the roles of the school health educator and the community health educator, (the former concerned with the health of the individual during a relatively short segment of the individual's' total life span and the community health worker focusing upon the years preceding and following this span), some colleges and universities have been expanding their graduate programs in health education in an attempt to encompass preparation for both types of position. For example, Teachers College and the Columbia University School of Public Health and Administrative Medicine are jointly sponsoring a 2-year program based upon the assump-

[7] Health Training for the 70's—Meeting To-day's Challenges. Pennsylvania's Health, Summer, 1970. *31*, No. 2, Page 2.

[8] Op. cit., p. 4.

tion that it is "possible and desirable in a 2-year program to produce a health educator who is qualified to work in either area."[9]

The Steps to Take

Actually the approach to the problem of exploring and meeting the need for health personnel has been well charted. A main obstacle to recruitment centers in the matter of communication: to find the possible recruit, to discover his point of interest and appeal, to help him understand the ramifications of possible suitable careers, and to help him take the proper initial steps. This implies adequately informed counselors, teachers, professional persons, parents, and others involved in the guidance of youth; definite available community sources of career information; and the wise and consistent use of mass media for education. The concrete suggestions regarding areas for action, made by vocational counselors during a National Health Forum were summarized as follows:

1. Health groups should produce recruitment materials more adroitly designed to influence and motivate young people to enter health fields.
2. Vocational guidance groups should be consulted on how to keep informative brochures objective and accurate, yet appealing.
3. Health material should be distributed from a central source instead of being, as now, hard to find and get.
4. Material should show the broad range of opportunities in health rather than presenting one or two of the better known areas.
5. Health groups should make greater effort to give young people first hand contact with health activities through individual conferences with persons actually engaged in the area of interest, more career-day field visits, and more opportunities to serve as volunteers.

Questions for Discussion

1. What are the specific health personnel needs in your community? What steps are being taken to meet them? By whom?
2. What are the different professional disciplines represented on the staff of your local health department? In view of the health problems of your community, do you consider this staff adequate in terms of types of professions and numbers of health workers?
3. Does the school system in your community conduct a planned program of career information? What is its nature? At what grade levels is it presented? Are health careers emphasized?

[9] Shimmel, Gilbert M., A Common Curriculum for School Health Educators and Public Health Educators, Am. J. Public Health, 59, No. 2, February, 1969, P. 315.

4. Do you know how many years of training are required to become (*a*) a general medical practitioner (*b*) a medical specialist (*c*) a nurse (*d*) a sanitarian (*e*) an engineer in public health (*f*) a veterinarian (*g*) a public health physician?
5. What is the typical training provided in the graduate schools of public health? Do you know where they are located? Are teachers eligible for admission?

Suggested Readings

1. *Career Opportunities,* New York, New York Life Insurance Company, 1958.
2. *Health Careers Guidebook,* Washington, D.C., U.S. Dept. of Labor, 1965.
3. Society of Public Health Educators: *Health Education as a Career,* New York, Metropolitan Life Insurance Company.
4. *New Careers in Health Science,* New York, The National Health Council, 1790 Broadway, 1961.
5. *Notes on Community Action for Health Careers,* New York, National Health Council.
6. *Partners for Health,* New York, National Health Council, 1955.
7. *Recruitment for Personnel in the Health Field,* New York, National Health Council, 1958.
8. *Some Perspectives on the Task Ahead in Health Careers,* New York, National Health Council, 1957.
9. Yahraes, Herbert: *What's in Your Future—A Career in Health?* New York, Public Affairs Pamphlet No. 281, 1959.
10. *Health Careers Recruitment: Progress; Problems; Project Suggestions for National, State and Local Action,* New York, National Health Council, 1963.
11. American Medical Association. *Horizons Unlimited.* General Handbook on Health Careers. Chicago: American Medical Association, 1966.
12. Health Information Foundation, Public Relations Director, 420 Lexington Avenue, New York, N.Y. 10017.
13. *Institutions Offering Programs of Specialization In Health Education.* 1970. School Health Education Study, 1507 M Street, N.W., Room 800, Washington, D.C. 20005.

PART IV
Epilogue

THE origins of community health are lost in the past. The achievements of its dynamic present have come from many cultures and many disciplines. The road to its future leads toward a chimerical horizon only vaguely discernable in the haze of as yet undetermined knowledge. We stand at a point in time which is significantly transitional. It would appear that we are passing from one major era of man's history and about to enter another. Great advances have been made which have solved many old problems. Meanwhile the everchanging world produces still other problems and the possibility of new advances. If the potential advances are to be realized, now more than ever we must demonstrate a willingness to change with changing times. We must seek out and discard our sacred cows and false gods.

This is symbolized in the accompanying figure. The old man in the foreground has seen great changes in his days. When he was born, he could anticipate a life of only a half century. Now nearing his end, and contemplating the future, he sees life extended beyond three score and ten. While the shadow of his life and time affects the new generation, the newborn child in turn casts his shadow before him. However, the shadow of things past must not be mistaken for the shadow of things to come.

False gods and sacred cows are symbolized by obstacles in the road. They represent outmoded measures such as placarding for disease and fumigation. There must be others to which we still blindly cling.

And what of the future? Symbolized also are new approaches to mental illness, addictions, accidents and the hazards of radiation. Our air and water become increasingly polluted, yet the potential of water as a medium for mass prevention is increasingly realized. Replacing empirical pills and placebos is an array of specific chemicals, biologicals and antibiotics. Limiting the full beneficial effect of these and other wonders yet to come are the apathy and prejudice of some people and the ignorance and misunderstanding of others. The fractionated human figure indicates the tendency to over-specialize rather than to consider the individual as a whole.

As the phoenix rises reborn from the ashes of its past, so too must we courageously discard the old and outmoded to allow the rebirth of vigorous new approaches to the achievement of even better health and more fruitful living for all.

Chapter 16

Where Have We Been? Where Are We Going?

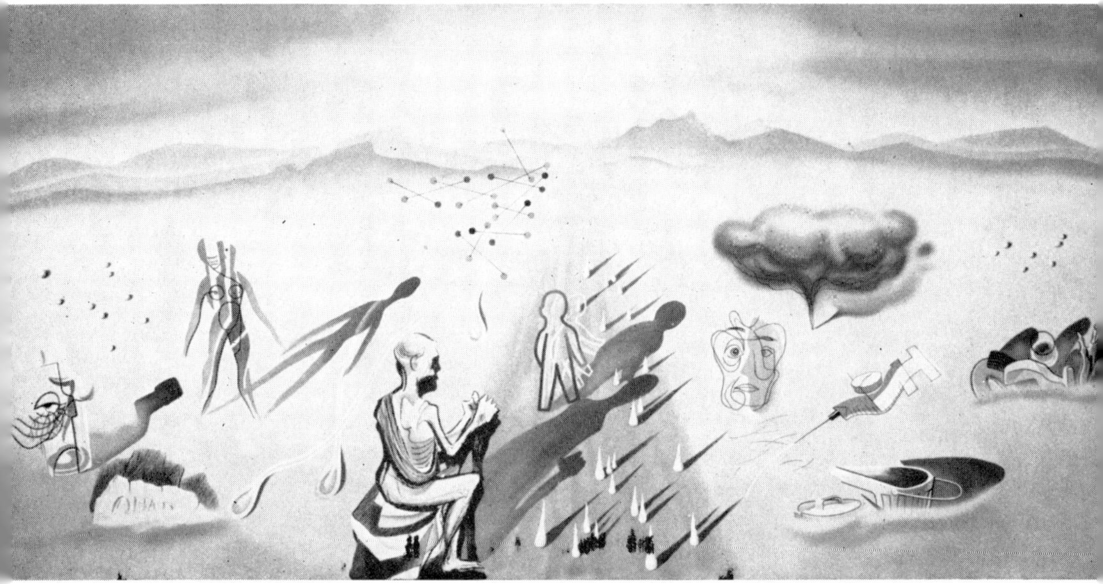

FIG. 61. The Time Dimension of Health.

THE past half century has encompassed some truly remarkable events. They have had more than their share of terrible strife and other catastrophes. On the other hand, they have witnessed the most amazing advances in the history of mankind. Within this short period, man has explored the recesses of his mind and of the atom, synthesized not only new complex compounds but even new elements, learned to preserve sounds and scenes, achieved the spanning of the oceans in the time it once took to drive to the county seat, and now is mightily engaged in exploring not only the depths of the seas and the earth, but also the mysteries of the living molecule and the reaches of interplanetary space.

Not the least of the great accomplishments of this period has been a first giant step toward the conquest of disease. The extent to which this goal has been achieved is exemplified by the 45 per cent drop in the general death rate from 17.2 per 1000 population in 1900 to 9.6 in 1969. This has resulted in a corresponding 43 per cent increase in the average life expectancy at birth from 49 years in 1900 to 70 years in 1969. During the same period, the risks of infancy have been reduced 75 per cent and the hazards to the lives of mothers have been almost completely removed as indicated by a drop of 96 per cent in the maternal mortality rate. At the beginning of the century, tuberculosis had the nickname, "Captain of the kings of death," and annually took away about 200 of each 100,000 of the population. That awesome death rate has now been reduced to about 3 per 100,000 persons, a drop of about 98 per cent. Many similar successes have been achieved with numerous other previously significant causes of death. Some of the most outstanding are shown in the accompanying table which presents the percentage reduction in their death rates between 1900 and 1969.

Offsetting these have been concurrent increases in the rates of death from some other conditions, notably certain of the chronic non-communicable diseases. Thus, the death rate from diabetes has increased about 40 per cent, from cancer about 130 per cent and, from cardiovascular diseases about 160 per cent. What can be done about these? Have we reached the zenith of our accomplishments and of our life expectancy? Must we now consider ourselves destined to acquire and succumb to these latter conditions? Not necessarily. There is really little reason for a diabetic to die from diabetes, and already the increase in deaths from certain malignancies and cardiovascular conditions has been retarded and, in a few instances, even turned back. That much remains to be learned and accomplished is quite true. But much is already being done, and much more can be done, even with our present knowledge. The goal is not merely longer life, perhaps over eighty years, but one in which advanced years are not synonymous with senility, suffering and illness. There is good reason to believe that this can be accomplished.

To understand better our role in this endeavor, it would be well to consider certain aspects of this remarkable period of transition in which we now find ourselves. We have all been aware of certain changes which have been occurring in the number and nature of our people. Indeed it would have been difficult in our time for them to have gone unnoticed.

Table 22. Percentage Reduction in Certain Causes of Death, U.S., 1900 to 1969

	Per Cent		Per Cent
Scarlet fever	100	Typhoid and paratyphoid	100
Erysipelas	100	Dysentery	99
Influenza and pneumonia	84	Diarrhea and enteritis	99
Tuberculosis	98	Diphtheria	100
Malaria	100	Measles	98
Poliomyelitis	100	Whooping cough	99

Measured by the chronometer of history, they have occurred with dramatic suddenness. They are evidenced by pressing needs and demands for more perambulators and rocking chairs, more pediatricians and geriatrists, more schools and hospital beds, more housing and household equipment, greater quantities and greater varieties of everything. There may be value in pinpointing a few of these changes and indicating their effects upon the necessarily related problems in public health and education and the programs devised to meet them.

Public health activities deal essentially with people. The extent to which they are concerned with things is only as they affect people. In recent years there have occurred very significant changes in the numbers and distribution of people. Much attention is now being given to the so-called "population explosion" or "protoplasmic deluge." The attention is well merited as this represents the single most critical issue confronting mankind and the planet in the long run. All other problems relate to it in one way or another. Overall it is alarming to note that it took man about 2 million years up to 1830 to reach his first billion, only 100 years from 1830 to 1930 to reach his second billion, a mere 33 years from 1930 to the mid 1960s, to reach his third billion and by 2000 A.D. will reach between 6 and 7 billions and be adding another billion every 5 years. This combined with the extent and rate at which we are using up our finite supply of planetary resources and polluting the earth's ecosystems spells inevitable eventual disaster unless a very significant change in man's value systems comes about. Our contribution to the population is interesting. While the population of the United States is not increasing at as rapid a rate as in many other parts of the world, notably Asia and Latin America, the fact that we are the most insatiable consumers more than makes up for any difference. Thus it has been validly pointed out that a baby born in the United States is the equivalent of five babies born in the rest of the world. He will consume five times as much of the world's goods and resources. Robert and Leona Rienow describe the case well in their book *Moment in The Sun.*[1] They point out that every 8 seconds a new American is born and begins to scream in a demanding voice that lasts for 70 years. "He is screaming," they indicate, "for 56,000,000 gallons of water, 21,000 gallons of gasoline, 10,150 pounds of meat, 28,000 pounds of milk and cream, 9,000 pounds of wheat and great storehouses of all other foods, drinks and tobaccos." In his lifetime he requisitions ". . . a private endowment of $5,000 to $8,000 for school building materials, $6,300 worth of clothing, $7,000 worth of furniture–and 200 pounds of peanuts . . ." He is a "prodigious consumer in a nation that accounts for one-fifteenth of the earth's people but consumes half of its total product."

Within the past 50 years, our numbers have approximately doubled. During most of this half century, however, the rate of natural growth

[1]Rienow, R. and Rienow, L.: *Moment in The Sun,* New York, Ballantine, 1967.

was actually slowing down. About 1940, it began to accelerate again and continued until 1960 when the trend was reversed. Now in 1970 it appears about to resume its increase. A seeming paradox is that, whereas until recently we were becoming more and more concerned with a rapidly aging population, we are now confronted with a population which is becoming both older and younger at the same time, that is, increasing in the numbers and proportions at both ends of the age scale at the expense of the proportionately ever smaller middle-aged group of producers.

The reasons are fairly clear. On the side of youth, we have never experienced such an increase in marriages, such a lowered average age at marriage and parenthood, and such an increase in births as has occurred since 1900. It is surprising to note that the average age at marriage and parenthood of girls in the United States is now among the lowest in the world and that our birth rate is now higher than in countries such as Italy or Japan which formerly were considered unusually fertile. On the side of aging, the spectacular successes in the fields of public health, medicine and nutrition have brought about an increase in the average life expectancy at birth from 47 years in 1900 to about 70 years at the present time. It is difficult to realize, for example, that a white girl born now has a better chance of living to age 60 years than she would have had of surviving to her fifth birthday in 1900! The same is true, of course, of boys and Negroes, although to a slightly lesser extent.

The result is that, while in 1900 only 13,000,000 persons or 18 per cent of the total population were in the age group over 45 years, by now the figures are about 50,000,000 persons and 30 per cent over 45 years of age. Meanwhile, due to the relatively recent sustained upsurge in birth rates, the median age of the population has begun a significant downward movement and is expected by 1975 to be almost back to the median age of about 25 years which prevailed at the beginning of the century.

With reference to the distribution of our population, we have been undergoing some significant changes. People are increasing in numbers and spreading to all parts of the country. However, the population increase is most marked along the east and west coasts, with lower absolute and proportionate increases in the great central heartland of the country. This has necessitated more new communities and the rejuvenation of many older communities. In the process, we have also been undergoing a remarkable degree of agglutination. In the past 60 years the urban population has increased to include most of the population, with only about 5 per cent now living on farms. Recently, a modified reversal of the process has occurred. A dual change in living and working has come about with the development of extensive suburbs on the one hand, and a number of vast metropolitan areas on the other. It is noteworthy that the 1960 and 1970 censuses showed that many of the largest cities of the nation had actually lost population during the previous two decades as a result of "the flight to the suburbs" where there have developed extensive self-contained decentralized living-shopping-recreation centers. This trend has been encouraged by the resettlement of large numbers of industries in previously undeveloped suburban or farm land, giving rise, in many instances, to the appearance of totally new communities in remarkably short periods of time.

As examples of the development of metropolitan complexes, one can point to those that extend from Boston to Washington, D.C., from San Diego to San Francisco, from Detroit and Windsor to Chicago and on down to Toledo and Cleveland, the Nashville-Atlanta complex, the group of Gulf Coast cities, the Saint Louis-Memphis axis, and various others.

Significant to this discussion is the change in the function of the city. Originally it developed as a center for trade, protection, and later manufacture. Then it became a convenient location for living, educational, and cultural pursuits. By now, the factors of protection and pleasant living have largely disappeared. Increasingly, facilities for trade and cultural activities are being decentralized from the truly urban situation. This leaves the city essentially a place for manufacturing and conducting business. With reference to inhabitants, the more affluent component of the population has tended to abandon the large central or core cities, leaving behind large residues of socio-economically disadvantaged groups, predominantly certain minorities, many chronically ill poor individuals and the aged. This has had very significant effects on many aspects of our culture and society, including increased needs in the core cities for social services, welfare, health and medical care, security provisions and the like.

Our mode of life has been changing significantly and rapidly. People are becoming increasingly mobile for the purposes of business, pleasure and residence. It is estimated for example, that at the present time about one-fifth of the population of the United States changes its address each year. With this mobility there has developed a more intermingled and cosmopolitan population, the latter also attributable in part to greater affluence and more education. Probably the most striking and significant cultural changes in our people, therefore, are the loss of the extended family, on the one hand, and an ever more intimate contact and interlinking among divers peoples on the other. In turn, these too have had fundamental effects on our mores, morals and ethics.

This, of course, is of great significance to public health, and is illustrated by considering some of the effects of many aspects of our late 20th century culture upon personal and community health and upon future public health programs. Businesses and industries, for the sake of economic and competitive efficiency, as well as in some cases on the basis of increased social and ecological ethics, must now actively search for and play an important role in the maintenance of healthy employees, and a healthy non-polluted environment. In fact, many go further and recognize the importance of contributing to the assurance of the health and well-being of the families of employees. These efforts in turn have been reflected in higher incomes and standards of living for longer periods of productive life. Industrial efficiency has also led to shorter working hours, hence, more time for leisure. Changes in food production and processing methods have had a marked effect upon the health and well-being of the population. While, as has been mentioned, only about 5 per cent of Americans now live on farms, they consistently produce ever greater surpluses of better and more nutritious food. The remarkable revolution which has taken place in food genetics and in the food processing and packaging industry has made possible better and more uniform foods of greater variety and availability in all parts of the nation at all times of the year.

Developments in the transportation industry through better highways and vehicles, including especially the refrigerated truck trailer, have played an important role in bringing foods, pharmaceuticals and many other products to the doorstep of the average citizen. These same improvements in transportation have also made it possible for those in health and related professions to function more widely and effectively. Almost daily the chemical industry has been producing materials and processes that greatly affect the well-being of people. Among these are insecticides, herbicides, pharmaceuticals, preservatives, synthetic fabrics easier to keep clean, new methods for disposal of waste, and many others. New methods of construction coupled with improved community planning have led to less drudgery, the elimination of the causes of some accidents, and fewer environmental hazards, particularly as they relate to the elimination of rats, vermin and fire hazards in housing.

A by-product of the advances in the field of communications has been some increase in public knowledge and information which has made people more aware of and concerned about matters of health and disease. The development and extensive use of insurance has long since proven its value in protection against the financial consequences of material risks. It has now been extended to cover the financial and other risks that arise from unpredictable illness on the one hand, and predictable aging on the other. In the field of medicine more and more emphasis is being placed upon prevention and it is interesting to note the increasing frequency with which mention of the need for better training in preventive medicine is made in important addresses by outstanding medical leaders.

What is the meaning of this for the future? It would seem obvious that the artificial barriers between therapeutic, preventive and promotive medicine must be broken down much further. The same applies to the parochial and rigid barriers and inadequate communication among various professions, especially those which relate to health, welfare, education and recreation. Each in our respective professions should seek means of more effective interprofessional communication, planning and action. This becomes particularly important when one considers the interrelationship of what earlier in this book has been called "The Syndrome of the Seven D's," disease, deficiency, destitution, dependency, despondency, delinquency and degeneracy. These, incidentally, may be applied not only in the social dimension but also in the age dimension, especially as it relates to the problems of the elderly, in the socio-economic dimension, and in the geographic dimension.

Reference has been made elsewhere to the basic fields of activity in public health. What do current trends do to them? A few random comments about certain aspects of them may serve to stimulate further thought and discussion.

Vital Statistics

The potentialities of the application of electronic data-processing in this field are enormous, especially in relation to the determination of truly accurate and detailed base-line data, and the provision of more accurate and rapid personal and community diagnosis upon which to base more efficient, rapid and effective health programs from the community on up to the national levels.

Maternal and Child Health

One of the most regrettable phenomena in our society is the continuing large number of deaths of newborn infants. It has been pointed out that to a considerable extent this is related to the failure of many expectant mothers to obtain prenatal care early, if at all. This in turn is related to inadequacies in personal health education especially during the secondary school period. From the natural, humanitarian, social and economic viewpoints, one may properly raise the question, "If parenthood is going to occur, is there anything more important and worth protecting?" Obviously much remains to be done in this area by teachers, public health workers and the medical profession working as partners. In another area, the intrinsic value of many of our customary activities in well-child supervision is increasingly subject to question, and needs re-evaluation. This is particularly true in view of the rapid and dramatic changes that have been occurring in our way and standard of living, the changing roles of schools, official and voluntary health agencies, and the practice of medicine. Increasingly, we are all becoming aware that we may be going through more or less stereotyped motions based upon concepts and standards which, while in earlier circumstances might have been valid, may no longer be so. Furthermore, with less professional time available in relation to the mounting numbers of those to be served, we can no longer afford the luxury of interagency or interprofessional jurisdictional competition. Such questions are really quite secondary, and in all probability have no single answer to fit all circumstances. Instead, we should and must focus more than ever upon needs and practicality, again on the basis of genuine interprofessional partnership. In addition, it would seem practical for communities to provide as much as possible of the disease preventive and health promotive services for their children from existing practicing physicians and other health professionals, as well as from a variety of community institutions rather than from employees and facilities of schools or health departments.

The large and increasing number and proportion of unwanted children, both legitimate and illegitimate, point to another very significant need;—a far more forthright, effective and universal approach to family planning and family planning education. A variety of quite effective methods of conception control are already available and considerable research is under way to improve them. Meanwhile, all citizens, including teachers, should be well versed in the problem of overpopulation, its implications for the family and the world, and what needs to be done to solve it.

Communicable Disease Control

Despite the great scientific advances of the past several decades, much time, effort and money is still being wasted on diseases which are now subject to eradication. For example, tuberculosis and the venereal diseases could and should be in the same category of practical extinction as smallpox. To the contrary, there has recently occurred a dramatic resurgence in the incidence of venereal diseases, predominantly among teen-agers. At the same time, studies have pointed to a surprising lack of health information among the adolescent and young adult population as one of the important causes of the increase in these serious diseases. Concurrently, while researchers have presented us with immunizing agents for an ever increasing list ol diseases, many people have yet to take advantage of them. This is one of the enigmas of human nature,—great clamor for practical preventatives, followed by inertia or carelessness concerning their use when they become available. Here indeed is a prime challenge to all those in education and in the social sciences.

Non-Communicable Disease Control

Successful application of existing knowledge and techniques concerning the communicable diseases would allow much needed accentuation of programs aimed at the more difficult and elusive non-communicable and addictive diseases. These various conditions, and especially the latter, offer excellent opportunities for inter-professional and inter-disciplinary partnership. It is clear that the greatest single obstacle to a successful attack upon these conditions is a widespread erroneous attitude of apathy and fatalism concerning them. While much remains to be learned, actually much could be accomplished just with the knowledge we presently have at hand. This includes not only early diagnosis and limitation of the consequences of disease processes already under way, but in many cases even prevention in the first instance. Many types of cancer, for example, can be prevented. The same is true of many types of cardiovascular conditions. Many addictions can be avoided. We don't have to wait. Much can be done now with what we have, if we work together and really try!

Environmental Health

Public health activity originated as a result of problems in the environment, specifically gross insanitation. Attention then swung away to other causes of concern. Interestingly, it is now returning to a renewed emphasis upon the environment but in a somewhat different sense than previously. As a result of our increased population, urbanization and technological development, there are steeply increasing demands placed upon our total environment. We still have essentially the same major resources to support us that we had 100 years ago, in terms of air, water, soil and raw materials. We are simply using them more intensively as the demand spirals. One result is that it now is necessary to place heavy emphasis upon such problems as air and water pollution, solid waste management, radiation control, accident prevention, housing, city planning and the like. In a very real sense we are running a race, not only with time but with our own technological development, with our own demands, and with man's capacity to adapt. If as a nation and a world we continue a laissez-faire policy in respect to these problems we will place man as well as increasing numbers of other species in serious jeopardy. Indeed, many scientists consider the continued survival of mankind subject to question as a result of the combination of rampant population increase and the ever more extensive and severe environmental abuse. Already we and many other nations have widespread serious problems from water unfit to drink, food unfit to eat, air unfit to breathe, and a resulting catastrophic medical bill. The schools and public health agencies share a great responsibility in the teaching of good environmental and ecological citizenship, and in the encouragement of and preparation for careers in the technical, scientific and other fields involved.

Mental Health

There are numerous great fields for exploration and extension in mental health. This is true not only in terms of pre- and post-institutional care and guidance, and in extra-institutional out-patient treatment, but also in terms of the prevention of mental illness and the promotion of mental health. Attacks upon addictive diseases, delinquency and the causes of senility have been mentioned. Significant advances are being made in relation to certain prenatal, genetic, environmental, nutritional and other causes of mental illness. Recent studies have shown that mental and physical fatigue as well as anxiety, two of man's most common complaints, are based to a considerable extent upon biochemical factors. Already, several new pharmaceuticals for the relief of fatigue due to mental and physical exhaustion, have been tested. They apparently relieve fatigue by increasing the efficiency of the metabolic processes of the body. On the other side of the coin are the problems generated by the stresses of life in a highly urbanized and industrialized society, as well as by automation, shorter work days, and early retirement. One thing is certain, inactivity is undesirable both for mind and body. Another challenge for the school is the encouragement of hobbies and avocations in the younger population, and of education and training for the older component of society in new fields of interest and second vocations.

The school has a particularly important role to play in teaching and counseling about narcotics and alcohol. All teachers should be familiar with the signs and symptoms which may result from the use of drugs and narcotics and thereby serve as an important link in early diagnosis and prompt treatment of situations which can affect an individual's entire future life and seriously affect others.

* * * *

As the end of this book is approached, it is important to emphasize the common interest and purpose which should be shared by the school and the community with regard to the goal of health. This is because the one environment is merely a part of the other. In fact, one might regard the community itself like a school. It is endowed by the citizenry, it has manifold institutional characteristics, and it certainly provides plenty of opportunities for learning. The satisfactory school and the satisfactory community must of necessity share a vast area of interest. It stems from, colors and is colored by the same culture, and serves the same ends,—the survival and improvement of the lot of their common membership.

It is well to remind ourselves of these relationships. All too frequently educational institutions regard the communities which contain them as crass and profane as against their own intellectuality and sacredness. On its part, the community may look upon schools and colleges as semi-penal institutions, places in which to park children, or as some sort of medieval alchemists' tower whence solutions to all sorts of social and scientific problems may be anticipated.

What then is or should be the role of the school in relation to the over-all health of the community? First is a concern with total community health affairs. This is given priority because it is so often ignored. If the health of the public is a community affair, and if the school is part of the community, and if the school constitutes a reservoir of greater than average knowledge and ability, then it is proper to assume that among its dominant responsibilities should be a significant share of participation and leadership in community health affairs. This may be accomplished by all the means available in a free society: keeping currently informed, engaging in public and private discussion, promoting and participating in civic surveys and studies, serving on boards and commissions, or as consultants and advisors. Community leadership may also take the form of the provision by the school of continued education classes, forums, seminars, and meetings relating to the health needs of the community. All such activities should be pursued in relation to the many voluntary health agencies as well as to the official health agency. It is unfortunate that all too many in the academic field forego the opportunities and satisfactions to be found in this type of service, either because they claim they are too busy or for the even weaker reason of it being none of their business.

The second concern of the school with community health is its traditional responsibility for student well-being. In general, this responsibility has been approached through the provision of school environments which in varying degrees are safe and sanitary, quite good medical and nursing services, sometimes only fair personal health education, and often rather poor or even no teaching of community health. Despite the latter shortcomings, by attacking the most evident need, that is the immediate personal health and physical problems of the individual student, the average school has chalked up a rather good record and in this sense seems to merit much credit. But there is danger that the successes may be more apparent than real, more temporary than permanent. For one thing, the school years constitute the healthiest period of life. In addition, schools and colleges have been riding the crest of a rising tide of general improvement in individual health and nutrition which has not been particularly of their making. Rather, it has resulted from the remarkable recent developments in environmental and public health, preventive medicine, medical research, improved medical practice, food technology, and a rapidly upward-spiralling economy. Furthermore, it is the group now in schools and colleges that has benefited the most from these advances. There can be only one conclusion. In view of the fact that the great threats to life come later and that the foundations for their cause or their prevention may be laid during the educational period, many schools and colleges appear to be falling somewhat short of their responsibilities and opportunities if they limit themselves essentially to individual health problems of the moment.

Here we are confronted with a truly great challenge. With an ever-increasing enrollment in schools and colleges there is a real opportunity to develop a broad community awareness and change in attitude with regard to the growing health problems of adulthood and later life. But the attitudes and patterns of living must be established prior to the achievement of adulthood. Where can this be done better than in the school situation? Unfortunately, however, too many educational institutions still regard health instruction either as body building, or as incidental rather than fundamental. Under the circumstances, it is not surprising that so many citizens give up or give in to the complex pressures, demands, and frustrations with which our modern competitive society confronts the individual on his emergence from his academic experience. It is not surprising that 1 in every 10 in the United States, suffers or will suffer from some form of mental illness.

The answer is not to be found in more and better books or more frequent and more difficult tests about health. There is a limit to how many facts may be retained for prompt use. Facts memorized or learned often have a tendency to change or be forgotten. It would be far better to develop the analytic abilities and problem-solving skills of the student in relation to personal and community health. Every student group experiences a wide variety of health problems because they form the very stuff of life. Given some basic facts and provocative teachers, students can gain much from opportunities to define, analyze, and solve everyday personal and community problems. The latter especially would provide a great fund of enjoyable and fruitful experience if the various community health agencies and the schools really got together and developed with students mutually advantageous arrangements for learning situations.

The third concern of the school with community health relates to career development which has been the subject of a separate chapter. Health in all of its aspects is a very personal thing. The product is personal service, its source is personal, and the recipient is personal. As a result, large numbers of many types of individuals are required. In terms of persons employed, the provision of health services already represents one of the largest occupational groups. Despite this serious shortages exist in practically all categories. The development of these health workers has been described as "America's most essential industry." However, as the President's Commission on the Health Needs of the Nation concluded, ". . . we have come to realize that the growth of this industry is taking place in fits and starts with no overall plan and only a limited amount of long-range planning."

Out of this problem come two great responsibilities and functions for our education system. On the one hand there is a need to encourage more students to aspire to the various professions and callings necessary to the community's health. On the other hand, perhaps the single most valuable contribution of the school to the solution of this problem takes the form of providing the pre-professional student with a very broad liberal education so that there is built into him not so much scientific and technical details, which he can obtain later, as a sound philosophy and a pattern for learning and living. The objective should be many-faceted and include the development of integrity, emotional stability, imagination, and capacity for growth, based upon an appreciation of human relationships and a sense of social responsibility. Its attainment involves the four basic academic ingredients so well outlined by Professor Theodore M. Greene, Professor of Humanities at Scripps College. "(1) Training in the accurate and felicitous use of *language,* as the essential condition of all reflection, self-expression, and communication with others; (2) Training in the acquisition of *factual knowledge* of ourselves, our society, and other societies, the physical world, and ultimate reality so far as it is humanly knowable; (3) Training in mature and responsible *evaluation and decision* in the controversial areas of social policy, morality, art and religion, and (4) Training in *synoptic comprehension, i.e.,* in the escape from the multiple provincialisms which bedevil mankind and in the attainment of larger and more inclusive perspectives."

Only thus can schools and colleges provide a breadth and elasticity of viewpoint which will enable the student to roll with the intellectual punch as new discoveries, needs, and demands appear in relation to his own and his community's health.

Appendix A

Some Commonly Used Rates and Ratios

$$\text{Crude Birth Rate} = \frac{\text{number of live births}}{\text{total population}} \times 1000$$

$$\text{Age Specific Birth Rate} = \frac{\text{number of live births to women 15 to 45 years}}{\text{number of women 15 to 45 years in population}} \times 1000$$

$$\text{Crude Death Rate} = \frac{\text{number of deaths from all causes}}{\text{total population}} \times 1000$$

$$\text{Age Specific Death Rate} = \frac{\text{number of deaths in an age group (ex. 10–19 yrs.)}}{\text{population in the age group (ex. 10–19 yrs.)}} \times 1000$$

$$\text{Cause Specific Death Rate} = \frac{\text{number of deaths from a specific disease}}{\text{total population}} \times 100{,}000$$

$$\text{Maternal Mortality Rate} = \frac{\text{number of maternal deaths}}{\text{total number of live births}} \times 1000$$

$$\text{Infant Mortality Rate} = \frac{\text{number of deaths under 1 year of age}}{\text{total number of live births}} \times 1000$$

$$\text{Neonatal Mortality Rate} = \frac{\text{number of deaths under 1 month of age}}{\text{total number of live births}} \times 1000$$

$$\text{Morbidity Rate} = \frac{\text{number of cases of a specific disease}}{\text{total population}} \times 100{,}000$$

$$\text{Case Fatality Rate} = \frac{\text{number of deaths from a specific disease}}{\text{number of cases of the specific disease}} \times 100$$

Life Expectancy = The number of years of life remaining to the average individual of a specified age at the time for which the life expectancy is stated. Thus, a life expectancy of 35 at age 40 in 1960 means that the average person who has reached age 40 in 1960 could look forward to 35 more years of life.

NOTES:

a) rates may be computed for any specifically stated period of time, *e.g.*, monthly, annually.

b) in computing maternal, infant and neonatal mortality rates, stillbirths are not included in the denominator because of the considerable variation in the extent to which they are reported.

Appendix B

Some Important Agencies, Organizations and Resources

Inextricably intermingled in the nation's design for health are the efforts and activities of a multitude of organizations and individuals functioning at local, state, national or international levels. An attempt to name in each category all of the many agencies, institutions and groups which, through participation by means of funds, grants, scholarships, personnel, services or programs, justly merit such recognition, would be impossible. Therefore, the lists which follow have been selected mainly in consideration of teachers and community leaders who wish to become familiar with some of the more important and pertinent organizations and agencies which might serve as resources in health and health education. For convenience, they are listed under five headings: philanthropic foundations, professional organizations, private or voluntary health agencies, official governmental agencies, and commercial organizations.

1. Philanthropic Foundations

Philanthropic foundations established for health or health education purposes, often dedicated to the solution or alleviation of a specific health problem as indicated by their founders—individuals, families, business, industrial or professional organizations, or cooperative groups of organizations:

Association for the Aid of Crippled Children, 345 East 46th Street, New York N.Y. 10017

Avalon Foundation, 713 Park Avenue, New York, N.Y. 10021 N.Y. 10022

The Samuel Bronfman Foundation, Inc., 375 Park Avenue, New York, N.Y. 10022

The Commonwealth Fund, One East 75th Street, New York, N.Y. 10021

The Ford Foundation, 477 Madison Avenue, New York, N.Y. 10022

The Fund for the Advancement of Education, 477 Madison Avenue, New York, N.Y. 10022

The Grant Foundation, Inc., 130 East 59th Street, New York, N. Y. 10022

The Harkness (William Hale) Foundation, Inc., 872 Madison Avenue, New York, N.Y. 10021

The John A. Hartford Foundation, Inc., 420 Lexington Avenue, New York, N.Y. 10017
Health Information Foundation, 420 Lexington Avenue, New York, N.Y. 10017
The W. K. Kellogg Foundation, 250 Champion Street, Battle Creek, Michigan 49017
The Joseph P. Kennedy Foundation, 230 Park Avenue, New York, N.Y. 10017
The Kresge Foundation, 2727 Second Avenue, Detroit, Michigan 48201
The Samuel H. Kress Foundation, 221 West 57th Street, New York, N.Y. 10019
Lasker (Albert and Mary) Foundation, Inc., 405 Lexington Avenue, New York, N.Y. 10017
The Life Extension Foundation, Inc., 11 East 44th Street, New York, N.Y. 10017
The Josiah Macy, Jr. Foundation, 16 West 46th Street, New York, N.Y. 10036
The John and Mary R. Markle Foundation, 511 Fifth Avenue, New York, N.Y. 10017
Milbank Memorial Fund, 40 Wall Street, New York, N. Y. 10006
The National Vitamin Foundation, Inc., 149 East 78th Street, New York, N.Y. 10021
New York Foundation, 61 Broadway, New York, N.Y. 10006
The Nutrition Foundation, 99 Park Avenue, New York, N.Y. 10016
Rockefeller Brothers Fund, 30 Rockefeller Plaza, New York, N.Y. 10020
The Rockefeller Foundation, 111 West 50th Street, New York, N. Y. 10020
The Russell Sage Foundation, 505 Park Avenue, New York, N.Y. 10022
Smith, Kline and French Foundation, 1500 Spring Garden Street, Philadelphia, Pa. 19130
The Social Research Foundation, 345 Park Avenue, New York, N.Y. 10022

2. Professional Organizations

Professional organizations whose interests and efforts center upon the establishment and maintenance of desirable standards, the promotion and upgrading of health programs in schools, colleges, community or international situations:

American Academy of Pediatrics, 1801 Hinman Avenue, Evanston, Ill. 60201
American Academy of Political and Social Science, 3937 Chestnut Street, Philadelphia, Pa. 19104
American Association for Health, Physical Education and Recreation, 1201 16th Street, N.W., Washington, D.C. 20036
American Association for the Advancement of Science, 1515 Massachusetts Avenue, N.W., Washington, D.C. 20005
American Association of School Administrators, 1201 16th Street, N.W., Washington, D.C. 20036
American College Health Association, Gannet Medical Clinic, Cornell University, Ithaca, N.Y. 14850
American Council on Education, 1 Dupont Circle, N.W., Washington, D.C. 20036
American Dental Association, 211 E. Chicago Ave., Chicago, Ill. 60611
American Dental Hygienists Association, 100 East Ohio Street, Chicago, Ill. 60611
American Dietetic Association, 620 North Michigan Avenue, Chicago, Ill. 60611
American Home Economics Association, 1600 20th Street, N.W., Washington, D.C. 20009

American Medical Association, 535 North Dearborn Street, Chicago, Ill. 60610
American National Council for Health Education, 800 Second Avenue, New York, N.Y. 10017
American Nurses Association, 10 Columbus Circle, New York, N.Y. 10019
American Occupational Therapy Association, 250 West 57th Street, New York, N.Y. 10019
American Orthopsychiatric Association, 1790 Broadway, New York, N. Y. 10019
American Osteopathic Association, 212 East Ohio Street, Chicago, Ill. 60611
American Pharmaceutical Association, 2215 Constitution Avenue, N.W., Washington, D.C. 20037
American Physical Therapy Association, 1790 Broadway, New York, N.Y. 10019
American Psychiatric Association, 1700 18th Street, N.W., Washington, D.C. 20009
American Psychological Association, 1200 17th Street, N.W., Washington, D.C. 20036
American Public Health Association, 1740 Broadway, New York, N.Y. 10019
American School Health Association, 107 S. Depeyster, P.O. Box 416, Kent, Ohio 44240
American Sociological Association, New York University, Washington Square, New York, N.Y. 10003
American Veterinary Medical Association, 600 South Michigan Avenue, Chicago, Ill. 60605
Association for Childhood Education International, 3615 Wisconsin Avenue, N.W., Washington, D.C. 20016
Association for Supervision and Curriculum, 1201 16th Street, N.W., Washington, D.C. 20036
Child Study Association of America, 9 East 89th Street, New York, N.Y. 10028
National Association of Social Workers, 95 Madison Avenue, New York, N.Y. 10016
National Catholic Conference on Family, 1312 Massachusetts Ave., N.W., Washington, D.C. 20005
National Congress of Parents and Teachers, 700 Rush Street, Chicago, Ill. 60611
National Council on Family Relations, 1219 University Avenue, S.E., Minneapolis, Minn. 55414
National Education Association of the United States, 1201 16th Street, N.W., Washington, D.C. 20036
National League for Nursing, 10 Columbus Circle, New York, N.Y. 10019
National Recreation Association, 8 West 8th Street, New York, N.Y. 10011
Society of Public Health Educators, 81 Hillside Rd., Rye, N.Y. 10580
World Confederation of Organizations of the Teaching Profession, 1330 Mass. Ave. N. W., Washington, D.C. 20005

3. Private or Voluntary Health Agencies

Private or voluntary citizen supported health agencies whose objectives, programs, services, and activities focus upon the health of the community, or a particular phase of health, or a special segment of the population; most of which have state and local affiliates:

Alcoholics Anonymous, General Service Headquarters, P.O. Box 459, Grand Central Annex, New York, N.Y. 10017
American Cancer Society, 521 West 57th Street, New York, N.Y. 10019
American Diabetic Association, 1 East 45th Street, New York, N.Y. 10017
American Hearing Society, 919 18th Street, N.W., Washington, D.C. 20006
American Heart Association, 44 East 23rd Street, New York, N.Y. 10010
American Hospital Association, 840 North Lake Shore Drive, Chicago, Ill. 60611
American National Red Cross, 17th & D Streets, N.W., Washington, D.C. 20006
American Social Health Association, 1790 Broadway, New York, N.Y. 10019
Family Service Association of America, 215 Park Avenue South, New York, N.Y. 10003
National Association for Mental Health, 10 Columbus Circle, New York, N.Y. 10019
National Association for Retarded Children, 386 Park Avenue South, New York, N.Y. 10016
National Council on Alcoholism, 2 East 103rd Street, New York, N.Y. 10029
National Epilepsy League, 208 N. Wells Street, Chicago, Ill. 60606
National Foundation, 800 Second Avenue, New York, N.Y. 10017
National Health Council, 1790 Broadway, New York, N.Y. 10019
National Multiple Sclerosis Society, 257 Park Avenue South, New York, N.Y. 10010
National Safety Council, 425 North Michigan Avenue, Chicago, Ill. 60611
National Society for Crippled Children and Adults, 2023 W. Ogden Avenue, Chicago, Ill. 60612
National Society for the Prevention of Blindness, 1790 Broadway, New York, N.Y. 10019
National Tuberculosis and Respiratory Disease Association, 1790 Broadway, New York, N.Y. 10019
United Cerebral Palsy Association, 66 East 34th Street, New York, N.Y. 10016

4. Official Governmental Health Agencies

Official governmental health agencies whose programs, activities or services have the primary over-all responsibility for the health and health education of the community, the school or of a segment of the population, or which focus upon a particular health problem:

State and local Departments of Health
Federal agencies: (unless otherwise indicated, Washington, D.C.
publications: Superintendent of Documents,
U.S. Government Printing Office
Washington, D.C. 20402)

U.S. Civil Defense Administration
U.S. Department of Agriculture: Bureau of Human Nutrition and Home Economics Research
U.S. Department of Commerce: Bureau of the Census
U.S. Department of Health, Education, and Welfare: Public Health Service, National Institutes of Health; Food and Drug Administration; National Office of Vital Statistics; Welfare Administration; Office of Education; Office of Vocational Rehabilitation

U.S. Department of Interior: Bureau of Mines; Bureau of Indian Affairs; National Parks Service
U.S. Department of State: Agency for International Development
International agencies:
World Health Organization, Palais de Nations, Geneva, Switzerland
Pan-American Health Organization, WHO Regional Office for the Americas, 525 23rd St. N.W., Washington, D.C. 20037
United Nations Children's Fund (UNICEF), United Nations, New York, N.Y.
United Nations Educational, Cultural, and Scientific Organization (UNESCO), United Nations, New York, N.Y.
International Union for Health Education, 3 Rue Viollier, Geneva, Switzerland

5. Commercial Organizations

Commercial organizations which through funds, products, materials, services, research or leadership contribute significantly to the advancement of human health or health education:

Aetna Life Insurance Company, Hartford, Conn.
American Institute of Baking, 400 East Ontario Street, Chicago, Ill. 60611
American Meat Institute, 59 East Van Buren Street, Chicago, Ill. 60605
Better Vision Institute, Inc., 630 Fifth Avenue, New York, N.Y. 10020
Blue Cross Association, 840 North Lake Shore Drive, Chicago, Ill. 60611
The Borden Company, 359 Madison Avenue, New York, N.Y. 10017
California Fruit Growers Exchange, Box 5030 Metropolitan Station, Los Angeles, Cal. 90055
Carnation Milk Company, Box 2035, Los Angeles, Cal. 90054
Cereal Institute, 135 La Salle Street, Chicago, Ill. 60603
Colgate-Palmolive Company, New York, N.Y.
Equitable Life Assurance Society of the United States, Box 580, General P.O., New York, N.Y. 10001
Evaporated Milk Association, 307 North Michigan Avenue, Chicago, Ill. 60601
Florida Citrus Fruit Commission, Lakeland, Florida
General Foods Corporation, 250 North Street, White Plains, N.Y. 10605
General Mills, Inc., 9200 Wayzata Blvd., Minneapolis, Minn. 55426
International Cellucotton Products Company, 919 North Michigan Avenue, Chicago, Ill. 60611
John Hancock Mutual Life Insurance Company, Box 111, Boston, Mass. 01401
Kimberly-Clark Corporation, Educational Department, Neenah, Wisconsin
Lever Brothers, 390 Park Avenue, New York, N.Y. 10022
Metropolitan Life Insurance Company, School Health Bureau, One Madison Avenue, New York, N.Y. 10010
National Association of Blue Shield Plans, 425 North Michigan Avenue, Chicago, Ill. 60611
National Dairy Council, 111 North Canal Street, Chicago, Ill. 60606
National Live Stock and Meat Board, Department of Nutrition, 407 South Dearborn Street, Chicago, Ill. 60605
Paper Cup and Container Institute, 250 Park Avenue, New York, N.Y. 10017
Personal Products Corporation, Milltown, New Jersey 08850
Procter and Gamble Distributing Company, Public Relations Division, Gwynne Building, Cincinnati, Ohio 45202

Prudential Life Insurance Company, Newark, New Jersey
Smith, Kline and French Laboratories, 1530 Spring Garden Street, Philadelphia, Pa. 19130
Tampax, Inc., 161 East 42nd Street, New York, N.Y. 10017
United Fruit Company, Education Department, Pier 3, North River, New York N.Y. 10006
Wheat Flour Institute, 309 West Jackson Blvd., Chicago, Ill. 60606

Appendix C

Some Pertinent Professional Periodicals

Key to symbols used:	m : monthly	q : quarterly	
	bi : bimonthly	nos. : number per year	

American Anthropologist, (bi): American Anthropological Association, 1703 New Hampshire Ave., N.W., Washington, D.C. 20009

American Journal of Nursing, (m): American Nurses Association, 10 Columbus Circle, New York, N.Y. 10019

American Journal of Public Health and the Nation's Health, (m): American Public Health Association, 1740 Broadway, New York, N.Y. 10019

American Journal of Orthopsychiatry (q): American Orthopsychiatric Association, 1790 Broadway, New York, N.Y. 10019

American Journal of Sociology, (bi): University of Chicago Press, 5750 Ellis Avenue, Chicago, Ill. 60637

American Psychologist, (m): American Psychological Association, 1200 17th Street, N.W., Washington, D.C. 20036

American Sociological Review, (bi): American Sociological Association, New York University, Washington Square, New York, N.Y. 10003

Annals, The, (bi): American Academy of Political and Social Science, 3937 Chestnut Street, Philadelphia, Pa. 19104

Childhood Education, (8 nos.): Association for Childhood Education International, 3615 Wisconsin Avenue, N.W., Washington, D.C. 20016

Human Organization, (q): Society for Applied Anthropology, Rand Hall, Cornell University, Ithaca, New York 14850

International Journal of Health Education, (q): International Union for Health Education, 3 Rue Viollier, Geneva, Switzerland

Journal of the American Dietetic Association, (m): American Dietetic Association 620 North Michigan Avenue, Chicago, Ill. 60611

Journal of Health and Human Behavior, (q): Leo Potishman Foundation, Texas Christian University, Fort Worth, Texas 76129

Journal of Health, Physical Education and Recreation, (9 nos.); *Research Quarterly,* (q): American Association for Health, Physical Education and Recreation, 1201 16th Street, N.W., Washington, D.C. 20036

Journal of Home Economics, (10 nos.): American Home Economics Association, 1600 20th Street, N.W., Washington, D.C. 20009

Journal of School Health, (10 nos.): American School Health Association, 107 S. Depeyster, P.O. Box 416, Kent, Ohio 44240

Marriage and Family Living, (q): National Council on Family Relations, 1219 University Avenue, Minneapolis, Minn. 55414

Mental Hygiene, (q): National Association for Mental Health, 10 Columbus Circle, New York, N.Y. 10019

National Catholic Educational Association Bulletin, (q): National Catholic Education Association, 1785 Massachusetts Avenue, N.W., Washington, D.C. 20036

National Parent-Teacher, (10 nos.); *National Congress Bulletin,* (10 nos.): National Congress of Parents and Teachers, 700 North Rush Street, Chicago, Ill. 60611

NEA Journal, (9 nos.): National Education Association of the United States, 1201 16th Street, N.W., Washington, D.C. 20036

Nursing Outlook (m): National League for Nursing, 10 Columbus Circle, New York, N.Y. 10019

Panorama, (q): World Confederation of Organizations for Teacher Preparation, 1330 Massachusetts Avenue, N.W., Washington, D.C. 20005

Public Health Reports, (m): Public Health Service, Department of Health, Education, and Welfare, Washington, D.C. 20203

Recreation, (10 nos.): National Recreation Association, 8 West 8th Street, New York, N.Y. 10011

Rural Sociology, (q): Rural Sociological Society, Department of Rural Sociology, College of Agriculture and Home Economics, University of Kentucky, Lexington, Kentucky 40506

Safety Education, (9 nos.); *National Safety News* (m): National Safety Council, 425 North Michigan Avenue, Chicago, Ill. 60611

The School Administrator, (m): American Association of School Administrators, 1201 16th Street, N.W., Washington, D.C. 20036

School and Society, (bi): The Society for the Advancement of Education, 1834 Broadway, New York, N.Y. 10023

School Health Review (q): American Association for Health, Physical Education, and Recreation, 1201 Sixteenth St., N.W., Washington, D.C. 20036

Science, (w): American Association for the Advancement of Science, 1515 Massachusetts Avenue, N.W., Washington, D.C. 20005

Social Health News, (m): American Social Health Association, 1790 Broadway, New York, N.Y. 10019

Social Work, (q): National Association of Social Workers, 95 Madison Avenue, New York, N.Y. 10016

Student Health, (q): American College Health Associatlon, Gannet Medical Clinic, Cornell University, Ithaca, New York 14850

To-day's Health, (m): American Medical Association, 535 North Dearborn Street, Chicago, Ill. 60610

WHO Bulletin, (q); *WHO Chronicles,* (m); *World Health,* (bi): World Health Organization Publications, Columbia University Press, International Documents Service, 2960 Broadway, New York, N.Y. 10027

Index